the fast
800
favourites

the fast
800
favourites

Over 100 best-loved recipes
for a healthy lifestyle

DR CLARE BAILEY MOSLEY

First published in Great Britain in 2025
by Short Books, an imprint of
Octopus Publishing Group Ltd
Carmelite House
50 Victoria Embankment
London
EC4Y 0DZ
www.octopusbooks.co.uk

An Hachette UK Company
www.hachette.co.uk

Some of this material previously appeared in *The Fast 800 Recipe Book*, *The Fast 800 Keto Recipe Book*, *The Fast 800 Treats Recipe Book* and *The Fast 800 Easy*.

The authorized representative in the EEA is Hachette Ireland, 8 Castlecourt Centre, Dublin 15, D15 XTP3, Ireland (email: info@hbgi.ie)

Text copyright © Parenting Matters Limited 2025

Recipe contributors: Dr Clare Bailey Mosley,
    Kathryn Bruton, Caroline Barton, Justine Pattison
    and Dr Sarah Shenker

Publisher: Jo Morrell
Commissioning Editor: Katie Forsythe
Editorial Assistant: Sarah Ramnath-Budhram
Project editor: Jo Roberts-Miller
Nutritional analysis: Fiona Hunter
Design and art direction: Smith & Gilmour
Cover design: Smith & Gilmour
Photography: Smith & Gilmour
Food styling: Phil Mundy, Annie Rigg and Lola Milne
Props Styling: Hannah Wilkinson and Olivia Wardle
Senior Production Manager: Katherine Hockley

ISBN 9781804193679
eISBN 9781804193686

A CIP catalogue record for this book is available from the British Library.

Printed and bound in China.

10 9 8 7 6 5 4 3 2 1

Publisher's note
The information contained in this book is provided for general purposes only. It is not intended as and should not be relied upon as medical advice. The publisher and author are not responsible for any specific health needs that may require medical supervision. If you have underlying health problems, or have any doubts about the advice contained in this book, you should contact a qualified medical, dietary or other appropriate professional.

Contents

Introduction

Michael's focus was always on helping people improve and transform their health and happiness. He truly was unique in the way he'd put his body on the line in the name of science, and was well known for having brought his own type 2 diabetes into remission, when everyone assumed it was a chronic and incurable condition. He did it by losing 9kg (10 per cent of his body weight) on an intermittent fasting diet that he called the 5:2 diet, where he cut down his calorie intake to 800cals, twice a week, and ate a healthy, lower-carb, Mediterranean-style diet the rest of the week.

As I sat down to write this introduction, a bar of chocolate fell from the back of the cupboard with an ironic clunk. Like many of us, Michael found it difficult to resist a sweet treat and had quite a chocolate addiction. He would ask me to hide it, and later, I'd find chocolate in forgotten places. But, by identifying his weaknesses and finding ways to work around them, Michael was able to share his knowledge to help thousands of people implement positive changes in their lives.

We loved working together and chatting about the latest research, and how we could share new medical information so others could benefit, too. In his many books, Michael followed the evidence and the principles remained the same. From *The 8-Week Blood Sugar Diet*, where Michael was 'alerting us to one of the greatest silent epidemics of our time – raised blood sugar levels', to *The Fast 800* and *The Fast 800 Keto*, which explain how to combine a lower-carb, Med-style diet with cutting down to 800–1000cals, so a 'fast day' is enough to give you the nutrients you need, while also burning fat.

There is compelling research that demonstrates that cutting back on sugar and starchy carbohydrates, and increasing protein, such as meat, fish, tofu and eggs, allows your body to 'flip the metabolic switch' and go from burning sugar for energy, to burning fat as your main fuel source. But, unlike traditional keto, which is more restrictive, having 800–1000cals 'fast days' means you can include healthy complex carbs, such as beans, pulses and wholegrains, and still achieve ketosis and burn fat. Going into ketosis not only leads to rapid weight loss, but it also promotes the release of your natural hunger-suppressing hormones, including GLP-1, while decreasing the hormones that make you hungry, such as ghrelin, so you don't feel ravenous all the time. What's more, you are likely to feel more energetic and alert.

Whether you want to lose weight fast, harness the many health benefits of intermittent fasting, or just slow the encroachment of middle-age spread, the Fast 800 plan provides a highly nutritious and extremely adaptable way of eating for better health. The recipes are also suitable for people taking weight loss drugs who need to make sure they are getting the right nutrients, particularly plenty of protein and fibre in every meal. Michael would have been incredibly proud of our son, Dr Jack Mosley, who has picked up the baton and written the bestselling book, *Food Noise* on this subject.

In the western world, chronic ill health affects over 50 per cent of us, primarily due to poor-quality ultra processed foods. These foods are addictive and keep us wanting more and more (and more...). They are highly accessible – quick to make and even quicker to consume. This is why it's so important to make your own nutritious and delicious dishes. The recipes in this book keep things simple and quick, and many of them can be cooked in batches.

Michael and I have long been passionate about helping people improve their metabolic health – how the body processes and regulates energy from food, such as maintaining normal blood sugar levels, normal blood pressure and a healthy waist circumference. There is now increasing awareness of the multiple chronic conditions caused by poor metabolic health such as inflammation, sleep apnoea, non-alcoholic fatty liver disease (NAFLD), polycystic ovary syndrome, poor skin, dementia and so many more. The principles of the Fast 800 and the recipes in this book can help you take control of your metabolic health and feel healthier and happier, which was always Michael's mission.

Here we share the recipes that became our favourites over the years. We have adapted as many of these as possible for those of you using an air fryer to make them even more accessible. All the dishes are simple to prepare, delicious and carefully balanced, to ensure you get all the necessary nutrients. As well as being extremely tasty, they will keep you full and well-nourished on your weight-loss journey! The recipes include many of Michael's favourites. He thoroughly enjoyed being my chief taster – and I'm sure you'll love the recipes, too.

Wishing you all the best on your Fast 800 journey!

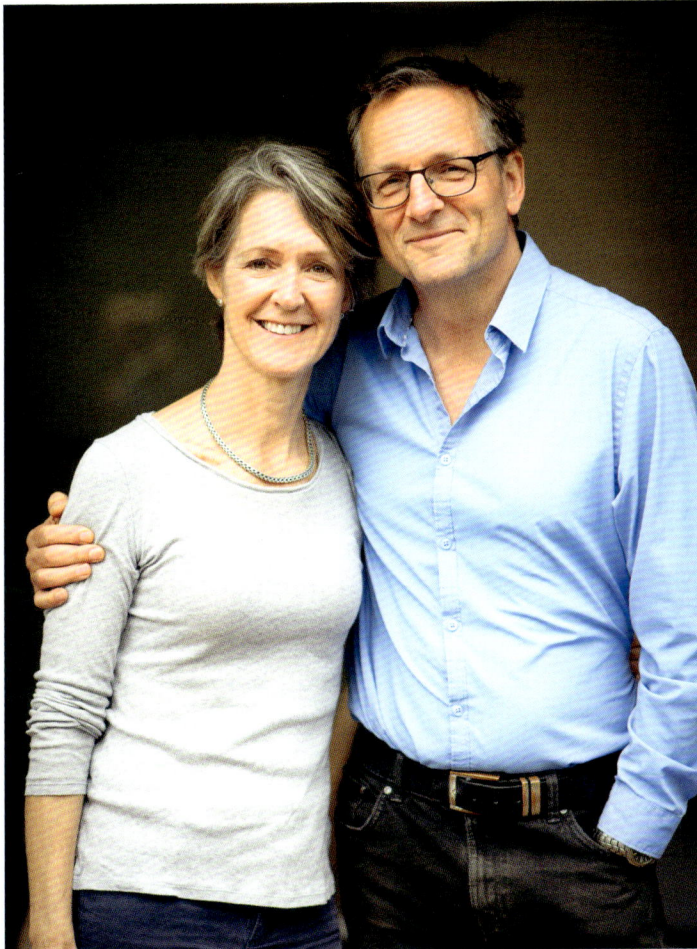

What is the Fast 800?

This diet is designed to be as flexible as possible, while incorporating the best science-based advice. All the meals are based on a lowish-carb Mediterranean-style way of eating, but how you manage the 800–1000cals days is down to you.

Most people choose to kickstart their diet with a fast-track plan of 800–1000cals a day, every day, for two or more weeks. If you do have a lot to lose – and if the diet suits – you can continue this for up to 3 months at a time.

If you don't have much weight to lose, or wish to do it more slowly, you can move on to the 5:2 – consuming 800–1000cals a day for two days a week and on the other days continuing to eat a healthy, Med-style diet, keeping carb intake low and controlling portion size.

You could add in a relatively new form of intermittent fasting called Time Restricted Eating (TRE), whereby you eat all your calories within a narrow time window each day – usually within 10–12 hours. This extends the length of your normal overnight fast (when you are sleeping and not eating), giving your body an opportunity to burn fat and do essential repairs (see page 12).

As with any diet, the Fast 800 may not suit everyone, so check with your health professional first (see page 14).

A Mediterranean-style diet

While 'lowish' in carbohydrates, this is not a restrictive diet, where you have to give up everything that contains carbs. However, it does mean reducing or avoiding sugary, starchy and ultra-processed foods (UPFs), such as white bread, white pasta, rice and potatoes, as well as most breakfast cereals, since these readily convert to sugars in your body.

As a general principle, the Med-style way of eating involves eating whole foods cooked from scratch and prepared in a more traditional way. Mindful of our time-poor lives, I've tried to keep the recipes as simple as possible.

We've also shared tips on how to create some of the recipes using an air fryer.

The great thing about eating a Med-style diet, rather than a low-fat one, is that you can enjoy plenty of olive oil, avocados, some full-fat dairy, lots of nuts, seeds and oily fish – all the kinds of ingredients that make food tasty and filling. They also have anti-inflammatory properties, as well as helping us absorb important nutrients and vitamins. The programme also includes recipes for luscious and colourful vegetables, fruit, wholegrains, beans and lentils for much needed extra fibre.

So, what's out and what's in?

For the past 50 years we have been told to keep our consumption of fat to a minimum for fear that it will block our arteries and cause a heart attack. To compensate for this, we were encouraged to eat at least a third of our calories as starchy carbohydrates, in many cases putting up blood sugars and driving obesity.

Likewise, the official line has commonly been to advise people to eat three meals a day, with snacks between meals and before bed if we got hungry. As a result, many of us are eating six times a day, leaving our metabolism constantly battling to keep sugar levels in the normal range. And given that most of us eat more than we burn, these extra calories usually end up getting stored as fat.

However, the good news is that in the past decade there has been a whole body of exciting new research that has turned standard dietary advice on its head. Studies have shown that, unlike the widely advocated 'slow and steady' approach, rapid weight loss helps people lose weight faster, get closer to their goal and help keep the weight off. By combining moderately low-carb, Mediterranean-style diet with a limit of 800–1000cals, you have a highly effective way to lose weight, restore blood sugars and re-set your metabolism.

What's out

❶ Sugary, starchy and processed foods

It is increasingly clear that we should avoid sweet, starchy and highly processed foods altogether. They will undo much of the health benefit you get from eating healthily and are often toxic for the important microbes living in our guts that produce substances to keep us healthy and boost our mood. Be kind to these vital bugs and they will take care of you...

We describe the Fast 800 as a lowish carbohydrate diet. This is because not all carbs are equal. Refined and starchy carbs, such as white bread or white rice, are very rapidly broken down, causing a spike in blood sugars and encouraging fat storage and weight gain. But not all carbs are bad. More complex carbohydrates, like wholegrains, beans or lentils, are slower to break down as they contain more fibre. As a result, they release less sugar and do so more slowly, leaving you feeling full for longer, while the fibre in them makes its way down to the large intestine, where those helpful microbes convert it into important substances that help keep us well.

❷ Hidden sugars

Sadly, we are surrounded by hidden sugars – they are found in all sorts of foods, including savoury snacks and takeaways, and can be very hard to spot. Check the ingredients in any ready-made convenience food, and the word 'sugar' may not appear at the top of the list, or indeed appear at all, despite it being included in significant quantities. Sugar often appears under alternative names, such as maltose, dextrose, fructose, glucose, lactose – of which there are 50–60 variations, many of which you won't even recognise. Add all these together and sugar can turn out to be the main ingredient.

Fruit, while it contains lots of health-promoting phytonutrients and fibre, is also a source of sugar. It's far better to eat the whole fruit than to have it in the form of juice, as the juicing process removes the fibre and turns a healthy food, where the sugar is released slowly, into a sugar hit. Do include a portion or two of fruit a day, but try to make it a low-sugar variety, such as berries, rather than sweet tropical fruits.

Alcohol is another challenge – it behaves like sugar, breaking down rapidly and causing a sugar spike. A single glass of wine can contain between 200–300cals and ends up stored in the liver as fat, causing inflammation. Spirits tend to contain slightly less sugar. But because alcohol disinhibits us, we are more likely to eat crisps or go for a takeaway when we've been drinking! So, for many reasons, we recommend moderation and to avoid alcohol on a fasting day.

❸ Sweeteners

The trouble with sweeteners is that most of them damage the good microbes in your gut microbiome. Sweeteners are many times sweeter than natural sugar, which means that, regardless of their low-calorie content, they maintain your sweet tooth and can increase your sugar cravings. Luckily, while on the Fast 800 diet, you will find your tastes change and you can enjoy treats with far less sugar as your palate adapts.

We use dried and fresh fruit, such as dates, figs, bananas and apricots, as natural sweeteners in some recipes. Unlike sugar, fruit adds fibre and a variety of important vitamins and nutrients. And although dates contain sugar, they are bound in fibre, releasing the sugar more slowly and reducing sugar spikes.

If you really must have a sweetener, particularly in the first week or two while you re-set your sweet tooth, then the best one to go for is probably stevia. Michael had a sweet tooth, but over time his sugar cravings reduced. Although, he still asked me to hide the chocolate!

And what's in

1 Protein

It has become increasingly clear that protein is key to regulating your appetite and your general health. Protein is required by every cell and organ in the body, including the immune system and brain. It maintains your muscle mass and metabolism, as well as helping you to feel full. However, unlike carbohydrates and fat, your body is unable to store protein. It also isn't able to tell you what you are lacking, so if you aren't getting enough protein, you will continue to feel hungry and are likely to go on eating until you have satisfied your body's protein needs – and this drives weight gain. This is known as the 'protein leverage hypothesis'. So, it's important to get enough on a daily basis: you should aim for a minimum of 50g a day and perhaps 10–20g on top of that, particularly if you are older or very active. It is especially important when on an 800–1000 calorie day to ensure you get the minimum requirement of protein if possible.

To help you do this, we have included the protein content in our recipes, which are carefully calibrated to help give you adequate amounts. We also offer suggestions for how to add protein top-ups (see page 271), so that you can adapt salads or veg dishes according to your own taste. Getting enough protein can be challenging for vegetarians, and even more so for vegans, who might be advised to take protein supplements or use a meal replacement protein shake on 800–1000 calorie days.

Using good-quality, protein-rich, meal replacement shakes with natural ingredients (see thefast800.com for options) will also help on days when you have to rush out the door with an instant breakfast, or as an alternative to grabbing a sandwich and crisps for lunch.

2 Non-starchy veg

We know that there are numerous benefits to eating more vegetables. This includes an impressive 16 per cent reduction in the risk of having a stroke for every added portion. When you are trying to lose weight or control your blood sugars, it is best to stick to non-starchy vegetables, i.e. those that are lower in carbs and hidden sugars, such as spinach, cabbage and broccoli. And we encourage you to embrace variety and enjoy generous portions. Ideally, pile your plate with steamed greens, salad, or any of the other vegetables on the list at the back of the book (see page 272). They are so low in calories that they can be eaten freely, without counting.

It's fine to add a dressing or sauce to your veg, but do remember to include those added calories in your daily tally.

That said, adding a little olive oil to your non-starchy 'free' veg is actually beneficial, as it can improve the absorption of nutrients. This is particularly important when it comes to the absorption of the fat-soluble vitamins A, D, E and K. In the big scheme of things, a little drizzle of olive oil here and there is fine. The message is: don't worry about occasional extra calories, if it helps you eat more veg…

And since we also know that variety is key to us getting the nutrients we need, you might take this opportunity to push the boat out and try new veg. By eating different phytonutrients (the health-promoting substances produced by plants), you will contribute to your metabolic health and to reducing inflammation. That's why we are encouraged to 'eat a rainbow'. Embrace as many different coloured vegetables as you can – red salad leaves, purple broccoli or beetroot, yellow peppers, dark aubergines, as well as plenty of greens…

3 Fruit

Although fruit is a great source of important nutrients and fibre, go easy on it. Sweet fruits like mangoes and pineapple can be irresistible but they tend to put your sugar levels up. It is striking to see how often people with type 2 diabetes have been told to eat lots of fruit as part of their 5-a-day, when in fact grazing through the day on sweet fruits causes their blood sugars to spike and blocks any chance of fat burning.

Try to choose low-sugar fruits, particularly berries or hard fruit that contain plenty of fibre, such as apples or pears – and make sure you eat the skin, too, as that's where most of the health-promoting nutrients are found. Fruit is also best eaten either with a meal or straight after, rather than as a snack, when it's more likely to spike sugars and be stored as fat.

4 Fibre

Most of us don't get anywhere close to eating enough fibre – the average in the Western diet is about half of the necessary 30g a day. To get what your body requires, you need to eat seven or more portions of fruit and veg a day, as well as some wholegrains, beans and lentils.

On a fasting day it can be a challenge to get enough fibre, but you will find that you get to love your veg, and a suitable meal replacement shake can also provide a top-up.

5 Natural unprocessed fats, mainly plant-based

When it comes to choosing oils, the least processed the better. Try and go for cold-pressed or virgin oils, as they are unrefined and retain their natural nutrients – although they are more expensive, so buy what you can afford.

For frying at high temperatures, you can use a good-quality rapeseed oil. Extra-virgin olive oil is good for gentle frying and ideal for salads. Coconut oil, a bit like butter, is fine in moderation. I like the flavour it can give to some stir-fries and curries, and it provides a slightly sweet and flavoured alternative for baking.

As part of a healthy, Mediterranean-style diet, there are plenty of other 'good' fats to be found in the likes of oily fish, such as mackerel and salmon, as well as nuts and seeds, all of which have been shown to lower your risk of stroke and heart disease.

6 Dairy

We include a fair amount of full-fat dairy in our recipes because the evidence suggests that in moderation this is beneficial – and does not, contrary to some reports, lead to diabetes. Fermented dairy is best and full-fat products are less processed. Full-fat Greek-style yoghurt, for example, doesn't usually contain the starchy thickeners and sugars or sweeteners that are added to enhance low-fat products. We love the creamy richness of it. I try to eat a variety of yoghurts and kefir to improve diversity.

7 Meat in moderation

Many of us are trying to eat less meat in general these days, particularly red meat, both for health and environmental reasons. But meat is an excellent source of good-quality protein and, as we have seen above, getting adequate protein can be a challenge on fasting days. So, we have included a number of meat-based recipes here, as well as some veg-based ones that contain small quantities of processed meat, such as bacon or chorizo, both to boost protein and add extra flavour. Try to buy better-quality, grass-fed varieties, if you can.

The Fast 800 – a quick recap

STAGE 1

Rapid weight loss

By combining calorie restriction (800–1000cals) with a low-carbohydrate, Mediterranean-style diet you are more likely to get into fat burning – ketosis. Along with rapid weight loss, you will probably feel better, more energetic and have more mental clarity.

We recommend you start with the intensive stage, if possible. By sticking to 800–1000cals a day, every day, for at least two weeks, you will kickstart your weight loss and improve your metabolic health. Why 800–1000? Because this is low enough to induce mild ketosis, which is associated with fat burning, but high enough to ensure you get the nutrients you need.

After two to three weeks, pause and reflect on how it is going. If you are losing weight and not struggling with the diet, then carry on. You can continue this approach until you reach your goal, or for up to 12 weeks.

For convenience, some people find it helpful during this stage to make up some of their meals as shakes. See pages 58–63 for recipes, or visit thefast800.com, where you will find a range of ready-made meal replacement shakes with a Med-style formation and decent protein content to help fill the gap. You can also find a variety of protein powders.

STAGE 2

Intermittent fasting with the New 5:2

When you get close to your target weight, or if you are struggling on the rapid weight loss stage, you can swap to an intermittent fasting pattern – eating 800–1000cals on just a couple of days a week. Your weight loss rate will be slower on this regime, but it has been shown to be highly sustainable, and one of the most effective ways to lose weight and keep it off. We now recommend that, instead of reducing your calories to only 500–600, as in the original 5:2 Fast Diet, you can stick to 800–1000cals on fasting days.

STAGE 3

The maintenance programme

Once you've hit your goal, you can continue with a healthy Mediterranean way of eating, not calorie counting but exercising portion control. For this 'maintenance phase', you can go on using most of the recipes in this book; just double up portions, add extra protein (see page 271) and a few tablespoons of high-fibre, unrefined carbs, such as beans, lentils or wholegrains (see page 273), here and there and you are set for life.

You can enjoy the occasional treat, but try to maintain a diet low in sugar and moderately low in starchy carbs to help prevent sugars creeping up or weight piling back on. The message is: relax a bit, but not too much! If your weight increases or your new outfit starts to feel tight, you know what to do…

Adding in Time Restricted Eating

TRE is a form of fasting whereby you extend your overnight fast to restrict your eating window during the day. There is evidence that going 12 or even 14 hours without food gives your body and metabolism a chance to recover and focus on other functions, such as 'spring-cleaning' old and damaged cells, and helping you switch from burning sugar to burning fat. So how do you do this? Well, if you stop eating by 8pm and don't start again till 8am – that is a 12-hour overnight fast (i.e. 12:12). You can then build up to a 14-hour fast, which means eating all your day's food in a 10-hour window (14:10). Many people find that eating in a narrower window makes it easier to manage a fast day. Either way, it is a good habit for all of us to get into, as calories eaten within a few hours of bedtime are more likely to be stored as fat.

	STAGE 1	STAGE 2	STAGE 3
	Rapid weight loss	**The New 5:2**	**Maintenance**
how TO FAST	**800 – 1000 cals a day** (for up to 12 weeks)	**800 – 1000 cals 2 days a week** (intermittent fasting)	**No calorie counting, but portion control** (consider a weekly fast day – 6:1)
what TO EAT	**Lowish-carb Mediterranean-style diet** (or replace up to half your calories with meal-replacement shakes)		**Lowish-carb Med-style diet** (watching portion size)
when TO EAT	**Optional TRE 12:12 or 14:10** (Time Restricted Eating)		

Getting started

❶ Write down what you want to achieve

Think about why you want to lose weight. What difference will it make? What changes do you want to see? And how important is it to you? What will success look and feel like? Your personal goal may be to lose the weight around your middle; or to bring about a general improvement in your overall health, energy and mood. Reminding yourself about what motivates you will help keep you on track.

❷ Kitchen hygiene

This isn't about how clean and tidy your kitchen is. It means clearing away temptation, hiding (or even getting rid of) all convenience foods, snacks, biscuits, white bread or whatever your weaknesses are.

❸ Tell people you are doing the diet

This helps you to hold yourself to account and increases commitment and success.

SAFETY: Exclusions and cautions

This diet is not suitable for teenagers, or if you're breastfeeding, pregnant or undergoing fertility treatment. Do not follow the diet if you are underweight or have an eating disorder. Discuss with your GP if you are on medication or if you have a medical condition, including diabetes, low or high blood pressure, retinopathy, gallstones or epilepsy. Nor should you do this if you are frail, unwell or while doing endurance exercise. (For more detailed information see thefast800.com/faqs/)

Side effects

Dehydration. The most commonly reported side effects are headaches, constipation, feeling light headed and fatigued. These are mainly due to not drinking enough added water. (For more on how to stay hydrated see page 18.) As for constipation, again, keeping well hydrated helps keep things soft – and make sure you are eating enough fibre-rich food. We try to include plenty of fibre in the recipes in the form of non-starchy vegetables and some beans, lentils and wholegrains.

Low blood pressure. Within days of embarking on a low-calorie diet like the Fast 800, you may see a drop in your blood pressure, which is a common benefit, but if you are on medication, particularly for blood pressure, or have a medical condition, it is important that you speak to your health professional before starting as your medication may need reducing (see SAFETY: Exclusions and cautions).

Feeling rough at first. Flicking the metabolic switch so that your body goes from burning sugar to burning fat can leave you feeling a bit off-colour for a few days, while your body's metabolism adapts. This is known as 'keto flu' and will pass within a matter of days. In fact, patients often tell me that they then feel better than they had done prior to starting the diet, with more energy, a sharper mind and fewer food cravings. Despite being on 800–1000 calories, they find they are no longer hungry all the time. If your symptoms are severe or last longer than a week or so, it would be wise to discuss this with your health professional before continuing the diet. See thefast800.com for more information.

8 WAYS TO HELP YOU REACH YOUR GOAL

1 Avoid snacking between meals or late-night grazing. The trouble with snacking is that it reduces fat burning. If you must snack on a fasting day, eat a small portion of non-starchy veg, such as some sliced cucumber, broccoli or celery. Alternatively, try a few nuts (one portion is the amount that will sit on the palm of your hand) or a sliver of cheese.

2 Plan ahead. Willpower is fickle. Sometimes you have it, sometimes you don't. So best to assume it doesn't exist. Instead, plan to make things easier for yourself by ensuring that you have healthy, delicious alternatives to help you resist temptation. Don't go shopping when you're hungry, and put any likely temptations out of sight or, even better, just don't have them in the house!

3 Enlist your friends and family to support you. Explain what you are doing and why; perhaps you are wanting to reduce your blood sugars, or just to lose the extra weight that has been creeping up on you for years. Whatever your motivation is, the more they understand what you are trying to achieve, the more they can support you. Be specific: 'Please don't offer me cake/ another helping/ice cream...'

4 Add in TRE. This will enhance the effect of fasting on your weight loss and metabolic health (see page 12 for details).

5 Be more active. This is really important for your general health – switch the TV off, get up and go outside, walk more and try some strength-building exercises, as this increases your metabolic rate. A word of caution, though: while exercise is great for cardiovascular health, mood, strength and sleep, it is unfortunately a lousy way to lose weight. You need to run 36 miles to burn off a single pound of fat. So, go easy on the hard stuff at first, especially on fasting days – save that marathon training for a non-fast day, or when you are closer to your target weight or have finished the programme.

6 Get enough sleep. We are increasingly aware of the impact that poor and disrupted sleep has on our brain and mood, leaving us irritable, with even less willpower than usual, and far more inclined to crave sweet and starchy foods. On average, people tend to consume around 350 extra calories after a poor night's sleep. Sleep deprivation creates a vicious cycle of weight gain, snoring and exhaustion. (See Michael's book, *4 Weeks to Better Sleep*, for the full lowdown on why we sleep and how to get more of it.)

7 De-stress. Do this where you can, and try meditation. (*The Fast 800* book has some great advice on this; or go to thefast800.com)

8 And if you fall off the wagon... Please be assured that all is not lost. We all have bad days when we return to unhealthy food choices! Just start again the next day. The sooner you get back on track, the better. Be kind to yourself, it's just a blip.

FAQs

Does it matter if I eat 2 or 3 meals a day on a fast day? On the whole, it is probably easier to do 3 meals a day, but it's a matter of what works for you. We would advise, however, that you don't go down to one meal a day, particularly if it's soon before retiring to bed, as your body is more likely to treat it as a feast and store more fat. See the meal plans on pages 276–9.

Can I do it with shakes or protein powder, too? Yes, absolutely. We take a pragmatic view of meal replacement shakes. Eating real food is best, but if you are dashing out in a hurry and grabbing toast and jam for breakfast, or snatching a processed starchy lunch on the hoof, good-quality shakes are definitely preferable. They give you the protein and nutrients you need, and leave you feeling full. Do choose carefully as many of those available are full of sugars and contain inadequate amounts of protein (see thefast800.com for suitable low-carb, Mediterranean-formula options).

Should I take multivitamins? Our recipes are carefully balanced to include all the nutrients you need, but on a low-calorie diet it is not always easy to combine your meals for maximum nutritional variety, so we recommend taking a good-quality multivitamin on your 800–1000cals days as a back up.

What can I snack on? We would encourage you to avoid snacking between meals as this will stop fat-burning and may put sugars up. But if you must, nibble a small handful of nuts (unsweetened as they become very moreish otherwise!) or a few berries, or munch on a handful of non-starchy veg, such as carrots, cauliflower florets or celery. Alternatively, try a hot or cold drink to help keep hunger at bay (see suggestions on pages 18).

Can I exercise on a Fast 800 day? Doing more exercise helps us in lots of ways, including improving health and mood, but it's not a good way to lose weight. If you are already doing exercise and feel comfortable sticking with it on a fasting day, carry on with your current regime. But don't start a new, heavy programme or do endurance exercise on a fasting day. For those of you who have not been regular exercisers, you will find that as you lose weight you will feel better and have more energy and can get more active. Remember, it's not all about the gym. A lot of people surprise themselves and find they enjoy simple outdoor activities like walking or cycling. Walking with brief brisk bursts of 30–60 seconds can be a great way to start. And adding in some strengthening exercises will increase your muscle mass and improve your metabolism.

I have lost weight but recently hit a plateau. What can I do? It is common for weight loss to happen in bursts. Initial weight loss can be deceptive, as early on it also includes fluid loss. But if you stick to 800–1000cals you are likely to go on losing weight. When the weight loss seems to stall, some people find adding in shakes as part of their daily quota on a fasting day can help. It's also worth checking that you are still in the 800–1000cals zone. However, we are all different and some people will find that their weight loss is slower.

Can I eat bread? When it comes to bread, it's about choosing carefully, as white bread and a slice of seeded wholemeal sourdough are like chalk and cheese. You can occasionally have a thin slice of wholegrain, seeded or sourdough bread on a non-fast day, but try to avoid it on a fasting day. When you are buying bread, try to make sure the fibre content is higher than 7g in 100g.

Will I feel hungry all the time? For the first few days you are likely to feel hungry, but most people find that this settles as their metabolism re-sets. My patients often tell me how surprised they are that, despite such a dramatic drop in their daily calorie intake, within a week or two, they are no longer hungry all the time.

Is it expensive? Our calculations of a random sample of fasting-day recipes show the food to be affordable and likely to be cheaper.

Should I tell my doctor/health professional that I am doing a low-calorie diet? It is always a good idea to keep your health professional informed about a major change to your diet, particularly if you have a medical condition and/or are on medication (see SAFETY: Exclusions and cautions on page 14). It may help to print out a letter advising them about the diet, so they can monitor and support you in the process. This can be found at thefast800.com/healthcareprofessionals. Most health professionals will be aware of the 800-calorie approach and will be supportive.

EXTRA SUPPORT
It can make a real difference to have a partner, family member or diet buddy doing the diet with you in some way. Try to enlist friends, family, colleagues and anyone interested to help keep you motivated. For more information, see our website www.thefast800.com where you can access the Fast 800 Online Programme to help you stay on track and integrate the Fast 800 into your life.

Some useful tools and tricks

● **A tape-measure** for measuring your waist and neck, and a set of scales; you might also consider investing in a blood pressure monitor.

● **Keto stix** (a urine dipstick to measure if you are in nutritional ketosis – i.e. burning ketones from fat instead of burning sugar); these can be helpful at first or if you hit a plateau. Please note that ketosis reduces after a few weeks, but weight loss continues, although at a slower rate.

● **A diet journal** – studies have shown that keeping a food diary can be hugely helpful when you are trying to lose weight. Try our book *The Fast 800 Health Journal* to help monitor your progress and to keep yourself motivated.

● **Cooking equipment – minimal!**
A stick blender, some digital kitchen scales, a set of measuring spoons, a small and medium saucepan, a flameproof casserole with well-fitting lid, a wide frying pan or wok, a metal baking tray, baking dish (optional), medium bowl, vegetable peeler, spiralizer (optional) and a good sharp knife.

Hydration

Good hydration with minimal calories

Most of us fail to drink enough fluid. But keeping well hydrated is especially important on a fasting day as you are taking in less liquid with food and losing fluid when you burn fat. As a result, it's easy to get dehydrated, leaving you feeling exhausted, feeble, light-headed or suffering headaches.

On a fasting day you should drink an extra 1–1.5 litres of calorie-free fluids, mainly as water (and more if you are very active or the weather is hot). Sipping fluids can also distract you from cravings and reduce hunger between meals.

Do avoid drinks with sweeteners, as they can upset the good bugs in your gut; they are also likely to maintain your sweet tooth, as they are so many times sweeter than sugar and can leave you feeling hungrier.

Here are some lovely ways to add flavour without significant calories – drinks that can be enjoyed any time, and will not interfere with fat burning.

Cold refreshing drinks

We like water and drink it straight from the tap or filtered, and keep a bottle of water in the fridge. If you are inclined to forget to increase your fluid intake, try keeping a jug or bottle in the kitchen or at work – one that needs to be finished by the end of the day. Or carry a bottle with you. If you are not a fan of plain water, here's how you can make it more enticing:

● Drink carbonated water for a bit of fizz.
● For added flavour, put in a few berries or some fresh herbs, like mint, rosemary or thyme.
● Or you might add a squeeze of fresh lemon or lime, and drop a twist into the bottle.
● A slice or two of cucumber or courgette looks and tastes refreshing.
● For a stronger brew, keep a bottle of cooled fruit or herbal tea in the fridge.

Hot comforting drinks

Try to avoid putting milk in your tea or coffee between meals, as this adds calories and interferes with fat-burning – although, straight after a meal, a dash of milk in your drink is OK. Between meals try taking your tea with a squeeze of lemon or drink black coffee.

For variety, try sipping fruit teas. Or make your own herbal infusions, adding a handful of fresh herbs, such as mint, thyme or sage, to boiled water.

I'm a big fan of **mint tea**, with its smooth feel and sweet scent. Mint grows wild in the garden or you can keep it in a pot and harvest the larger leaves. Steep some leaves in hot water for 5 minutes. A generous handful of mint leaves contains a surprising amount of nutrients, including iron, vitamin and antioxidants, which may help protect your cells from damage. Peppermint is also thought to improve digestion.

Green tea, meanwhile, has been shown to be one of the healthiest drinks on the planet. Thanks mainly to its antioxidant properties, it is thought to reduce the risk of heart disease, improve brain function, protect against some cancers, as well as support weight loss.

However, green tea is an acquired taste, as it can be slightly bitter (that is part of what makes it so beneficial). We like to drink green tea with some finely sliced fresh root ginger (1cm unpeeled) and ½ teaspoon ground cinnamon stirred in to add a delicate sweetness. Allow the tea leaves and ginger to steep for 3–5 minutes, then remove them before you drink.

Tips for using this book

● **Calorie counts:** These refer to one individual serving, unless stated otherwise. That said, please be aware that we include calorie counts as a rough guide only. There are significant variations between different nutritionists, counters and apps, so don't be too concerned by a few extra calories here or there.

● **Increase non-starchy veg and reduce calorie counting:** We encourage you to enjoy low-calorie non-starchy veg without counting calories. Pile half your plate with 'free' vegetables, such as leafy greens, salad leaves or celery, which have minimal calories but huge nutritional benefits (see page 272 for non-starchy greens and veg). Unless, of course, you want to add a dressing or a teaspoonful of extra-virgin olive oil – in which case, see page 272 for calories.

● **Suggestions for non-fast days:** We offer plenty of tips if you are on the New 5:2 or have moved on to a maintenance stage to adapt the recipes to make them more substantial. These might involve simply increasing or doubling the portion size, or adding a few tablespoons of brown rice or lentils, an extra glug of olive oil, a slice of seeded bread or extra vegetables.

● **Make the recipes suit you:** These recipes are based on a Med-style way of eating, but can be adapted to fit different cuisines and tastes. Feel free to adjust them by using alternative flavours, or adding different herbs and spices – all of which have minimal impact on calories. The tastier and more satisfying your food, the more likely you are to stick to this way of eating.

SYMBOLS

We have added the following symbols to the bottom of each page, so you can quickly spot which recipes might suit you best. These are guidelines only and you should always consult your doctor if you are unsure which foods are best for you.

Michael's favourites.

Either do not contain any animal-derived substances, or are optional.

Vegetarian.

Do not contain gluten.

Do not contain nuts.

Do not contain dairy products, or have a non-dairy alternative given.

Freezer-friendly.

Quick and easy recipes for a super-speedy dish.

You will also find nutritional information above each recipe, including calories (cals), for each individual serving.

Although some of the recipes included here are vegan, the Fast 800 is not designed for vegans.

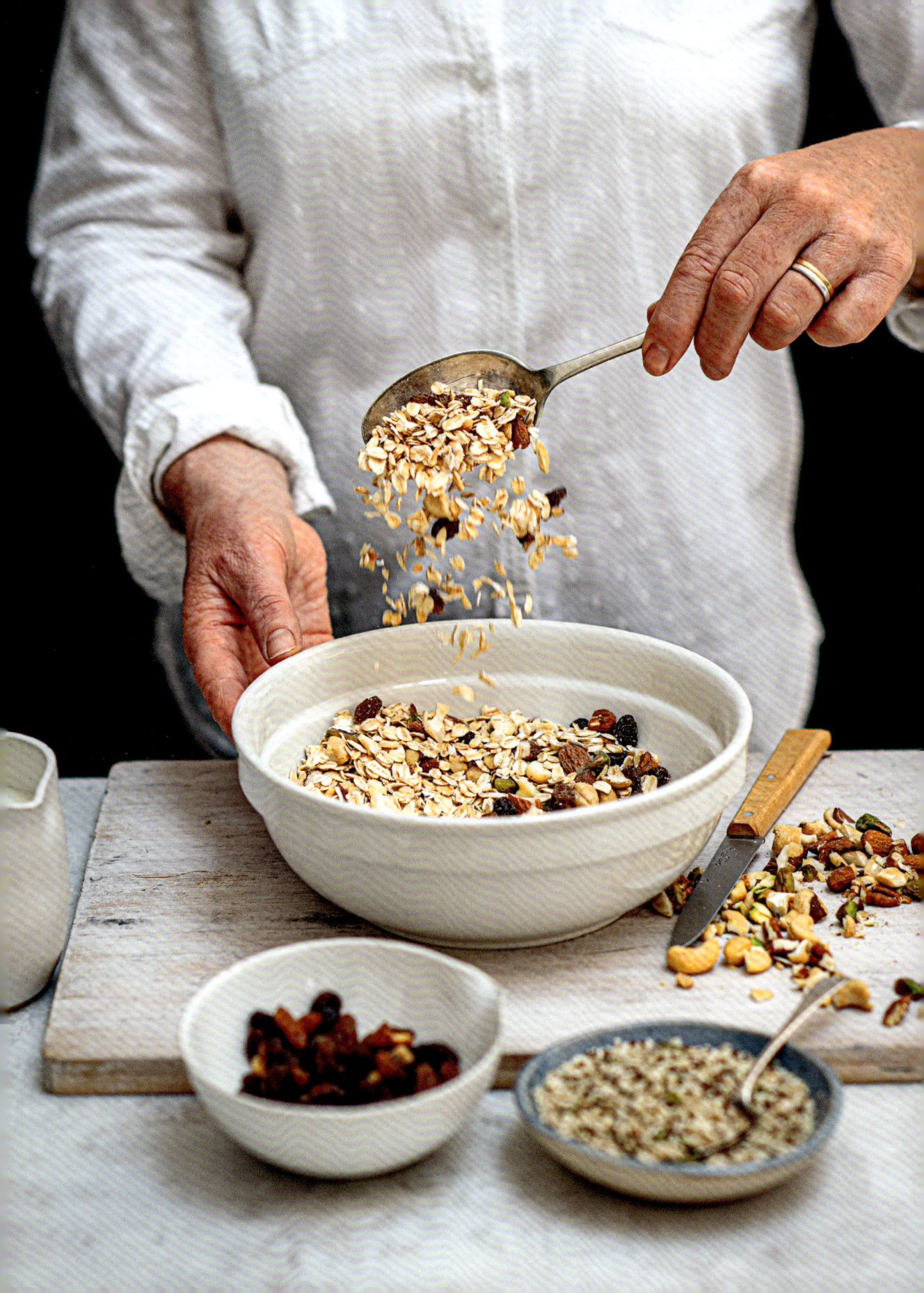

Breakfast and Brunch

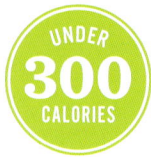

PER SERVING | **209cals** | PROTEIN **6.8g** | CARBS **18.1g**

Blueberry Bircher Muesli

SERVES **1** | PREP **5** mins

1 level tbsp rolled oats
1 level tbsp chia seeds
1 heaped tbsp frozen
   blueberries
3 tbsp full-fat live Greek
   yoghurt (around 45g)
1 tbsp full-fat milk
½ tsp ground cinnamon

NON-FAST DAY
Add a handful of chopped nuts
and/or serve a larger portion.

A nice little overnight muesli that can be easily thrown together using a tablespoon measure and some frozen blueberries. There is no need to defrost frozen blueberries prior to making this, as they will defrost in the fridge overnight. The chia seeds add protein, fibre and a creamy texture.

1. Place all the ingredients in a bowl, mix well and refrigerate overnight.

2. Stir to break up the blueberries before serving. Add an extra tablespoon of milk, if the mixture is too thick.

VEGGIE · GLUTEN FREE · NUT FREE

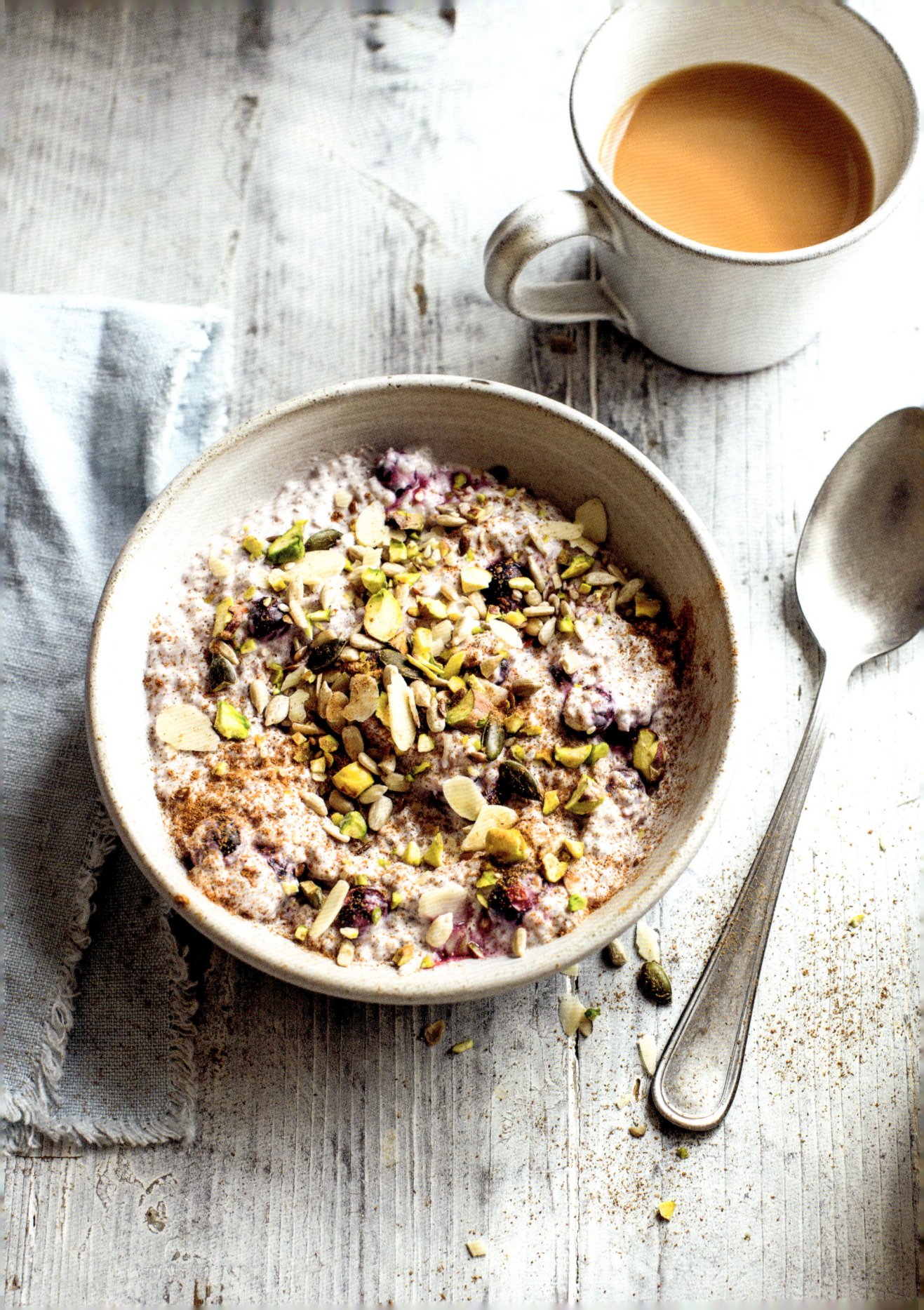

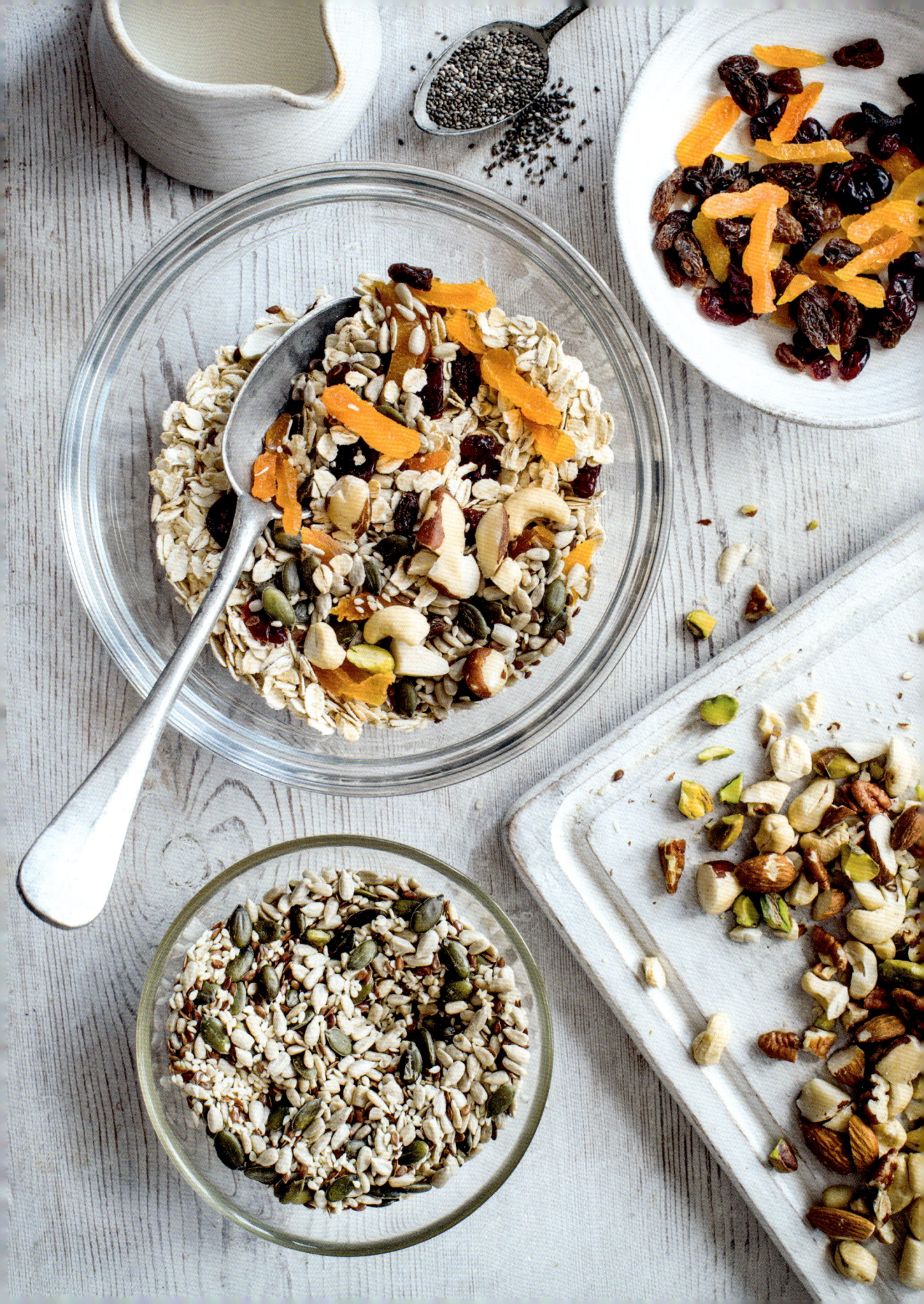

PER SERVING | **294cals** | PROTEIN **11.5g** | CARBS **23g**

UNDER 300 CALORIES

Nutty Seedy Porridge

SERVES 6 | PREP 10 mins | COOK 6 mins

100g plain mixed nuts, roughly chopped
100g rolled jumbo oats
50g mixed seeds
50g mixed dried fruit
100ml full-fat milk or dairy-free alternative, to serve

COOK'S TIP

For a creamier porridge, add 1 teaspoon chia seeds to each serving as you add it to the pan. Add an extra 2 tablespoons water and cook as directed. With the additional chia, each serving will contain 324cals and 12g protein.

A high-protein, fruity porridge. The rolled jumbo oats are minimally processed, giving you slow-release energy, while the nuts and seeds provide the protein and fibre you need to feel full for longer.

1. Tip the nuts, oats, seeds and dried fruit into a large bowl. Mix well together then transfer to a jar or other lidded airtight container.

2. For one serving of porridge, take 50g of the mix and place it in a non-stick saucepan. Add the milk and 100ml water, place over a medium heat and simmer for 5–6 minutes, stirring, until thick and creamy. Alternatively, put the porridge, water and milk in a large microwaveable bowl and cook on HIGH for 3 minutes. Stir and cook for a further 30–60 seconds, or until thick and creamy.

3. Spoon into individual bowls and leave to stand for 2–3 minutes to allow to thicken before serving.

VEGAN · GLUTEN FREE · DAIRY FREE

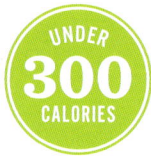

Pear and Cinnamon Porridge

SERVES | PREP | COOK
1 | **4** mins | **6** mins

30g jumbo porridge oats
1 Conference pear (around
    135g), peeled, cored and
    roughly chopped
¼ tsp ground cinnamon
75ml full-fat milk, or
    dairy-free alternative
5g toasted flaked almonds
    (around 2 tsp)

NON-FAST DAYS
Increase the portion size.

COOK'S TIP
If you can't find ready-toasted
almonds, toast your own
(see page 33) or use an
untoasted kind.

A comforting and filling breakfast. You can substitute
the pear with grated apple, if you like. Michael loved
a simple bowl of porridge sweetened by cinnamon.

1. Place the oats, pear and cinnamon in a small
saucepan. Pour in the milk and 120ml water, and cook
over a low–medium heat for 5–6 minutes, stirring
constantly, or until the oats are softened and creamy.

2. Pour into a deep bowl and scatter with the flaked
almonds to serve.

VEGAN   GLUTEN FREE   DAIRY FREE

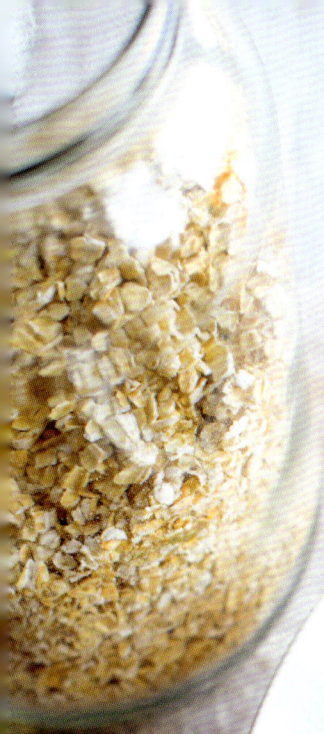

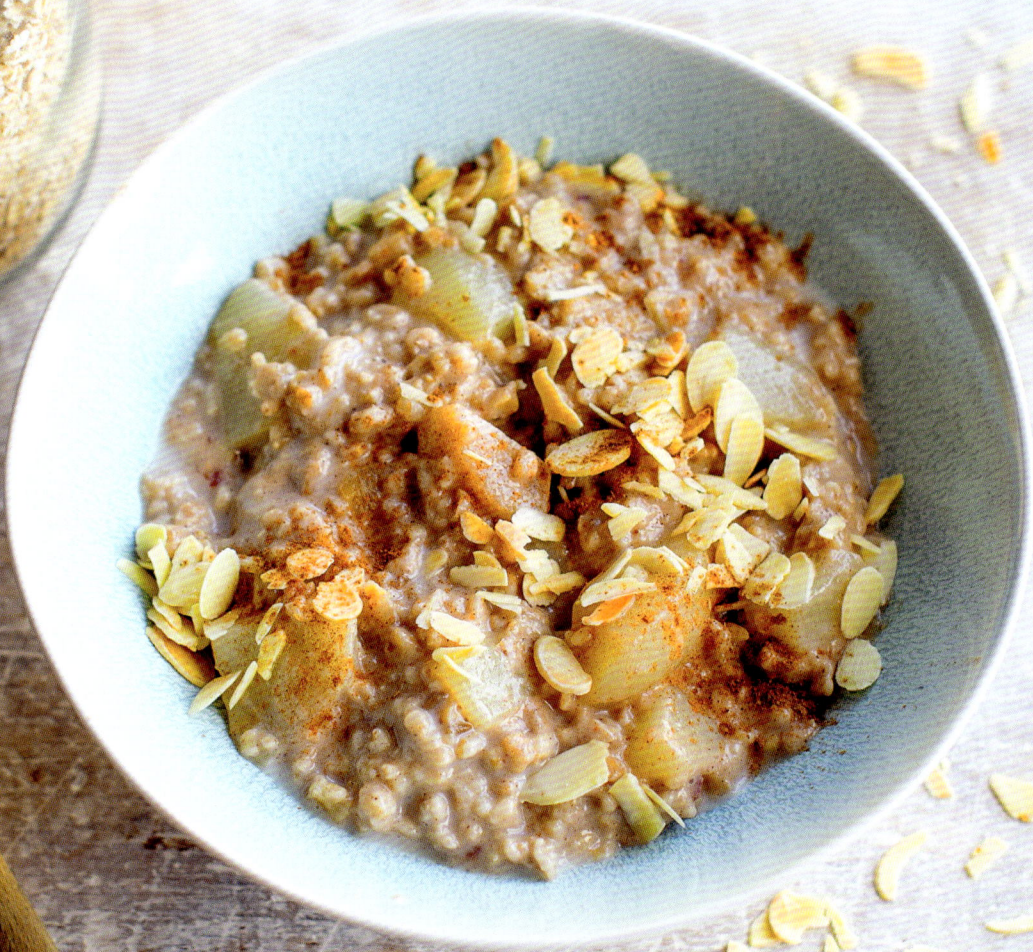

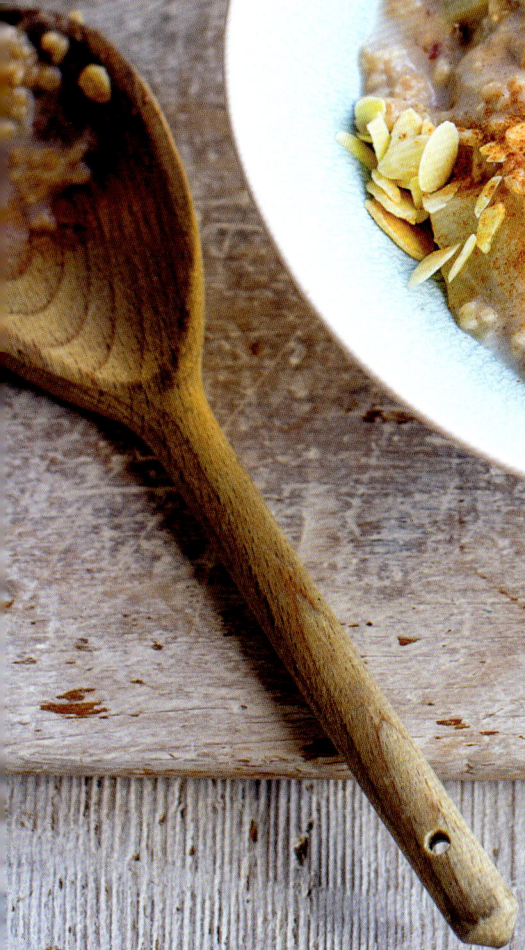

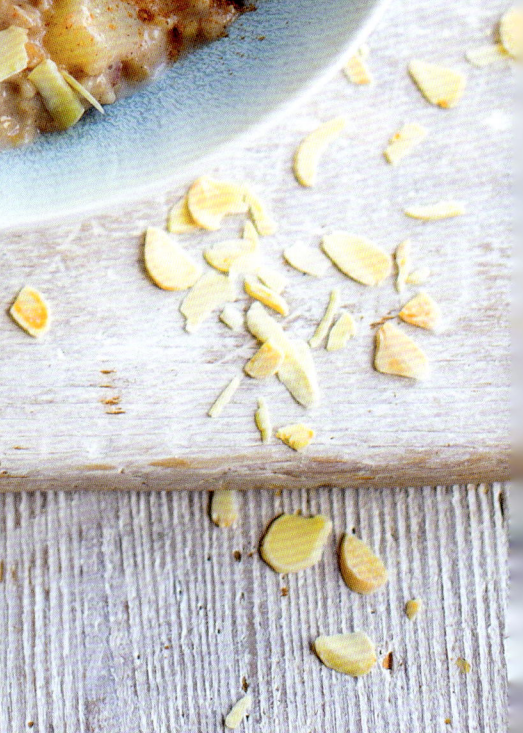

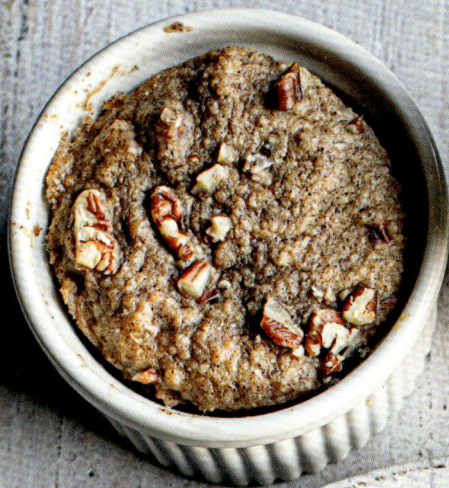

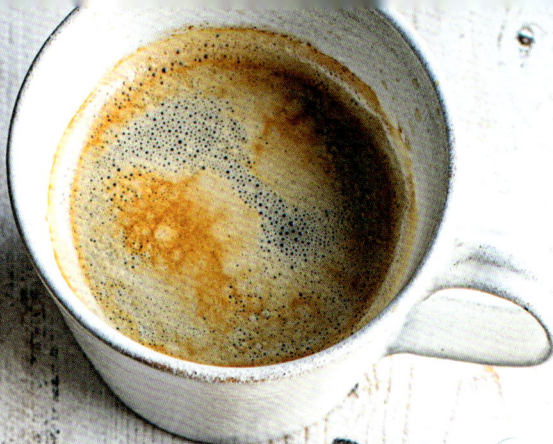

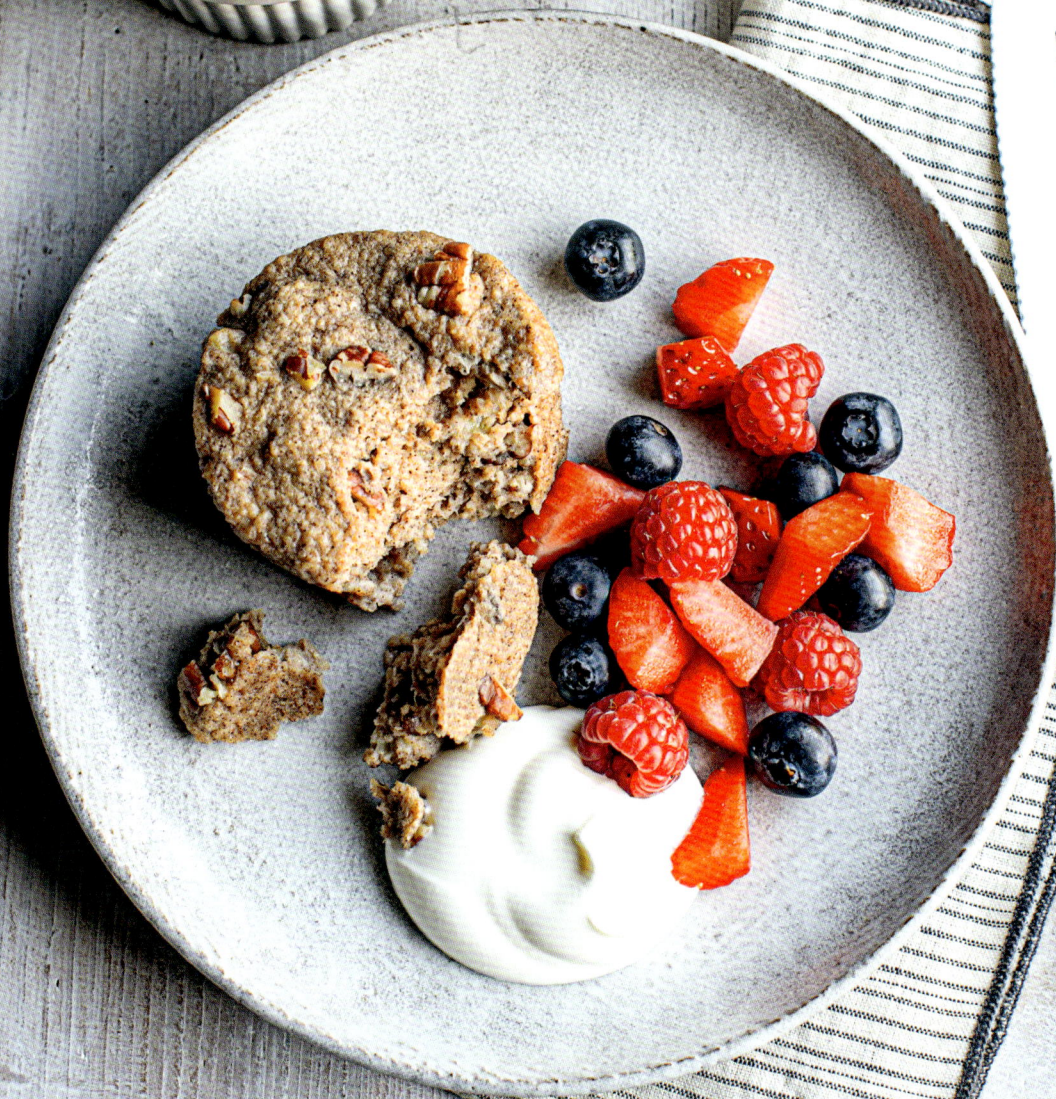

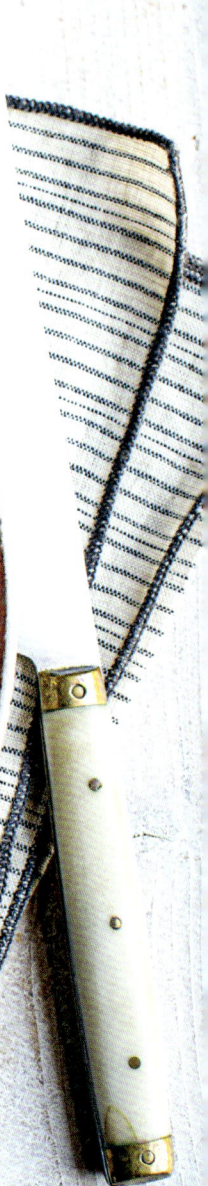

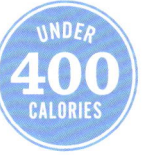

Banana and Pecan Muffin

SERVES
2

PREP
2
mins

COOK
2
mins

1 tbsp melted coconut oil
  or rapeseed oil
1 medium free-range egg
1 small ripe banana,
  peeled and mashed
  with a fork (around
  65g prepared weight)
20g ground almonds
20g wholemeal
  self-raising flour
¼ tsp baking powder
8 pecan halves,
  roughly chopped
½ tsp ground cinnamon

NON-FAST DAYS
Serve the muffin with a dollop
of full-fat live Greek yoghurt.

A warm, fluffy breakfast treat that is a healthy
alternative to a coffee-shop muffin. Serve with a
handful of fresh berries, if you like (25g will add 11cals).
You can melt the coconut oil in the microwave, but don't
let it overheat. We divided the mixture between two
small ramekins, instead of using a mug, and cooked
them together for the same amount of time – no need
to cut it in half, if you do this. Michael loved a good
muffin, especially when it contained plenty of
protein to keep you full for longer.

1. Use a tiny amount of the oil to lightly grease
a microwave-proof mug (to hold around 350ml).

2. Break the egg into the mug and beat really well
with a fork.

3. Add the banana, ground almonds, flour, baking powder,
pecans, cinnamon and the remaining oil, and mix well.

4. Place in a microwave and cook on high for about
1½ minutes, or until risen and firm (the time will vary
according to the wattage of your oven). The muffin should
have just begun to shrink back from the sides of the mug.
Leave to stand for 1 minute.

5. Loosen the sides of the muffin in the mug, then tip it out,
cut it in half and serve warm.

VEGGIE   DAIRY FREE

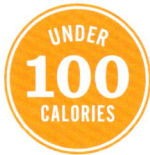

PER SERVING | **79cals** | PROTEIN **3.4g** | CARBS **1.4g**

Blueberry Protein Pancakes

MAKES	PREP	COOK
8	**5** mins	**8** mins

30g ground almonds
60g full-fat cream cheese,
   or dairy-free alternative,
   softened
2 medium free-range eggs
½ tsp vanilla extract
80g blueberries, plus
   extra to decorate
15g butter or coconut oil

COOK'S TIP
The pancakes freeze well. Store them with non-stick baking paper between each pancake so that it is easy to remove one at a time. Thaw them in the fridge and warm gently in a medium oven or for a short burst in the microwave to serve.

Easy and delicious – these pancakes are lovely served with yoghurt and more fresh blueberries. Partial to a pancake, Michael loved this high-protein, low-carb version, as it doesn't send sugars soaring.

1. Place the ground almonds, cream cheese, eggs and vanilla in a bowl and mix with an electric whisk until smooth. Stir in the blueberries.

2. Melt half the butter or coconut oil in a large non-stick frying pan over a medium heat. Pour in 4 tablespoons of batter to make 4 small pancakes. Cook for about 2 minutes, or until golden, then flip and cook on the other side for the same amount of time. Transfer to a plate and continue with the rest of the butter or coconut oil and batter.

3. Serve the pancakes warm with extra blueberries and full-fat live Greek yoghurt, if you like (don't forget to add the calories).

VEGGIE · GLUTEN FREE · DAIRY FREE

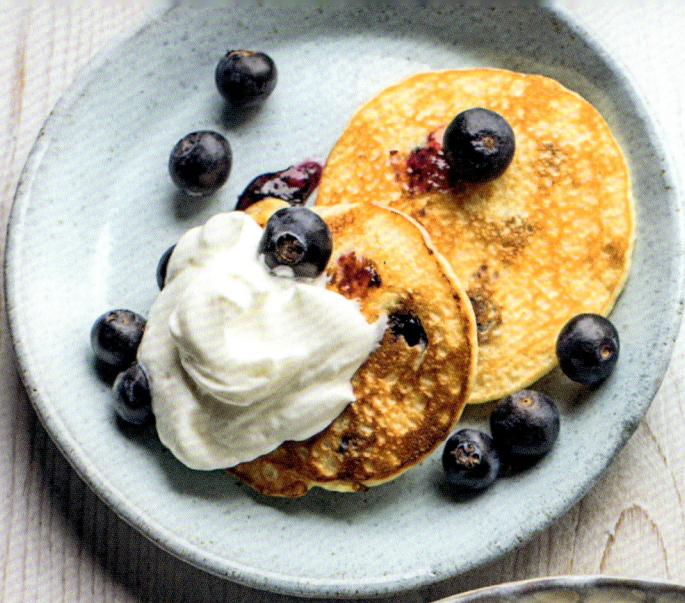

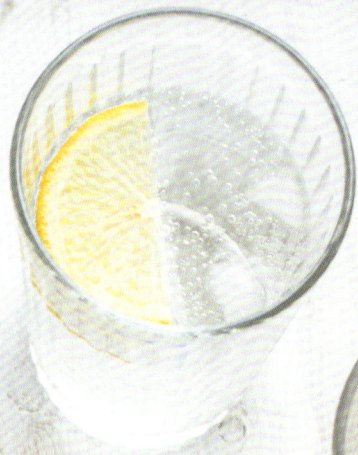

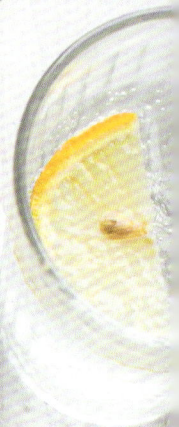

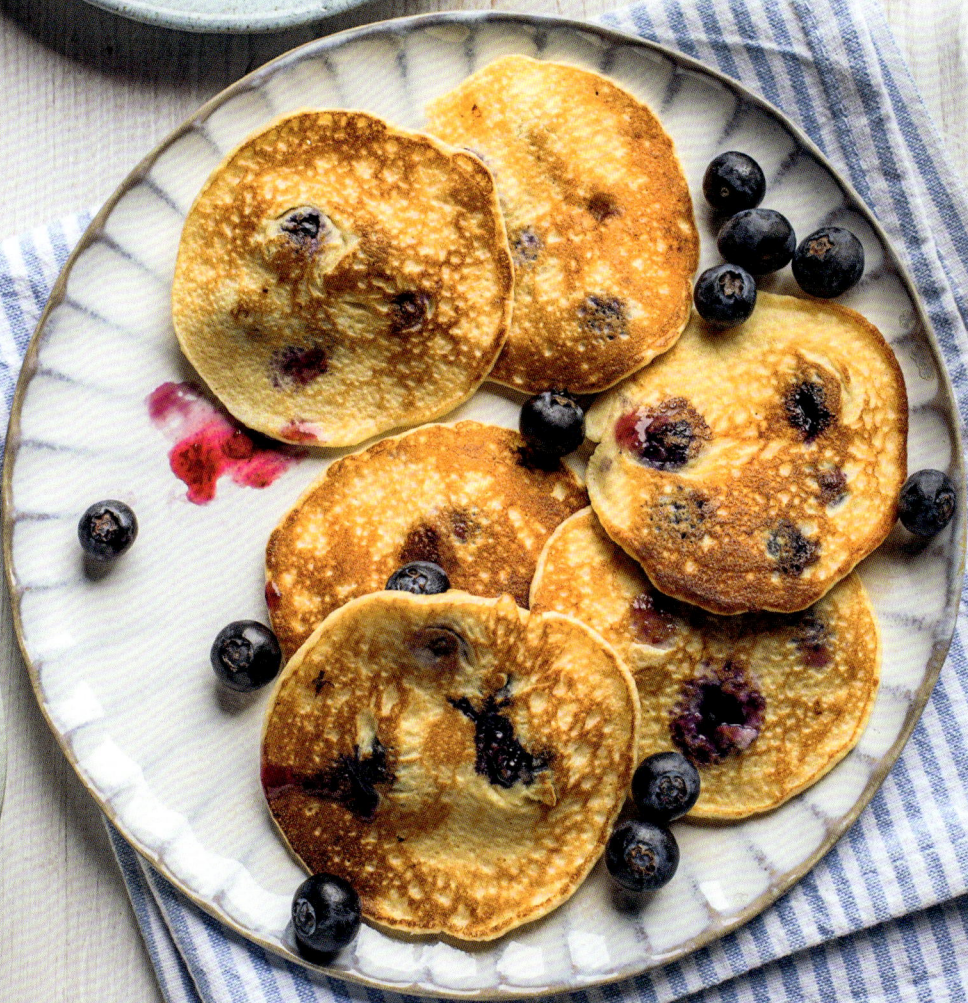

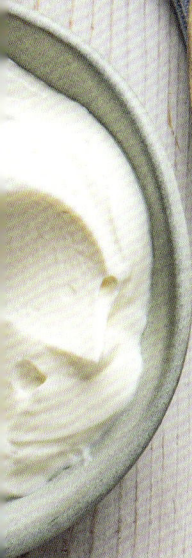

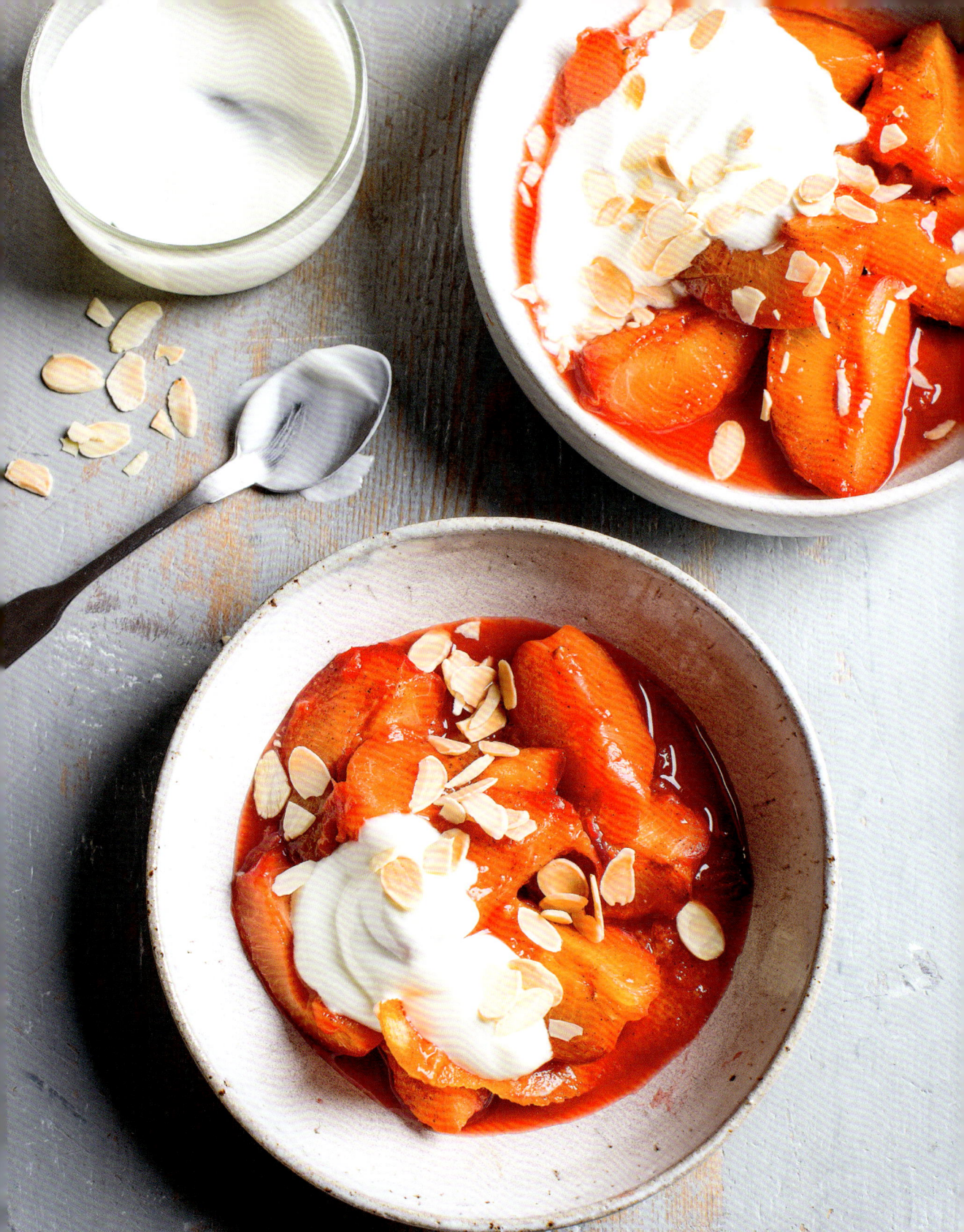

Spiced Breakfast Plums

SERVES **2**

PREP **5** mins

COOK **15** mins

4 plums (around 275g),
  halved and stoned
2 × 10–12cm strips of orange
  zest, removed with
  a vegetable peeler
juice of 1 large orange
  (around 100ml)
¼ tsp ground cinnamon
100g full-fat live Greek
  yoghurt, or dairy-free
  alternative
15g toasted flaked almonds

NON-FAST DAYS
Add extra toasted nuts.

COOK'S TIP
If you can't find ready-toasted
almonds, toast your own in
a dry frying pan over a low
heat for 1–2 minutes, stirring
regularly; or simply top with
the untoasted kind.

Delicious served warm or cold. This would also
make a refreshing dessert.

1. Put the plums in a saucepan. Add the orange zest and
juice, 150ml water and the cinnamon, and stir lightly.
Bring the liquid to a simmer, then cover with a lid, reduce
the heat to low and cook for 10–15 minutes, or until the
plums are soft but still holding their shape.

2. Divide the plums between two bowls and serve
warm or cold with the Greek yoghurt and a sprinkling
of toasted almonds.

AIR-FRYER TIP

Preheat the air fryer to 160°C, if needed. Place the
plums, cut-side down, in an even layer in a small baking
dish or directly into the air fryer. Add the strips of orange
zest, juice, water and cinnamon and stir until combined.
Air fry for 7 minutes, then turn the plums, spooning
the juices in the dish over them, and air fry for another
6–8 minutes until they are soft but hold their shape.
Serve as Step 2.

VEGAN   GLUTEN FREE   DAIRY FREE

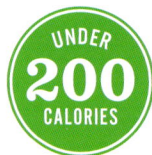

PER SERVING | **189cals** | PROTEIN **4.7g** | CARBS **13.1g**

Super Seeded Flapjacks

MAKES	PREP	COOK
16	**10** mins	**20** mins

200g rolled oats
200g mixed seeds
15 soft pitted dates,
    diced (about 115g)
125g butter, cubed,
    or coconut oil
2 tbsp honey
1 tsp ground cinnamon

COOK'S TIP
The flapjacks will keep
in an airtight container
for up to 7 days.

When the kids were young, I made mounds of flapjacks, with gallons of golden syrup, which is essentially refined sugar with water. Yes, they were popular, but with a few simple tweaks, such as adding seeds for extra fibre and protein, they still wolfed them down. Michael enjoyed making these simple, fibre-rich treats, with slow-release sugar from the dates.

1. Preheat the oven to 190°C/Fan 170°C/Gas 5 and line a 18cm square tin with non-stick baking paper.

2. Combine the oats and seeds in a mixing bowl.

3. Place 1 tablespoon of water in a small pan over a gentle heat. Add the diced dates, then use the back of a spoon to soften them and make a paste.

4. Add the butter or coconut oil, honey, cinnamon and a generous pinch of salt to the pan, then bring to a gentle simmer.

5. Stir the date mixture into the oats and seeds until coated. Press the mixture firmly into the prepared tin and bake in the preheated oven for about 15–20 minutes until golden.

6. Remove from the oven and leave to cool before cutting into 16 squares.

AIR-FRYER TIP

Preheat the air fryer to 170°C, if needed. Prepare the flapjack mixture as above, then cook in the air fryer for 15 minutes until golden.

VEGGIE | GLUTEN FREE | NUT FREE | DAIRY FREE

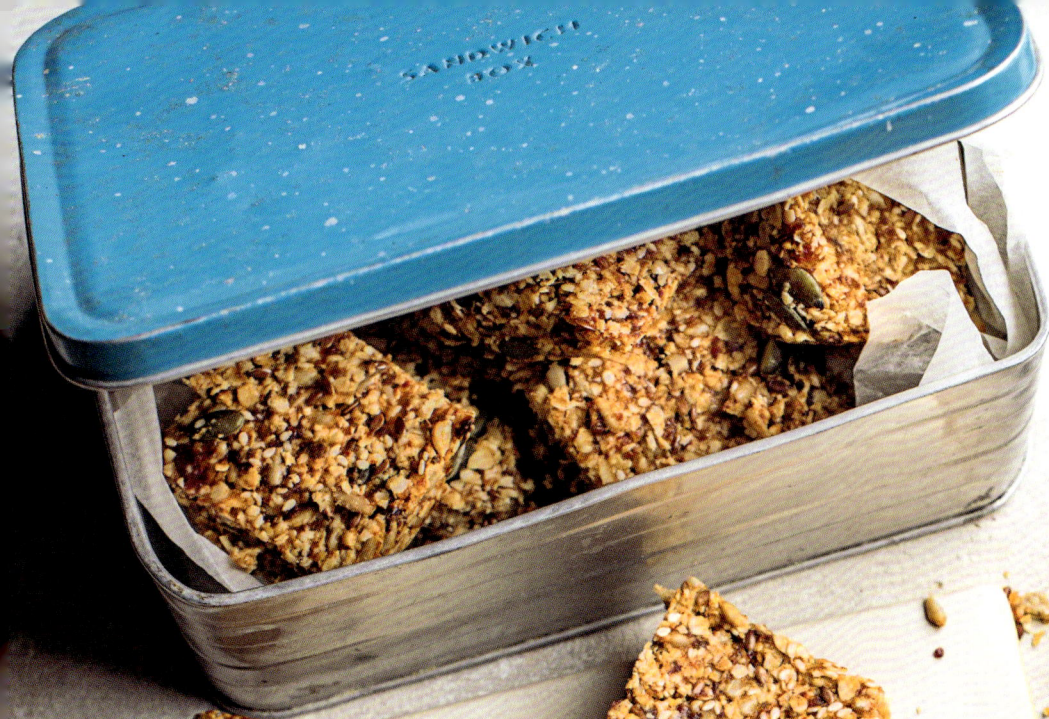

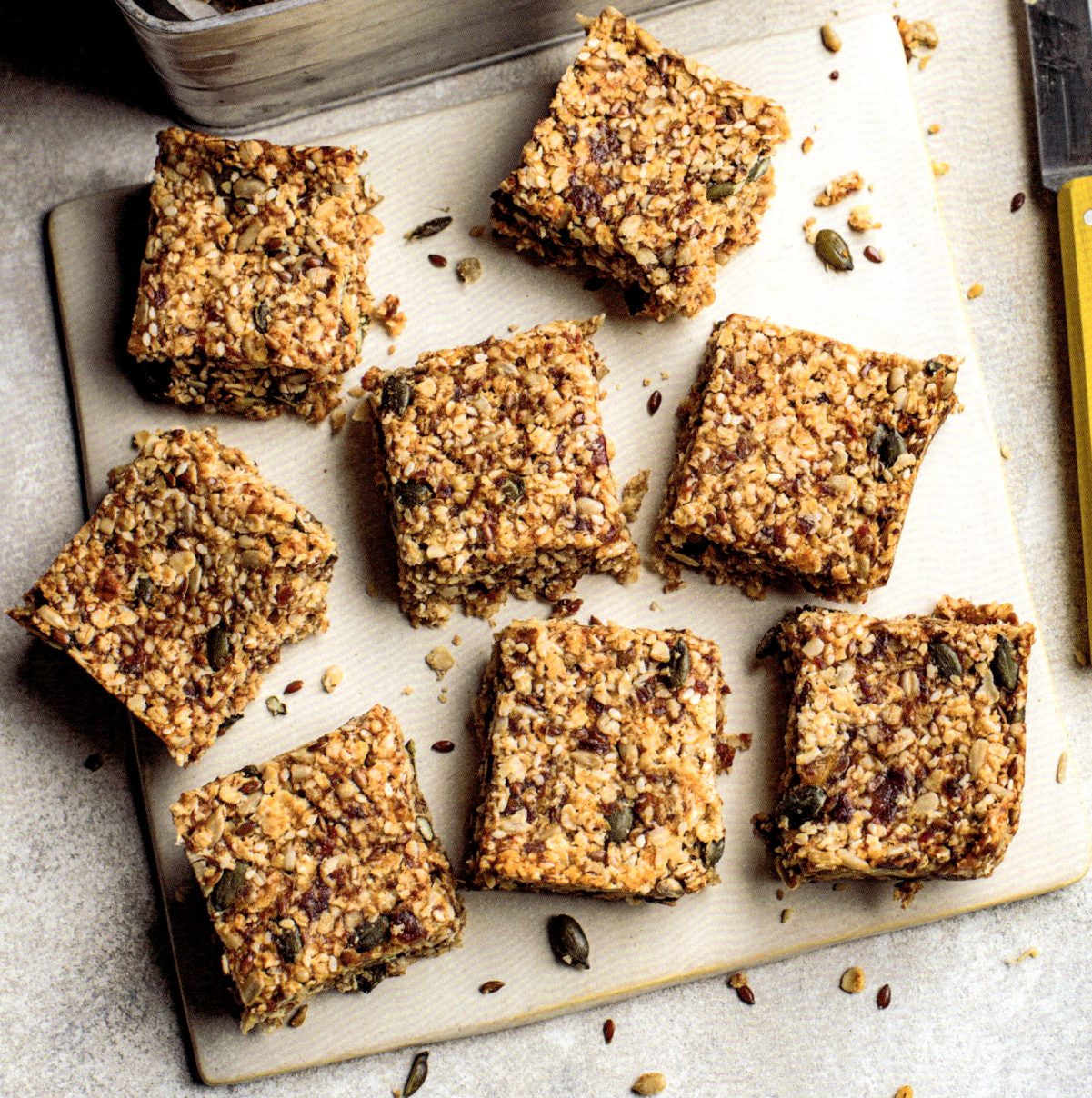

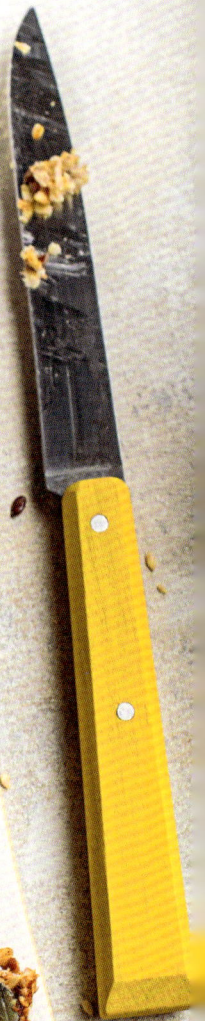

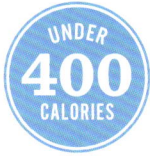

PER SERVING | **312cals** | PROTEIN **19.5g** | CARBS **17.5g**

Shakshuka

SERVES | PREP | COOK
2 | **5** mins | **20** mins

1 tbsp olive oil
1 red onion, finely chopped
1 red or yellow pepper,
   deseeded and thinly sliced
2 garlic cloves, crushed
1 tsp ground cumin
½–1 tsp hot smoked paprika
   (to taste)
1 × 400g can chopped tomatoes
1 tbsp tomato purée
4 medium free-range eggs
small handful fresh coriander
   or flat-leaf parsley, leaves
   roughly chopped, to serve
   (optional)

NON-FAST DAYS
Crumble feta over the top after
adding the eggs and serve with
warmed wholemeal pitta bread.

COOK'S TIP
If your frying pan doesn't
have a lid, use a heatproof plate
or a large piece of kitchen foil.
Covering the pan helps the eggs
cook and prevents the tomato
sauce from becoming too thick.

A hugely popular brunch dish from the Middle East
and North Africa made with eggs poached in a lightly
spiced tomato sauce. We often enjoyed a shakshuka
for brunch on a Sunday with the family.

1. Heat the oil in a medium non-stick frying pan or
shallow flameproof casserole that has a lid. Add the
onion and pepper and gently fry for 5–6 minutes,
or until softened, stirring regularly.

2. Add the garlic, cumin and smoked paprika and cook
for 20–30 seconds, stirring.

3. Tip the tomatoes into the pan, add the tomato purée,
a good pinch of salt and lots of ground black pepper.
Bring to a simmer and cook for about 4 minutes, or
until the tomato sauce has thickened, stirring regularly.

4. Make four holes in the vegetable mixture and break
an egg into each one. Cover the pan with the lid and
cook very gently for 3–5 minutes, or until the whites
are set but the yolks remain runny.

5. Sprinkle with the fresh herbs, if using, and season
with more ground black pepper to serve.

VEGGIE | GLUTEN FREE | NUT FREE | DAIRY FREE

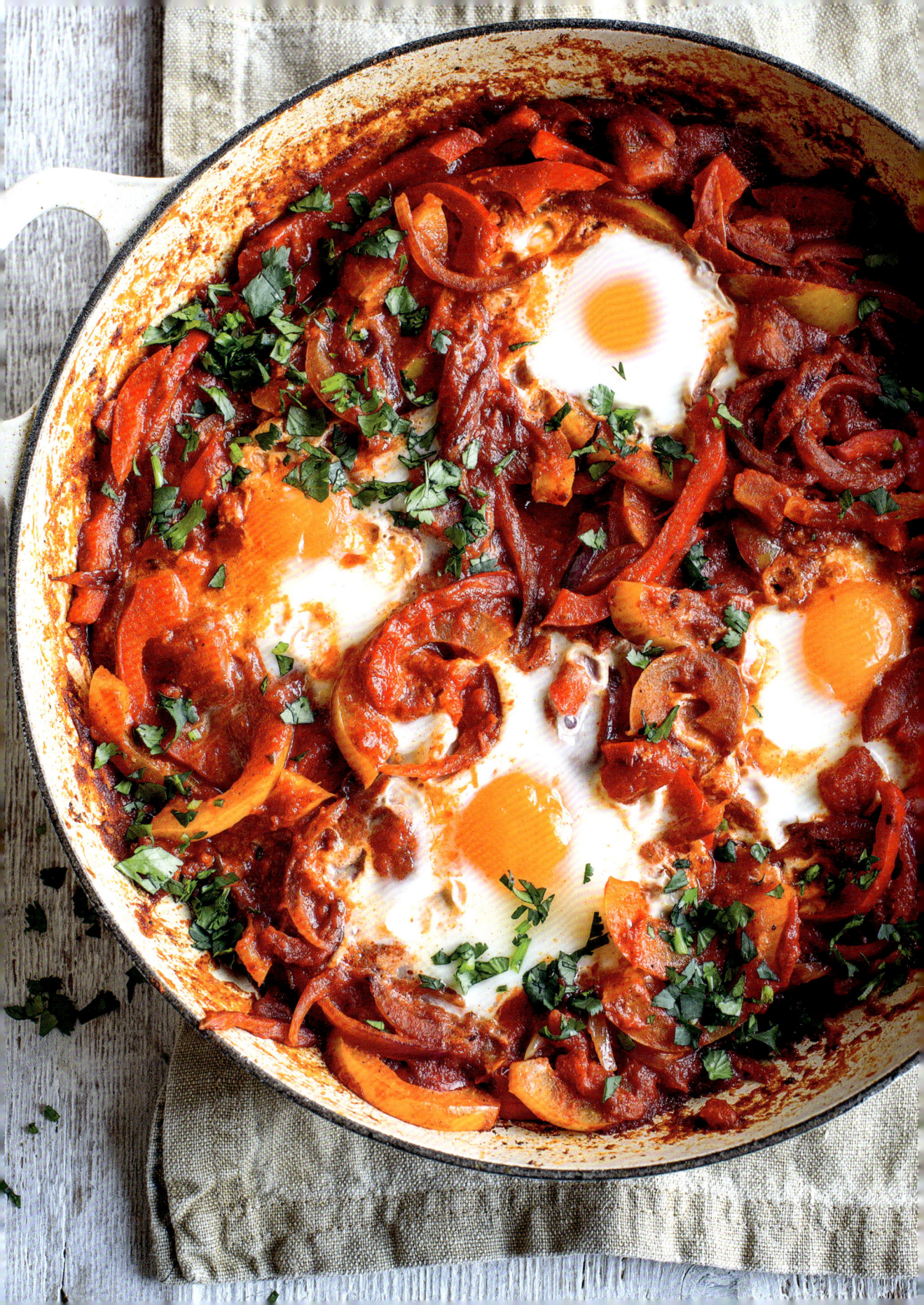

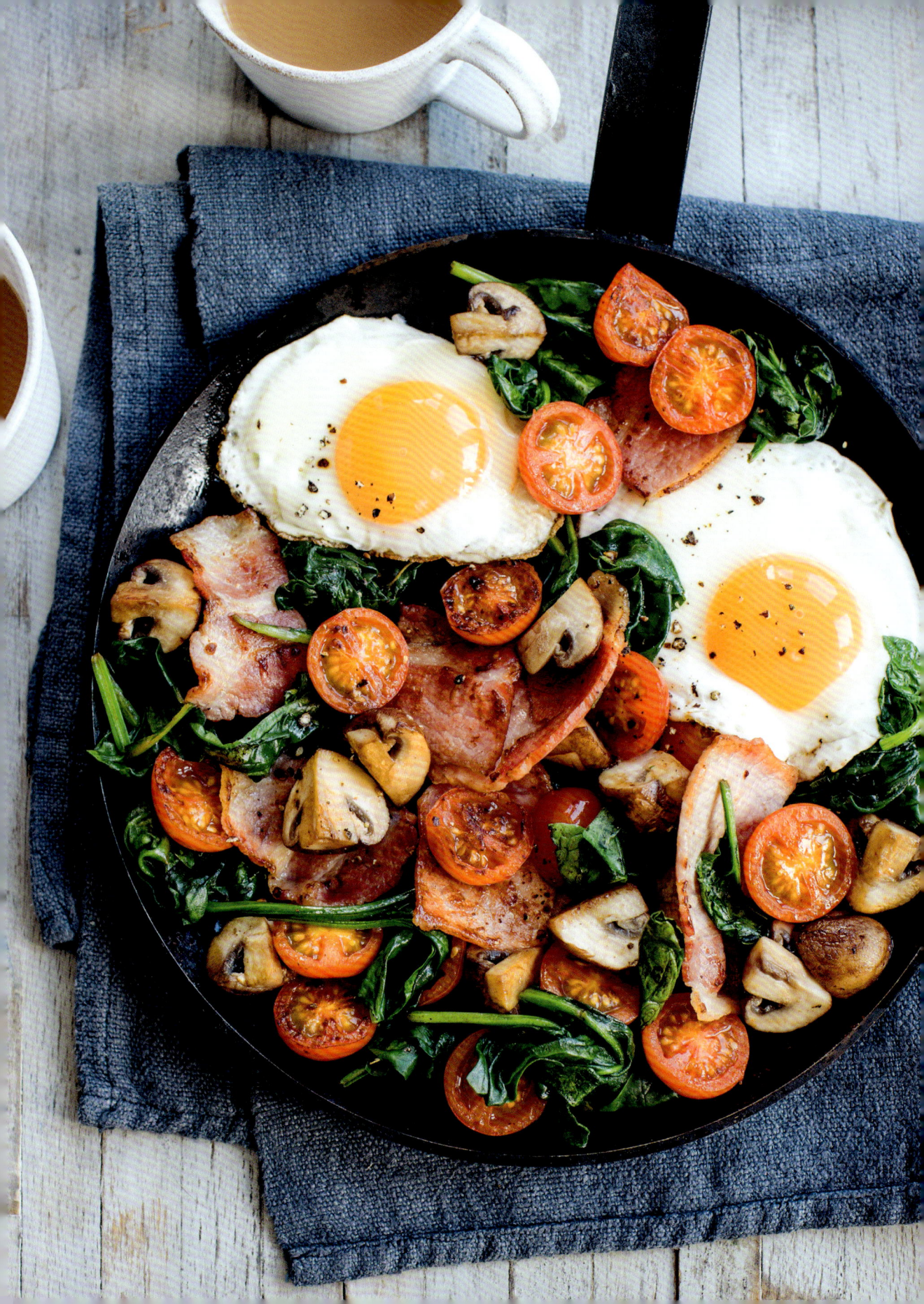

PER SERVING | **227cals** | PROTEIN **15.7g** | CARBS **2.1g**

UNDER 300 CALORIES

One-pan Breakfast

SERVES 2 | PREP 10 mins | COOK 7 mins

1 tbsp rapeseed or olive oil
2 rashers smoked back bacon, each cut into 3–4 slices
6–8 chestnut mushrooms, quartered or halved
10 cherry tomatoes, halved
50g young spinach leaves
2 medium free-range eggs

NON-FAST DAY
Serve with a thin slice of wholegrain toast.

The occasional fry-up at the weekend was right up Michael's street and is so satisfyingly filling. Breakfast was his favourite meal, and there are health benefits to eating ealier in the day.

1. Heat the oil in a large, non-stick frying pan over a medium heat. Add the bacon and mushrooms, and fry for 2 minutes, or until lightly browned.

2. Add the tomatoes and stir fry for a further 2 minutes, or until the tomatoes soften.

3. Fold in the spinach and move the whole mixture to the side of the pan.

4. Gently crack the eggs into the cleared space, reduce the heat to low and cook for 2–3 minutes, or until lightly set.

5. Spoon the bacon, tomatoes and mushrooms on to two warmed plates and top with the eggs. Season with ground black pepper and serve immediately.

GLUTEN FREE · NUT FREE · DAIRY FREE

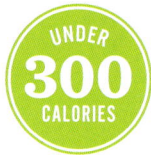

PER SERVING | **228cals** | PROTEIN **20.6g** | CARBS **2.1g**

Harissa Yoghurt with Soft-boiled Eggs and Spinach

SERVES	PREP	COOK
1	**2** mins	**6** mins

2 medium free-range eggs
100g young spinach leaves
2 tbsp full-fat live Greek
  yoghurt
1 tbsp rose harissa pesto
  or ½ tbsp harissa paste
small pinch crushed dried
  chilli flakes (optional)
1 tsp mixed seeds, toasted

COOK'S TIP
If you prefer less heat,
substitute sun-dried tomato
pesto for the harissa.

NON-FAST DAY
Serve with a thin slice of
wholemeal bread, sourdough,
or 2–3 tablespoons of quinoa.

A quick, easy breakfast with North African flavours. The creamy yoghurt adds extra protein and a tangy contrast to the crunchy seeds.

1. Bring a small saucepan of water to the boil and carefully lower in the eggs. Simmer for 5½ minutes. Using a slotted spoon, transfer the eggs to a bowl of iced water. Carefully peel the eggs and slice each one in half.

2. Remove the saucepan from the heat and plunge the spinach into the hot water. Stir for 30 seconds, then drain thoroughly and squeeze as much liquid as possible from the spinach.

3. Meanwhile mix the yoghurt and harissa together in a wide bowl.

4. Mix the drained spinach into the yoghurt and season generously with salt and freshly ground black pepper. Top with the eggs, chilli flakes, if using, and a sprinkling of mixed seeds to serve.

VEGGIE   GLUTEN FREE   NUT FREE

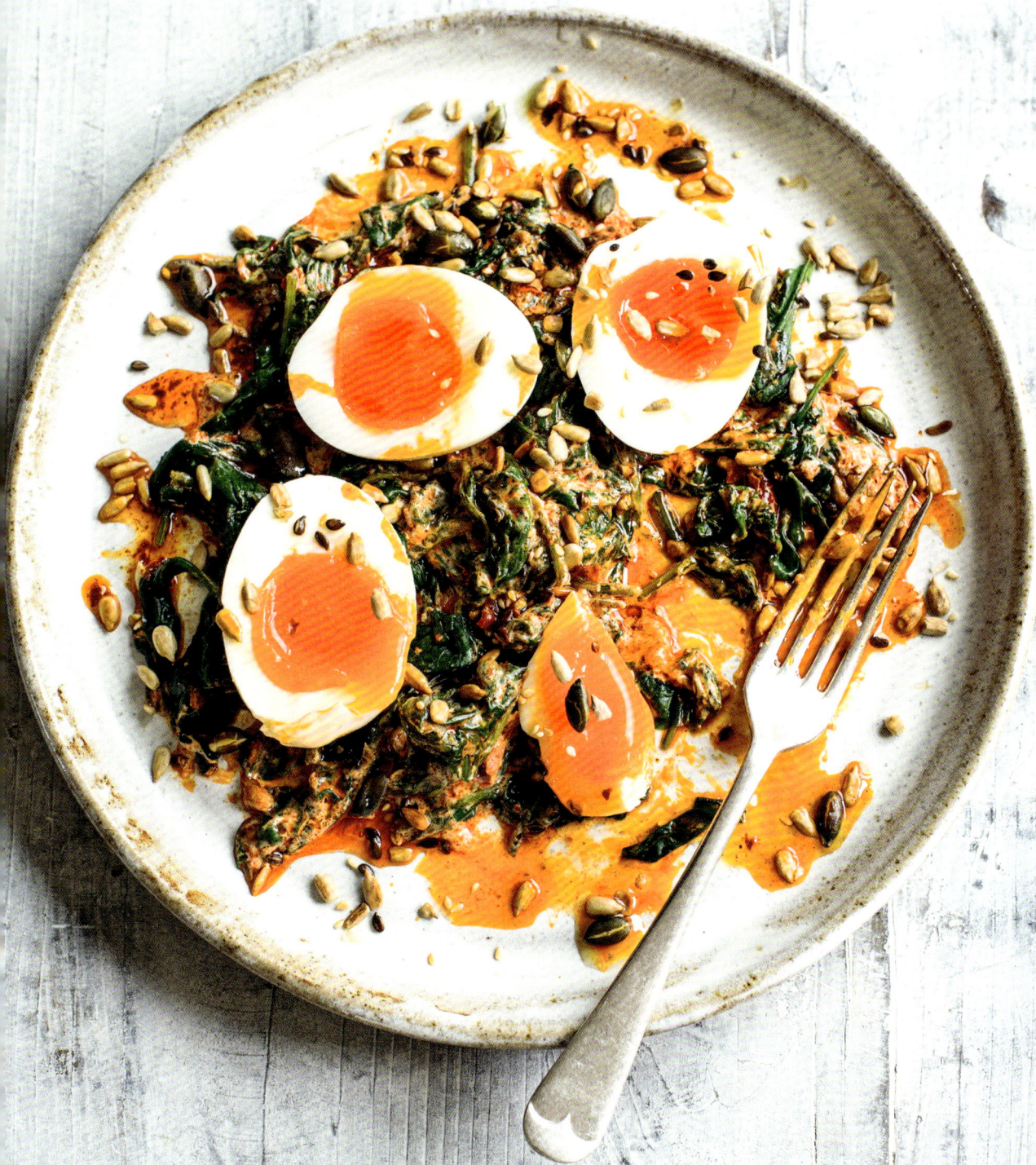

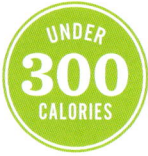

Chorizo Omelette

SERVES	PREP	COOK
2	**5** mins	**7** mins

½ tbsp olive oil
½ small onion, diced
4 medium free-range eggs
3cm piece cured chorizo,
   sliced and quartered
30g mature Cheddar, grated
60g cooked or leftover greens
½ tsp crushed dried chilli
   flakes (optional)

NON-FAST DAY
Have a larger portion.

This was one of Michael's go-to omelettes, which he cooked to perfection. It has fabulous Spanish flavours, is high in protein and is easy to make. It's even better topped with fermented veg, like sauerkraut (see page 225), which adds a delicious sweet, salty and tangy flavour, and is so beneficial to your health that you don't need to count the calories.

1. Place a non-stick frying pan over a medium heat. Add the oil and onion and sweat for 2 minutes.

2. Crack the eggs into a small bowl and whisk with a fork. Season well with freshly ground black pepper, then pour over the onion. Leave for 30 seconds to start to set, then use a spatula or wooden spoon to pull the egg into the centre of the pan, allowing the runny mixture to flow out into the empty space. Do this 4 or 5 times, working quite quickly.

3. When the omelette has started to set, add the chorizo, cheese and greens. Cook for another 2 minutes, then scatter over the chilli flakes, if using. Fold one half of the omelette over the other and slide onto a plate to serve.

GLUTEN FREE · NUT FREE

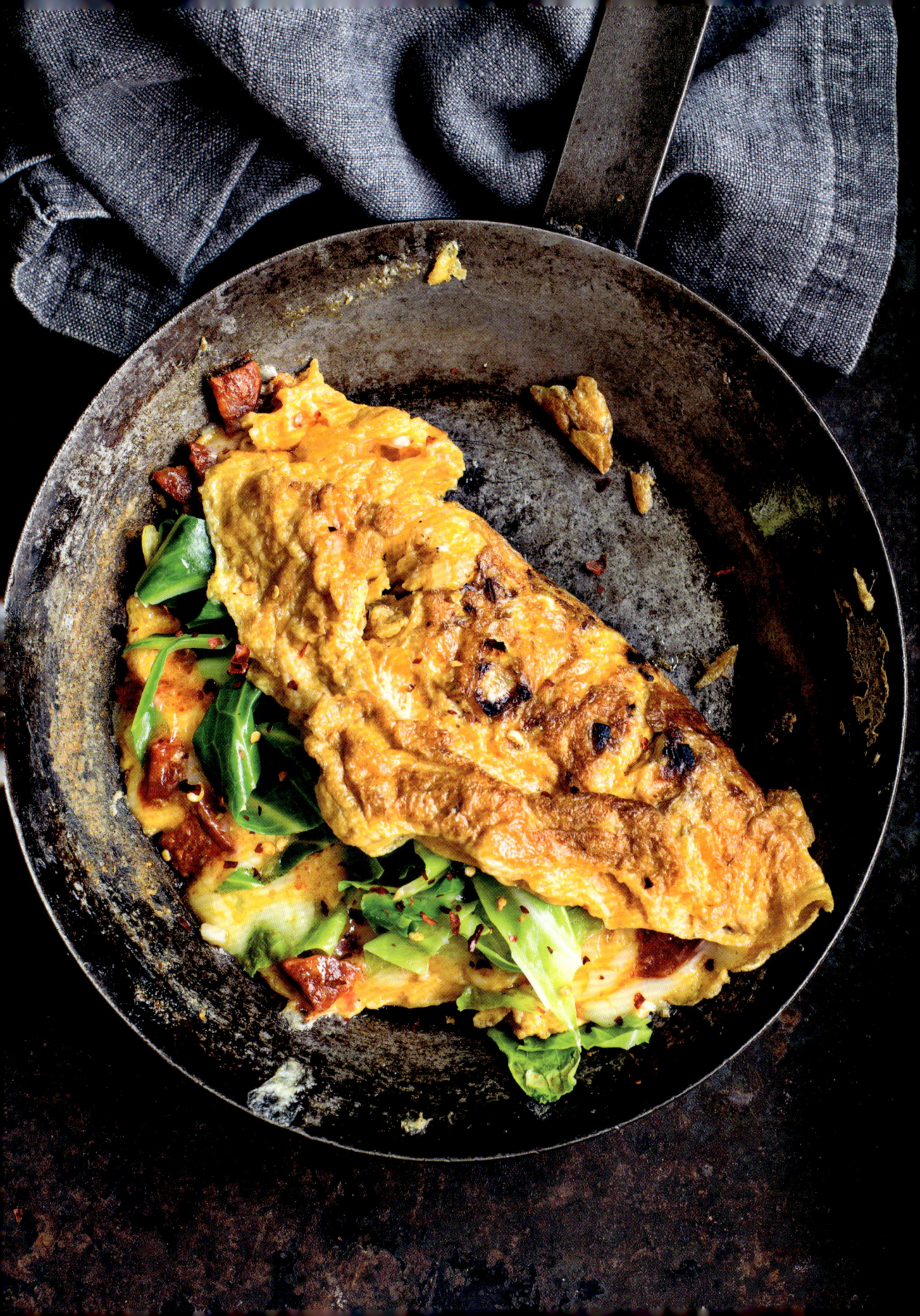

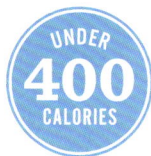

Breakfast Burrito

SERVES	PREP	COOK
1	**5** mins	**15** mins

1 chipolata sausage,
   halved lengthways
2 rashers smoked
   streaky bacon
1 large mushroom,
   thinly sliced
2 cherry tomatoes, halved
1 tsp olive oil
1 medium free-range egg
2 large iceberg lettuce leaves
½ tsp full-fat mayonnaise
½ tsp sriracha (optional)

NON-FAST DAY
Serve a double portion.

A Mexican-inspired burrito cleverly served in
crunchy lettuce.

1. Preheat the oven to 200°C/Fan 180°C/Gas 6 and line
a baking tray with non-stick baking paper.

2. Place the sausage, bacon, mushroom and tomatoes on
the prepared tray. Drizzle the mushrooms and tomatoes
with the oil, season with salt and freshly ground black
pepper and roast in the oven for 12 minutes.

3. Remove the tray from the oven and make some
space. Crack in the egg and return to the oven for
a further 3 minutes.

4. To assemble, layer the iceberg leaves on top of
one another, then spread with the mayo and sriracha
(if using). Stack the cooked ingredients on top, roll
tightly and serve.

AIR-FRYER TIP

Preheat the air fryer to 180°C, if needed. Place the
sausage, bacon and mushrooms on a lined tray in the air
fryer. Drizzle the mushrooms with oil and season. Cook
for 9 minutes. Remove the tray, turn the sausage, bacon
and mushrooms, and make some space for the egg and
tomatoes. Crack the egg into the space, add the tomatoes,
and air fry for another 3–4 minutes. Assemble the
burrito as Step 4 to serve.

GLUTEN FREE · NUT FREE · DAIRY FREE · ✓

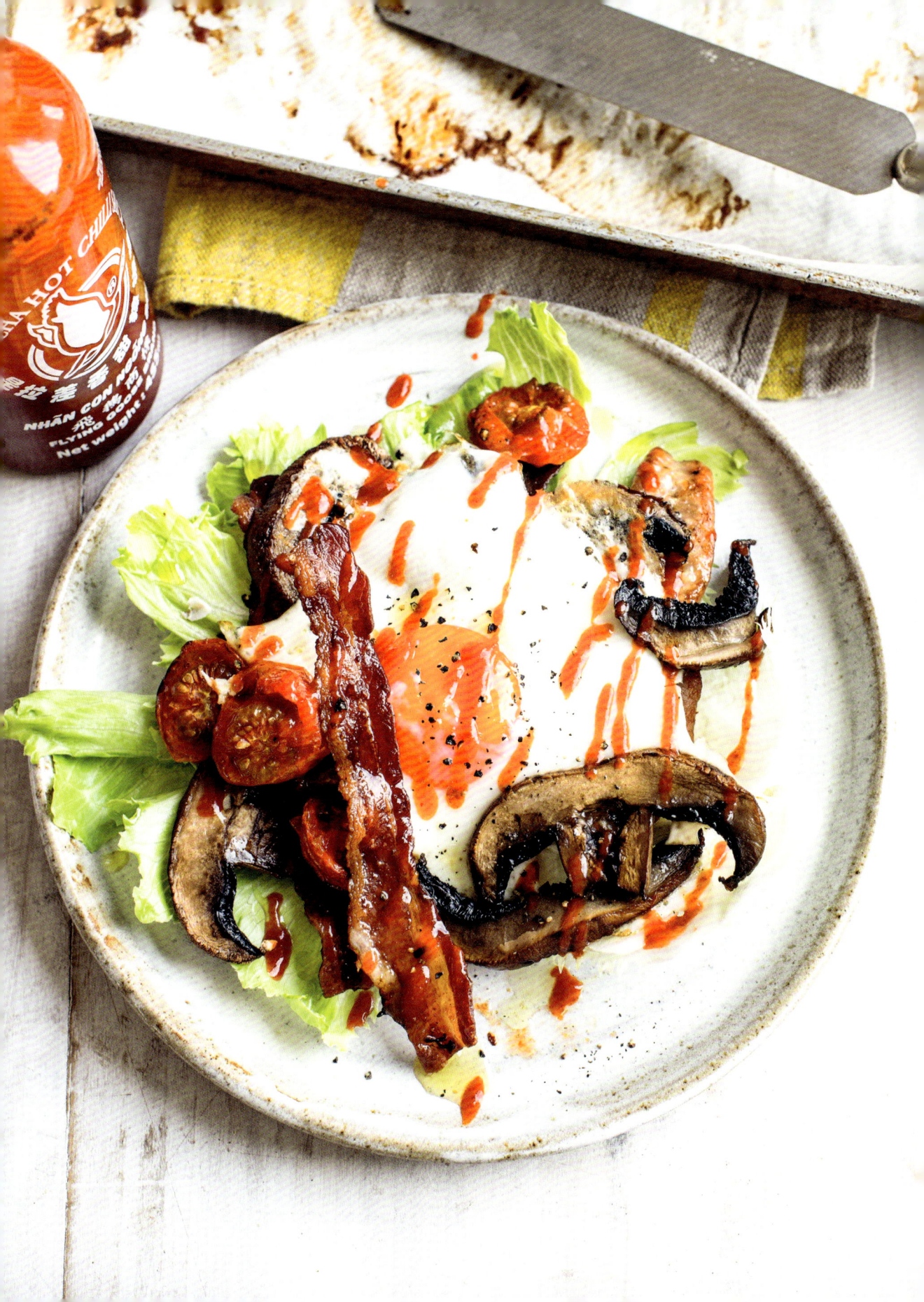

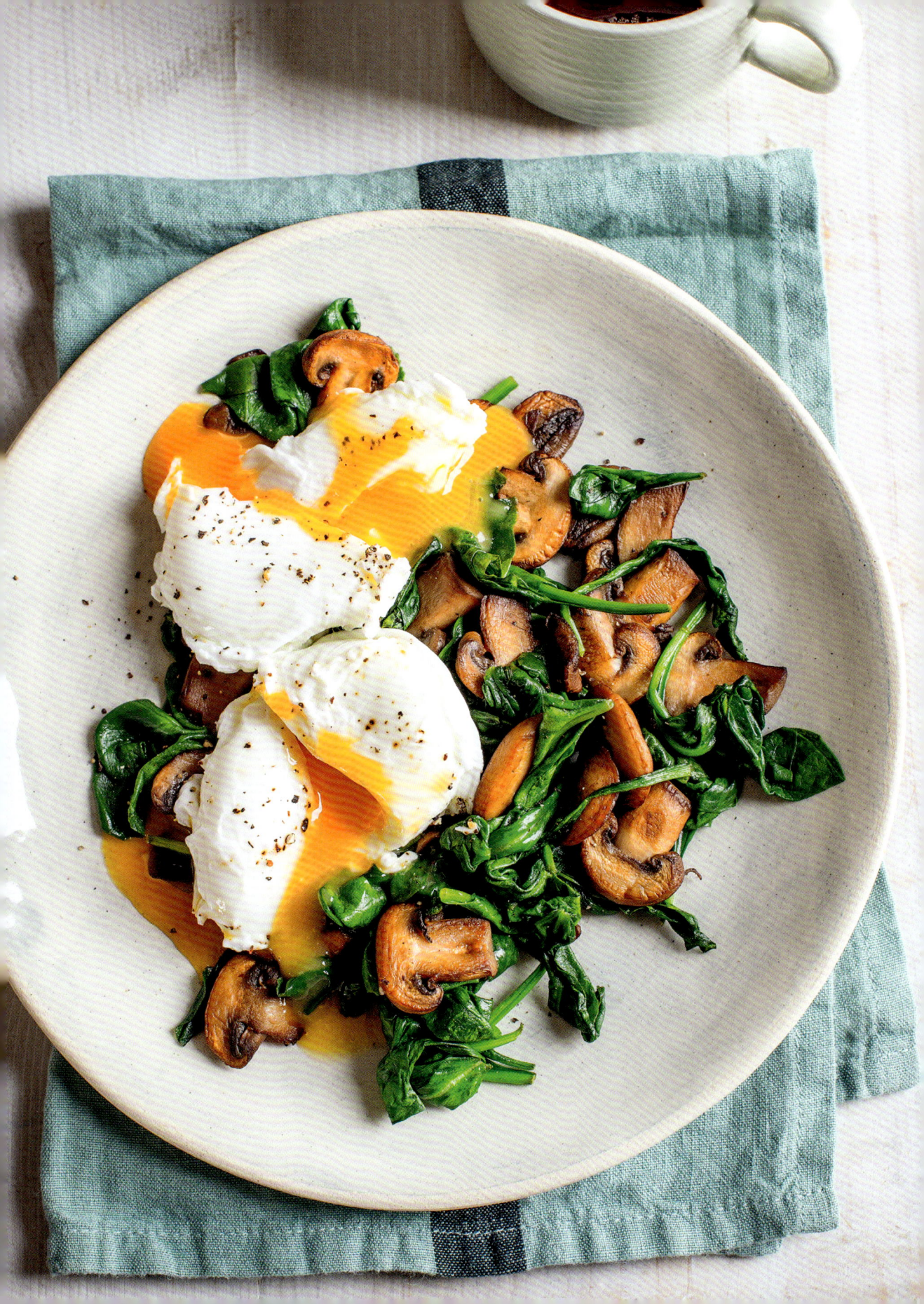

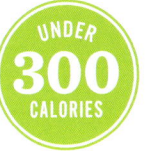

Poached Eggs with Mushrooms and Spinach

SERVES	PREP	COOK
1	**3** mins	**3** mins

2 medium free-range eggs,
    fridge cold
5g butter or 1 tsp olive oil
75g small chestnut
    mushrooms, sliced
large handful young
    spinach leaves

NON-FAST DAYS
Serve on top of a slice of
wholegrain sourdough toast.

COOK'S TIP
If you aren't using
fridge-cold eggs, reduce
the cooking time slightly.

A quick, low-calorie but filling breakfast for
one. Make sure you use eggs that are very fresh.

1. Third fill a saucepan with water and bring to
a gentle simmer.

2. Break each egg into a cup, then carefully tip one
at a time into the pan. Cook over a very low heat,
with the water hardly bubbling, for about 3 minutes,
or until the whites are set but the yolks remain runny.

3. While the eggs are poaching, melt the butter or oil in
a non-stick frying pan over a medium heat and stir fry the
mushrooms for 2–3 minutes or until lightly browned.

4. Add the spinach and toss with the mushrooms until
just wilted. Don't over-cook the vegetables, or lots of
liquid will be released. Season with a pinch of salt and
a good grinding of black pepper.

5. Spoon the mushrooms and spinach on to a warmed
plate. Drain the eggs with a slotted spoon and place on
top of the veg. Season with a little more ground black
pepper to serve.

VEGGIE | GLUTEN FREE | NUT FREE | DAIRY FREE

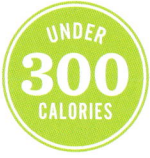

PER SERVING | **239cals** | PROTEIN **15.5g** | CARBS **18.4g**

Sardines with Tomatoes on Sourdough

SERVES | PREP | COOK
2 | **8** mins | **7** mins

2 thin slices wholemeal
or seeded sourdough bread
(each around 40g)
1 × 120g can sardines in olive
oil, drained
1 heaped tsp capers, drained
(optional)
8 cherry tomatoes, halved
large handful young spinach
leaves or rocket
2 tsp extra-virgin olive oil
dash balsamic vinegar
or Tabasco

This is a store-cupboard staple, and another great source of omega-3. For breakfast or lunch, Michael loved his super-healthy, oily fish.

1. Preheat the grill to high and line the grill pan with foil.

2. Place the bread on the foil and grill it until lightly browned on both sides; or use a toaster.

3. Mash the sardines roughly on to the toast and scatter with the capers, if using. (Make sure you completely cover the toast so it doesn't burn when it goes under the grill.) Place the tomatoes on top and season with a little salt and ground black pepper.

4. Place under the grill for about 2 minutes, or until the sardines are hot and the tomatoes have softened.

5. Transfer to two plates and serve with the leaves alongside, dressed with the oil and a little balsamic vinegar or Tabasco, to taste.

NUT FREE   DAIRY FREE

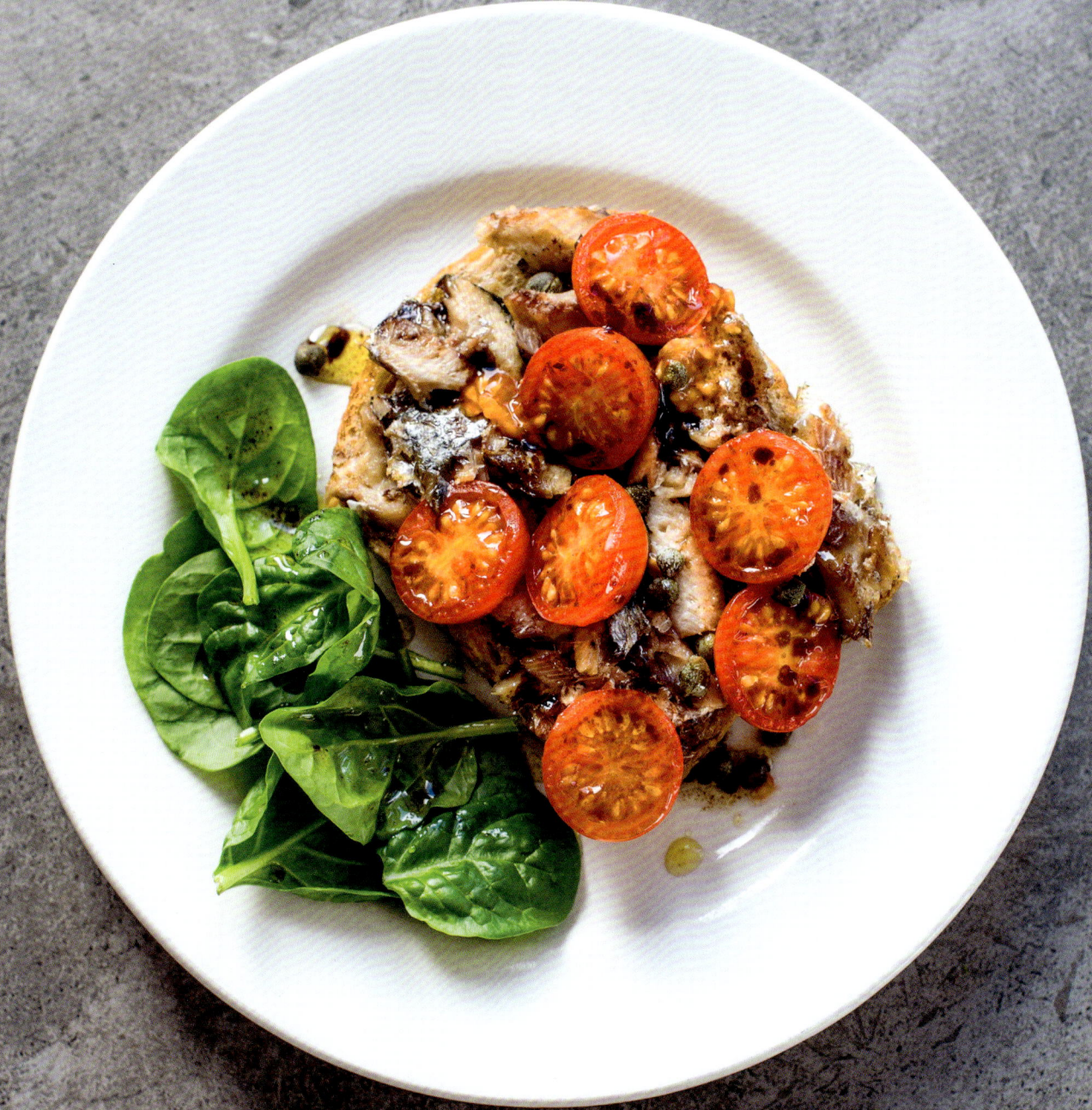

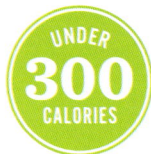

Smashed Avocado on Toast

SERVES **2** | **PREP** **6** mins

2 thin slices wholegrain
   sourdough bread
   (each around 20g)
1 ripe avocado, peeled, stoned
   and roughly chopped (about
   75g prepared weight – see
   tip below)
25g walnuts, roughly chopped
1 plump red chilli, deseeded
   and sliced, or a pinch of
   crushed dried chilli flakes
   (optional)
2 tsp balsamic vinegar

NON-FAST DAYS
Top the avocado toast with
one or two freshly poached
eggs, or some crumbled feta.
A tablespoon of toasted mixed
seeds is also a lovely addition.

COOK'S TIP
We've found the best way to
prepare an avocado is to cut
it in half, remove the stone,
and then, using a large serving
spoon, scoop between the skin
and the flesh and lift the half
avocado out in one piece.

This super-fast breakfast is a great way of using
up avocados that are over-ripe. If you can't get
hold of sourdough bread, any wholegrain will do.

1. Toast the bread and divide between two plates
(or serve on one plate to share).

2. Place the avocado and walnuts in a small bowl
and mash with a fork.

3. Spread the avocado mixture on to the hot toast,
sprinkle with the chilli, if using, and drizzle with
the balsamic vinegar. Season with salt and ground
black pepper to serve.

VEGAN   DAIRY FREE

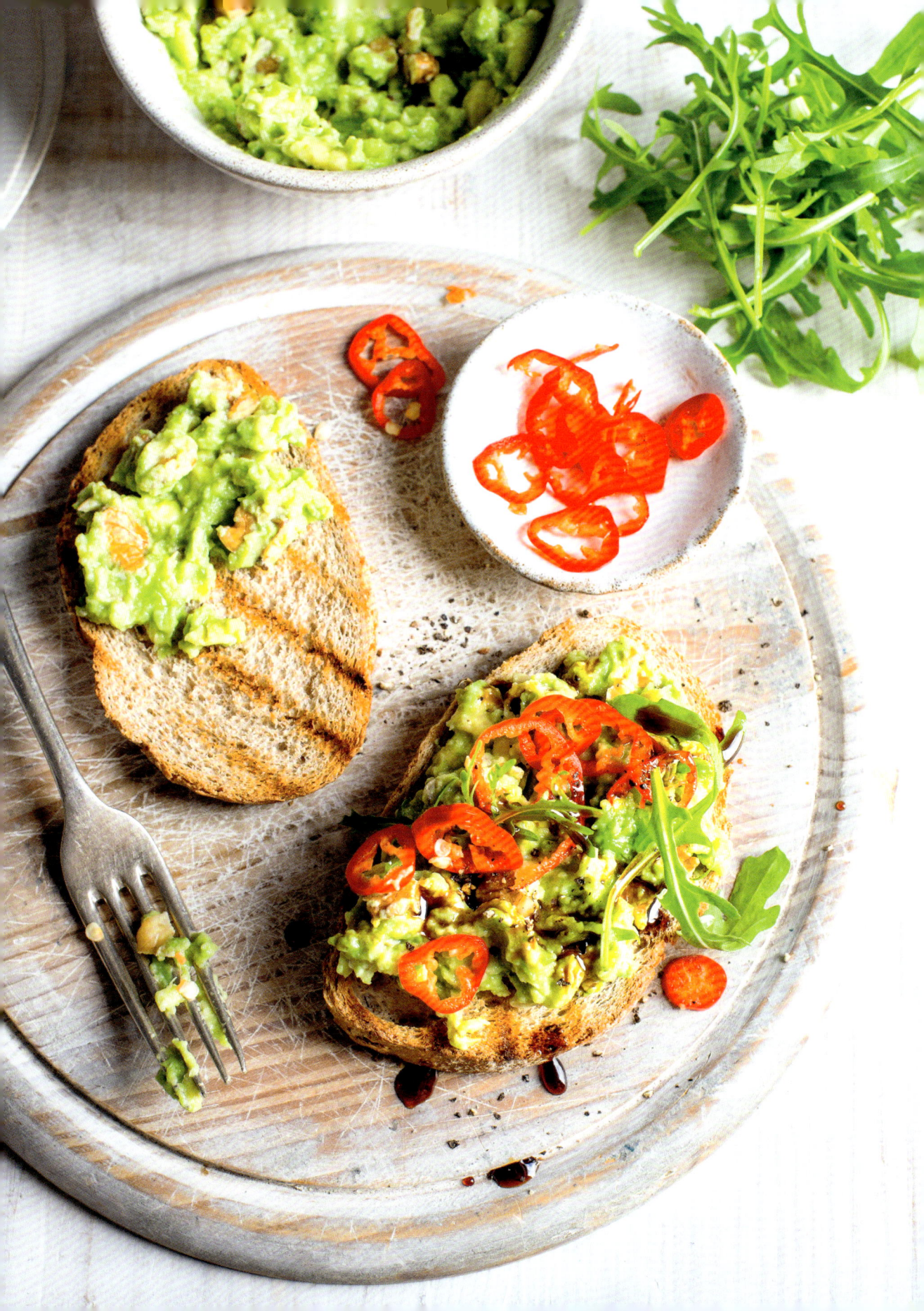

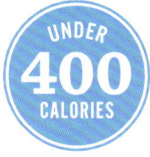

Cowboy Baked Beans

SERVES 2 | **PREP** 5 mins | **COOK** 10 mins

1 tbsp olive oil

1 small onion, very
   finely chopped

1 garlic clove, peeled
   and crushed

1 tsp smoked paprika,
   hot or sweet, to taste

1 × 400g can haricot
   beans, drained

350g passata

1 tbsp Worcestershire sauce,
   or vegan alternative

2 thin slices wholegrain
   bread (each around 20g)

NON-FAST DAYS
Serve with an extra slice
of wholegrain toast and a
generous drizzle of olive oil.

COOK'S TIP
You can use any canned
beans you like; just keep
the quantities the same.

Homemade baked beans are a favourite of ours. This simple version can be served at breakfast or as an accompaniment to grilled chicken or meat. It's also lovely topped with crumbled cheese for a quick supper. Michael loved a classic meal of beans and good-quality sausages, often without the toast on a fast day.

1. Heat the oil in a saucepan over a medium heat. Add the onion and fry gently for 3–4 minutes, or until soft.

2. Add the garlic and smoked paprika, and cook for a few seconds, stirring.

3. Tip the beans into the pan, add the passata and Worcestershire sauce, and season with salt and feshly ground black pepper. Bring to a gentle simmer and cook for 5 minutes, or until the sauce is thickened, stirring regularly, especially towards the end of the cooking time.

4. Meanwhile, toast the bread and place on two plates. Spoon the beans over the top and serve.

VEGAN | NUT FREE | DAIRY FREE

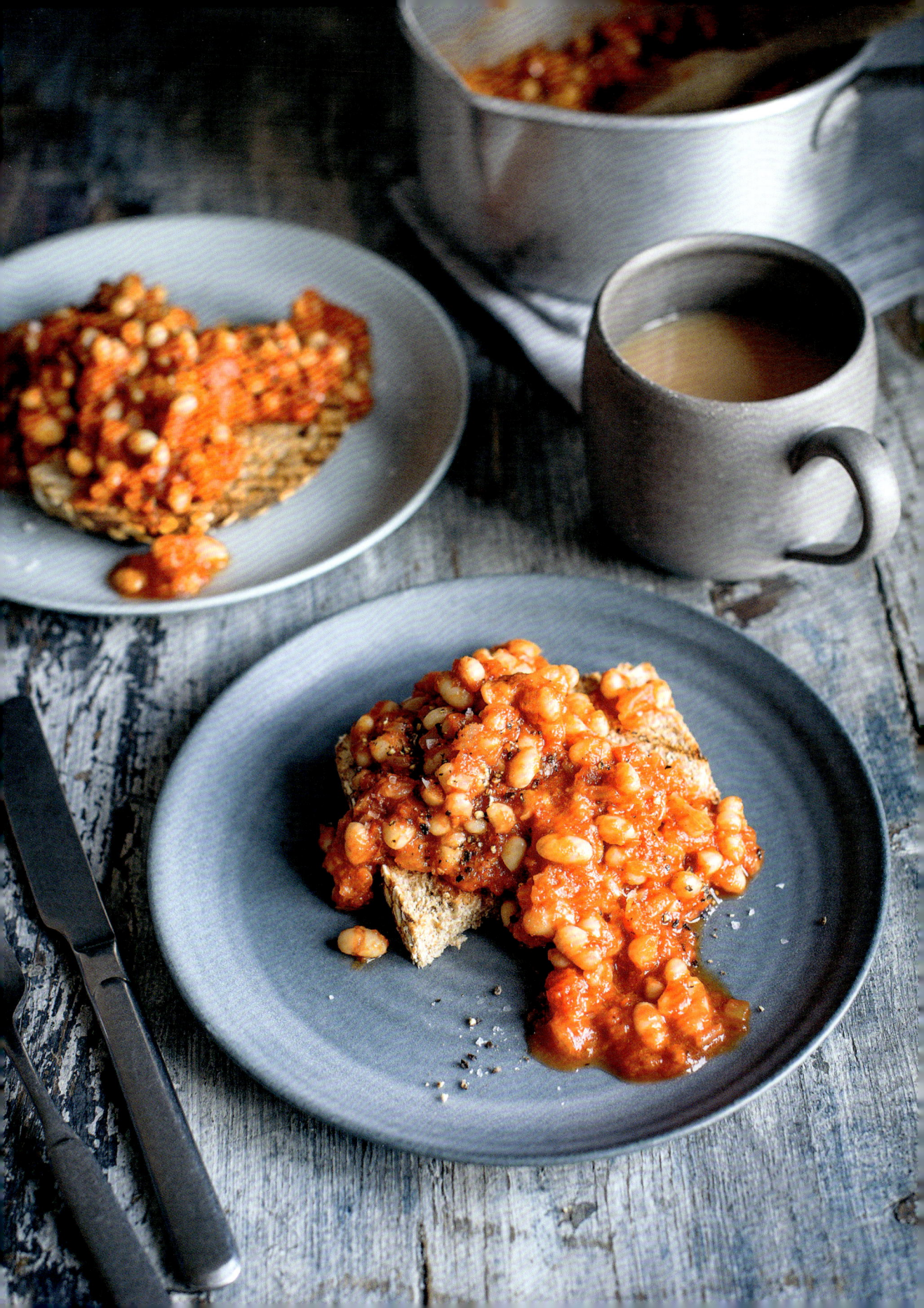

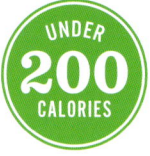

PER SERVING | **181cals** | PROTEIN **11.4g** | CARBS **1.2g**

Chorizo and Parsley Muffins

MAKES	PREP	COOK
6	**10** mins	**15** mins

70g chorizo, finely chopped
55g full-fat cream cheese
4 medium free-range eggs
30g ground almonds
1 tsp baking powder
¼ tsp salt
40g mature Cheddar, grated
10g parsley, leaves picked
   and roughly chopped
finely grated zest of ½ lemon
   (optional)

Even a small portion of chorizo packs a punch, bringing a garlicky, paprika-flavoured kick, and making these high-protein muffins delicious and satisfying.

1. Preheat the oven to 190°C/Fan 170°C/Gas 5. Line a 12-hole muffin tin with 6 cases (use silicone muffin cases, if possible).

2. Place the chorizo in a dry frying pan over a medium heat and fry for 3–4 minutes, stirring occasionally, until the chorizo is crispy. Transfer to a plate lined with kitchen paper and set aside.

3. Place the cream cheese, eggs, ground almonds, baking powder and salt in a medium bowl and whisk until smooth.

4. Stir in the Cheddar, parsley, cooked chorizo and lemon zest, if using, and divide the mixture between the muffin cases. Bake in the oven for 15 minutes until risen, golden and cooked through.

5. Serve warm or leave to cool on a wire rack.

AIR-FRYER TIP

Preheat the air fryer to 170°C, if needed. Line a 6-hole muffin tin with paper cases (make sure the tin fits in the air fryer) or place the paper cases in individual dariole moulds. Prepare the muffin mixture as above. Spoon the mixture into the paper cases and air fry for 15 minutes (you may need to do this in batches).

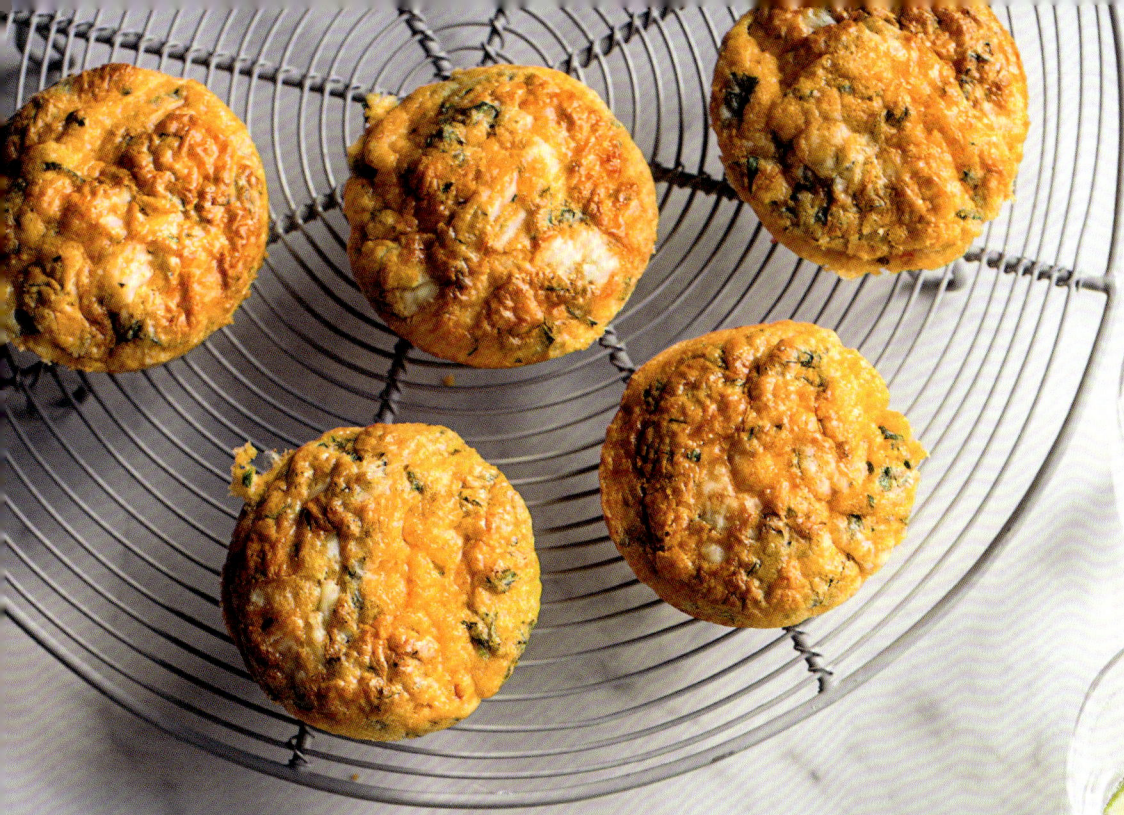

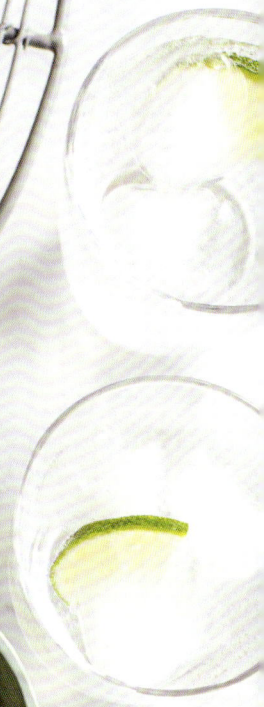

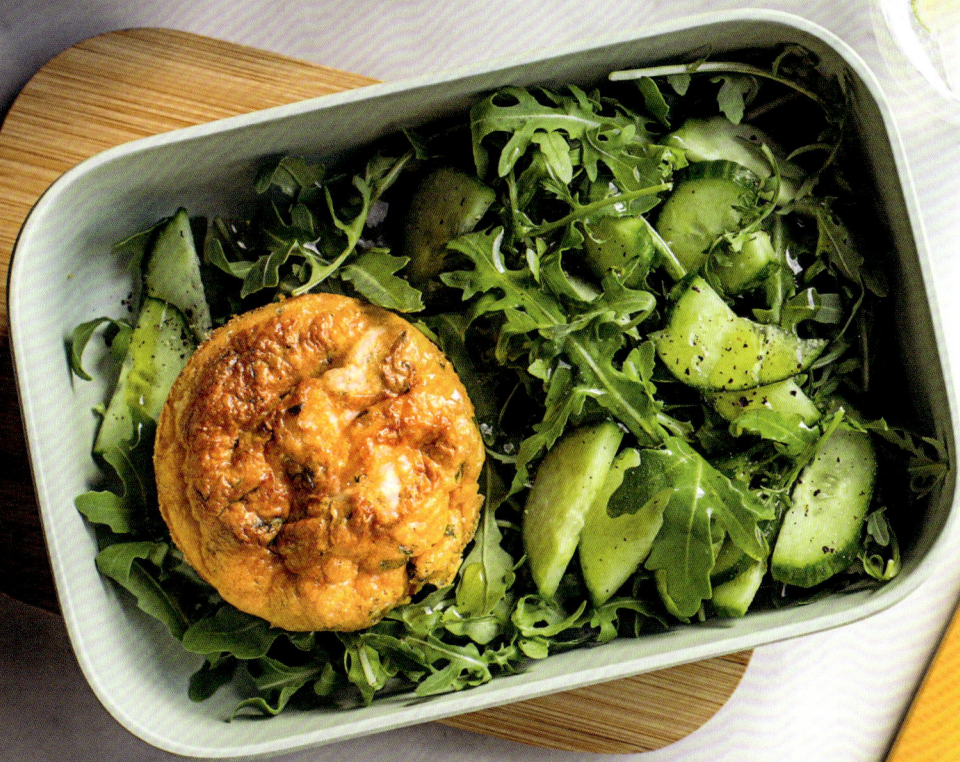

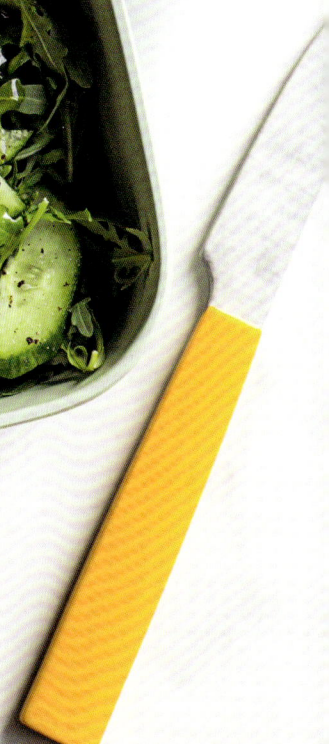

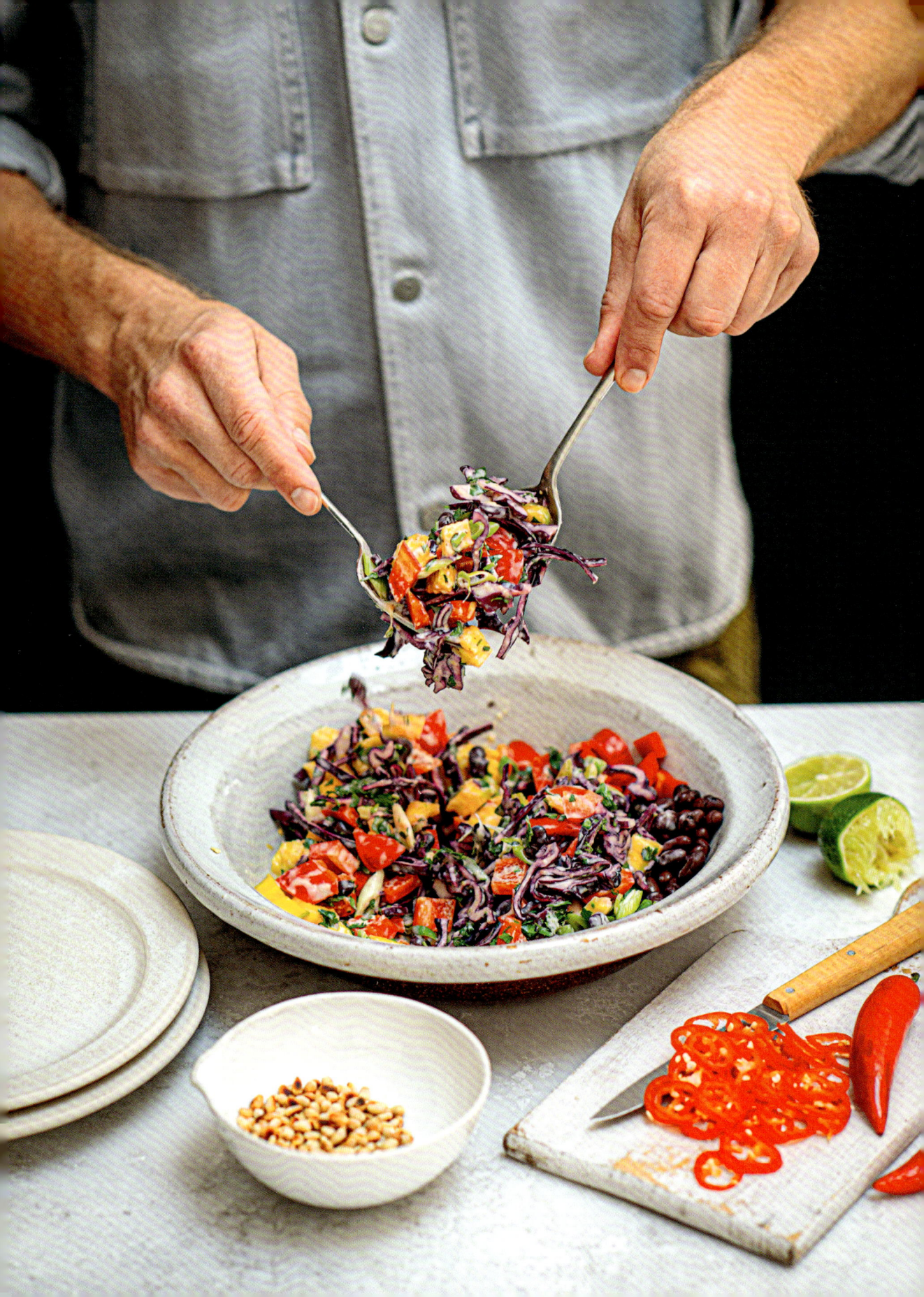

Shakes, Soups and Salads

EASY WAYS WITH SHAKES

Shakes are a super-easy and tasty addition to your fast day. They can help you get out of the door in a hurry knowing you will feel full, with the nutrients you need. They are also a great way to increase your daily protein. Here we offer a couple of basic recipes, with a choice of fruit and protein additions, so you can design a shake yourself. The fruit shake is higher in sugar than the green shake, so probably best to enjoy in moderation. For Michael, a low-sugar, protein-rich shake was useful when out and about. He also often used thefast800.com protein and meal-replacement shakes to ensure adequate protein, fibre and minimal sugars.

Fruit Shake

SERVES 1

2 tbsp full-fat live Greek yoghurt or dairy-free alternative (40cals/1.6g protein)

100ml full-fat milk or dairy-free alternative (63cals/3.3g protein)

½ banana, peeled and roughly chopped, around 50g prepared weight (43cals/0.6g protein)

1 tbsp jumbo porridge oats, around 7g (28cals/0.8g protein)

Add **1** fruit:

50g strawberries, hulled and halved (19cals/0.3g protein)

50g raspberries (16cals/0.7g protein)

50g cubed mango (33cals/0.3g protein)

60g frozen pineapple (27cals/0.2g protein)

50g frozen mixed berries, such as strawberries and blueberries (20cals/0.4g protein)

Add **1** protein source:

1 tbsp ground almonds (44cals/1.8g protein)

1 tbsp chopped mixed nuts (60cals/2.7g protein)

1 tbsp mixed seeds (61cals/2.7g protein)

1 tbsp whey powder (25cals/5.5g protein)

1 tbsp chia seeds (71cals/1.9g protein)

Add **1** optional extra:

1 tsp vanilla extract

½ tsp ground cinnamon

1 tsp finely grated fresh root ginger

finely grated zest of ¼ lemon or lime

squeeze lemon or lime juice

1. Put all the ingredients for the basic fruit shake in a blender.

2. Add one fruit and one protein source. Add an optional extra, if you like.

3. Add 3–4 tablespoons water or 3–4 ice cubes. Blitz until smooth. Add more water, if needed, to reach your preferred consistency.

4. Serve immediately.

Green Shake

SERVES 1
½ avocado, peeled, stoned and quartered
   (160cals/1.6g protein)
200g cucumber, trimmed and cubed

Add ❶ green vegetable:
25g young spinach leaves
25g young kale leaves, tough stalks removed
25g rocket leaves
25g watercress

Add ❶ protein source:
1 tbsp ground almonds (44cals/1.8g protein)
1 tbsp chopped mixed nuts
   (60cals/2.7g protein)
1 tbsp mixed seeds (61cals/2.7g protein)
1 tbsp whey powder (25cals/5.5g protein)
1 tbsp chia seeds (71cals/1.9g protein)
2 tbsp full-fat live Greek yoghurt
   (40cals/1g protein)

Add ❶ or ❷ optional extras:
small handful fresh mint leaves
small handful fresh basil leaves
1 tsp finely grated fresh root ginger
finely grated zest of ¼ lemon
squeeze lemon juice
good pinch crushed dried chilli flakes
splash Worcestershire sauce
splash Tabasco or sriracha sauce

1. Put both ingredients for the basic green shake in a blender.

2. Add one green vegetable and one protein source. Add an optional extra or two, if you like.

3. Pour in 150ml cold water and season with a little salt and lots of ground black pepper. Blitz until smooth. Add more water, if needed, to reach your preferred consistency.

4. Serve immediately.

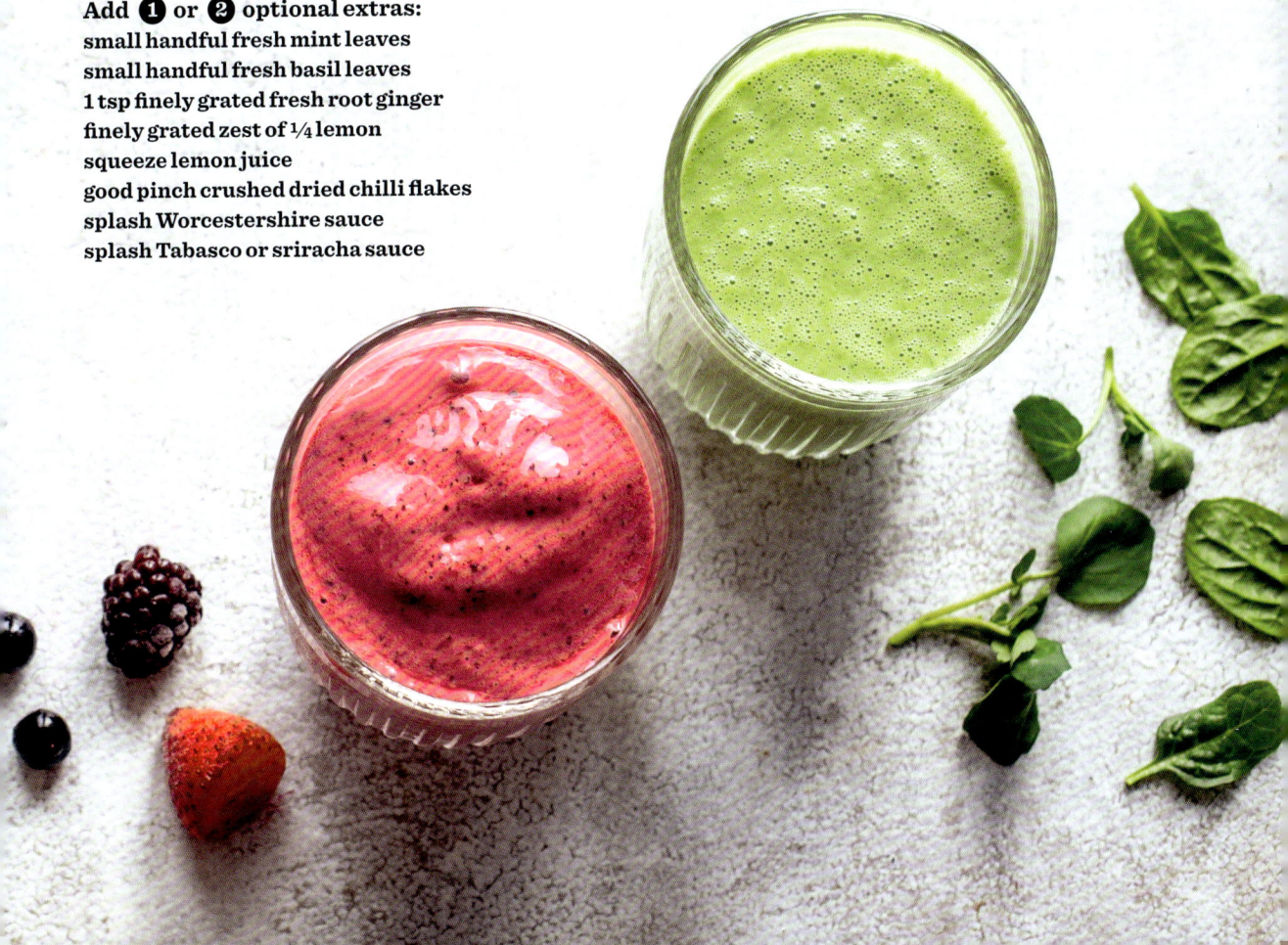

Shakes

Making these shakes is easy. Make sure your blender is sturdy enough to crush frozen berries, if using.

1. Put all the ingredients in a blender and blitz until smooth. Add more water, if necessary, to reach your preferred consistency.

2. Serve immediately.

Iced Berry Shake

Choose any frozen fruit you like for this shake.

SERVES 1
25g full-fat live Greek yoghurt
75ml semi-skimmed milk
40g frozen mixed berries
½ banana (50g peeled weight), peeled and roughly chopped
1 tbsp jumbo porridge oats
5g ground almonds
2 tbsp cold water

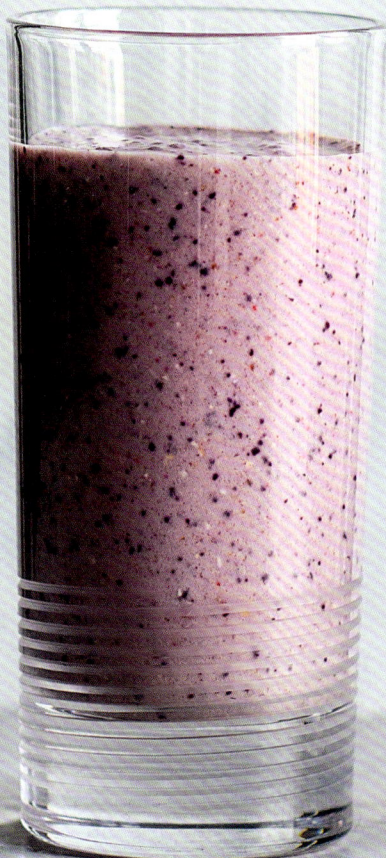

VEGGIE · GLUTEN FREE

Nutty Banana Shake

Use no-added-sugar nut butter for this creamy-tasting shake.

SERVES 1
20g full-fat live Greek yoghurt
100ml semi-skimmed milk
½ banana (50g peeled weight),
   peeled and roughly chopped
15g no-added-sugar cashew
   or almond nut butter
2 tbsp cold water

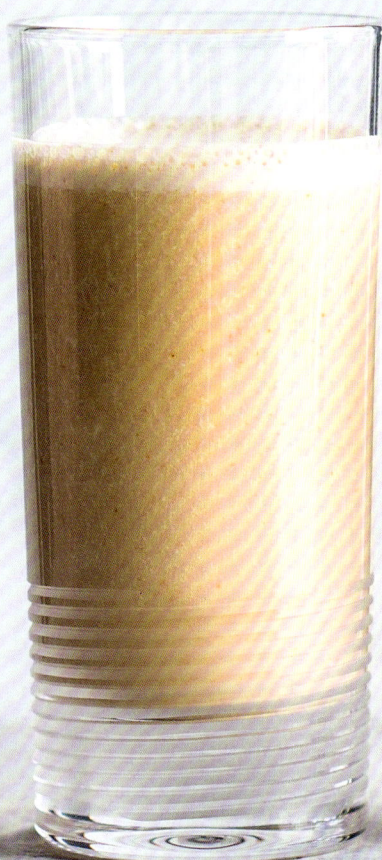

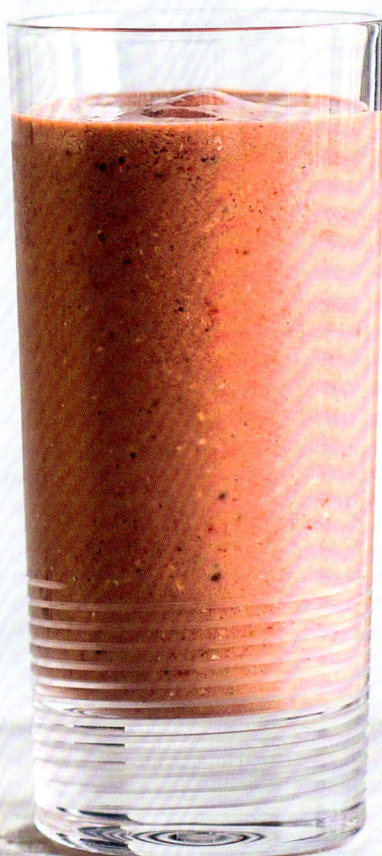

VEGGIE GLUTEN FREE ✓

Chocolate and Strawberry Shake

A delicious and filling chocolatey hit.

SERVES 1
25g full-fat live Greek yoghurt
100ml semi-skimmed milk
100g fresh or frozen strawberries
15g jumbo porridge oats
1 soft pitted date
1 tsp unsweetened cocoa powder
2 tbsp cold water

VEGGIE GLUTEN FREE NUT FREE ✓

Minted Avocado and Cucumber Shake

A creamy shake with a refreshing hint of mint.

½ avocado, peeled, stoned
    and quartered (about 75g
    prepared weight)
200g cucumber, thickly sliced
25g young spinach leaves
12 fresh mint leaves
15g full-fat live Greek yoghurt
100ml cold water

VEGGIE · GLUTEN FREE · NUT FREE · ✓

Orange, Carrot and Cashew Shake

This makes a zingy drink with a vibrant orange colour. Make sure your blender is sturdy enough to cope with the carrot slices.

2 carrots (around 170g),
    trimmed and sliced
½ orange, peeled and
    cut into chunky pieces
15g no-added-sugar cashew
    nut butter or almond butter
125ml cold water

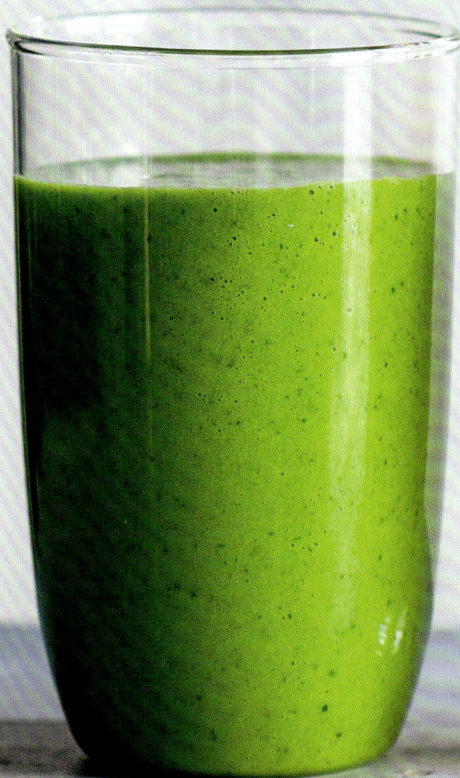

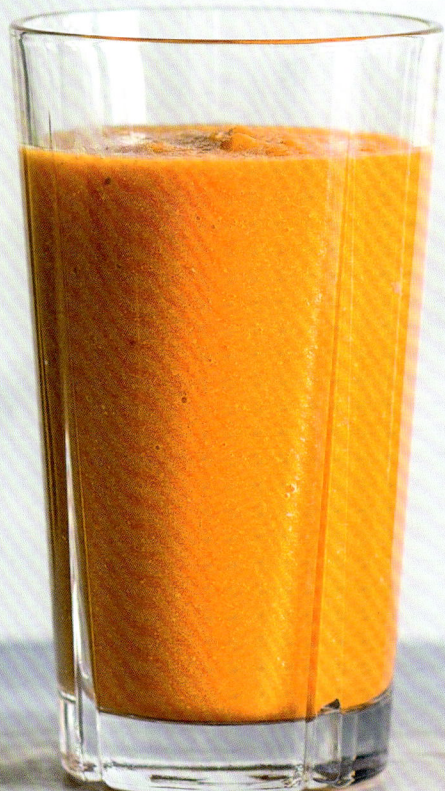

VEGAN · GLUTEN FREE · DAIRY FREE · ✓

Green Ginger Shake

Crisp green apple adds fibre and sweetness to this gorgeous green shake. Use a red-skinned apple if you prefer.

1 green apple, quartered and cored
½ courgette (around 65g), trimmed and thickly sliced
8g fresh root ginger, roughly chopped
½ tsp ground turmeric
10g mixed seeds (such as sunflower, pumpkin, sesame and flax)
2 tsp extra-virgin olive oil
100ml cold water

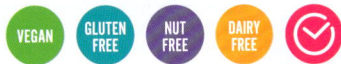

VEGAN · GLUTEN FREE · NUT FREE · DAIRY FREE

Gazpacho-style Shake

Seasoned with salt and freshly ground black pepper, this is lovely served cold with a couple of ice cubes.

100g cucumber, roughly chopped
2–3 ripe vine tomatoes (around 125g), quartered
½ red pepper, deseeded and sliced
¼ small red onion (around 20g), peeled
25g full-fat live Greek yoghurt
10g ground almonds
1 tbsp tomato purée
1 tsp extra-virgin olive oil
2 tbsp cold water

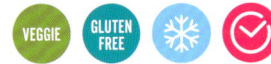

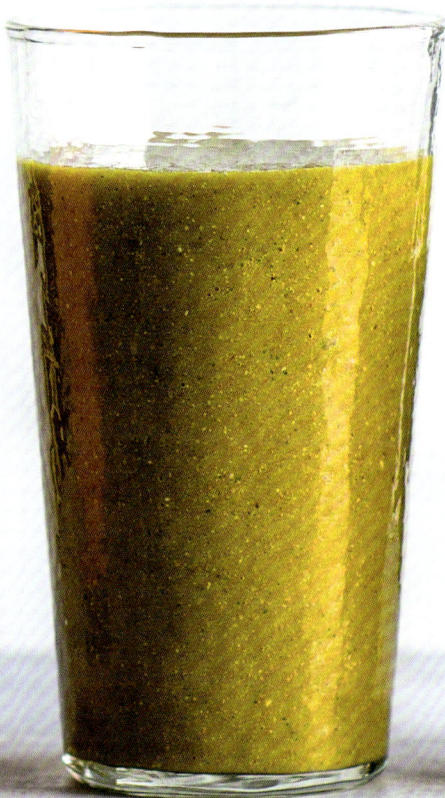

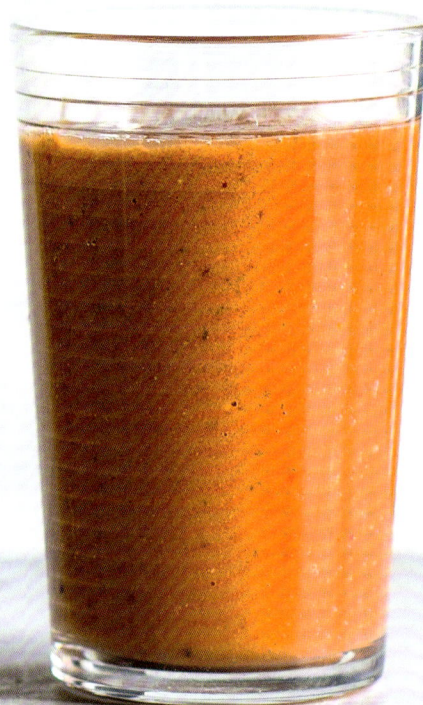

VEGGIE · GLUTEN FREE

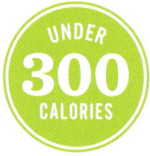

Blueberry and Chocolate Protein Smoothie

SERVES | PREP
1 | **4** mins

100g silken tofu
100g full-fat live Greek yoghurt
50g frozen blueberries
1 medjool date, stoned
1 tsp vanilla extract
1 tsp unsweetened
   cocoa powder

This creamy smoothie gives a protein boost thanks to the tofu, while the cocoa not only adds flavour but is surprisingly high in fibre. Ideal for taking to work or for breakfast in a hurry.

1. Place all the ingredients in a food processor or blender and blitz until smooth.

2. Serve immediately.

VEGGIE   GLUTEN FREE   NUT FREE

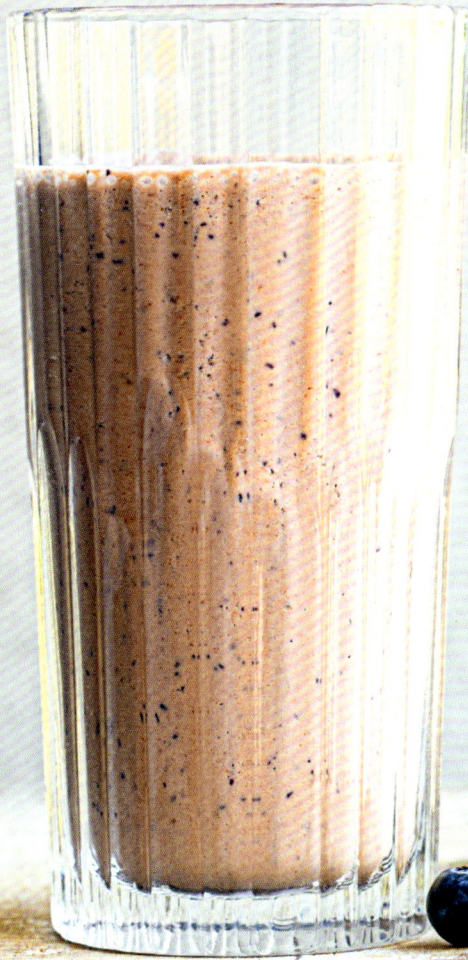

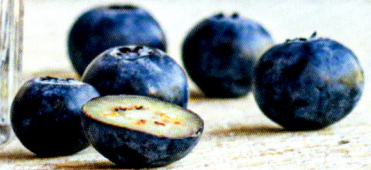

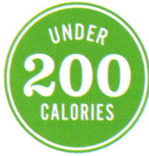

PER SERVING | **185cals** | PROTEIN **7.1g** | CARBS **15.6g**

Kiwi, Pineapple and Spinach Smoothie

SERVES
2

PREP
5
mins

1 kiwi, peeled
50g frozen pineapple
25g young spinach leaves
15g cashew nuts
50g full-fat live Greek yoghurt
   or dairy-free alternative
200g full-fat milk or
   dairy-free alternative
1 tsp honey
8 ice cubes

This smoothie is deliciously refreshing and packed with goodness.

1. Place all the ingredients in a food processor or blender and blitz until smooth.

2. Serve immediately in two tall glasses.

VEGGIE   GLUTEN FREE   DAIRY FREE

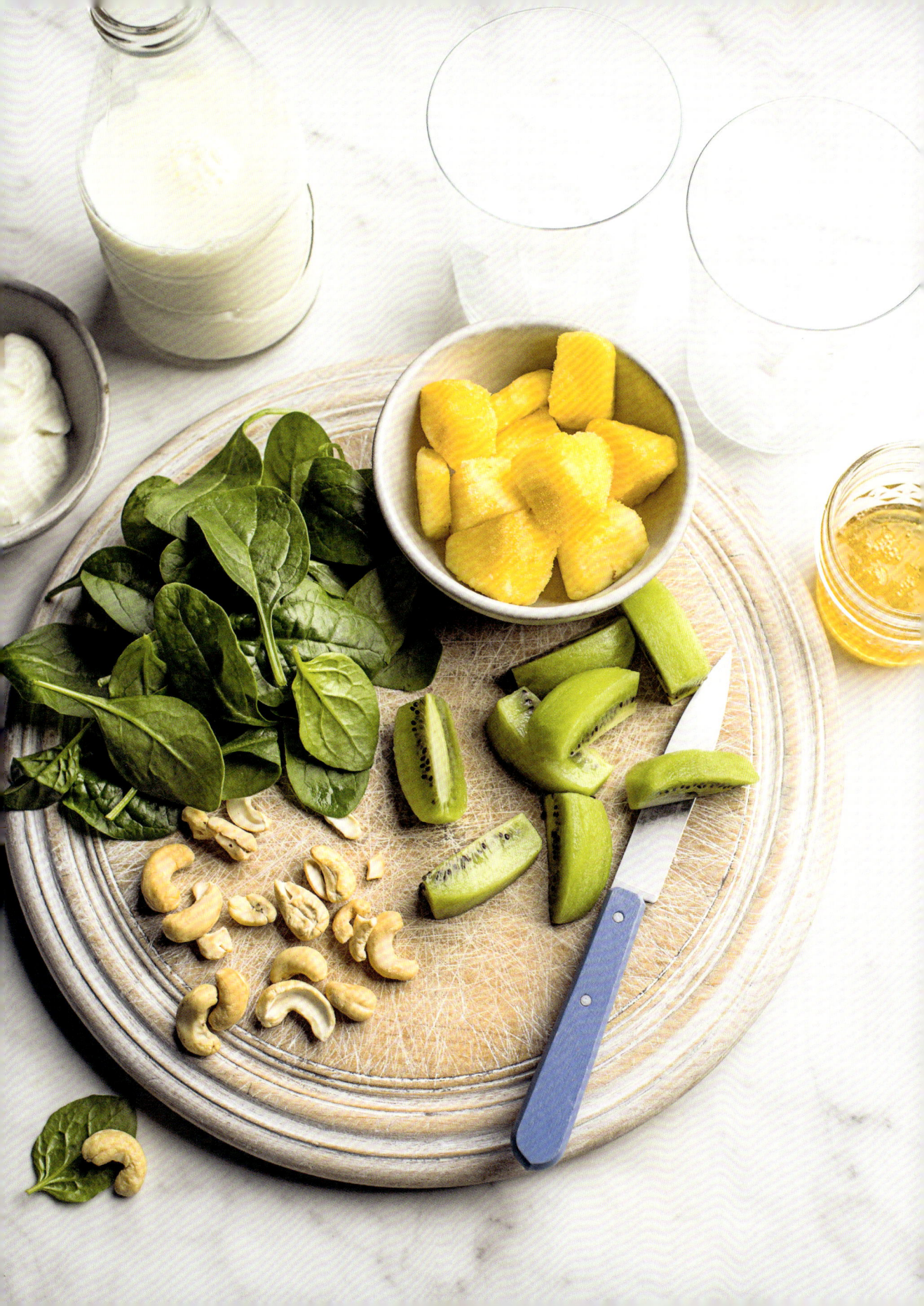

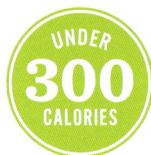

Almost-instant Noodle Soup

SERVES **2** | PREP **8** mins | COOK **8** mins

50g dried wholewheat noodles
or soba buckwheat noodles
4 tsp miso paste
20g fresh root ginger,
peeled and finely grated
2 tbsp dark soy sauce
4–6 chestnut mushrooms
(around 75g), finely sliced
large handful young
spinach leaves
4 spring onions, trimmed
and finely sliced
½ tsp crushed dried
chilli flakes
25g roasted cashew nuts,
roughly chopped
2 large handfuls fresh
coriander, leaves
roughly chopped

NON-FAST DAYS
Add extra protein, such
as shredded cooked chicken
or cubes of tofu.

COOK'S TIP
The just-boiled water will warm
the ingredients but they won't
be hot, so you could give the
soup a blast in a microwave
to heat it further. Make sure
your container is suitable for
microwave cooking. You could
also heat the soup in a pan.

A delicious, Asian-inspired soup, which works
particularly well as a lunch on the go. Dry noodles
come in different-sized bundles – do your best to
keep as close to 50g as possible.

1. Half fill a saucepan with water and bring it to the boil.
Add the noodles, return to the boil and cook for 3–4 minutes
until tender, or according to the packet instructions. Drain
the noodles and rinse under cold running water. Drain again.

2. Divide the miso paste, ginger and soy sauce between two
large heatproof jars (or other heatproof lidded containers).

3. Place the mushrooms on top, then add – in the following
order – the cooked noodles, spinach, spring onions, chilli
flakes, cashews and coriander. Cover and keep chilled.

4. When ready to serve, add 250–300ml just-boiled water
from a kettle (roughly a mug full) to each jar. The water
should rise about halfway up the ingredients. Cover loosely
and leave to stand for 2 minutes to allow the vegetables
to soften and the noodles to heat.

5. Stir well, leave to stand for a further 1–2 minutes,
then serve immediately.

VEGAN   DAIRY FREE

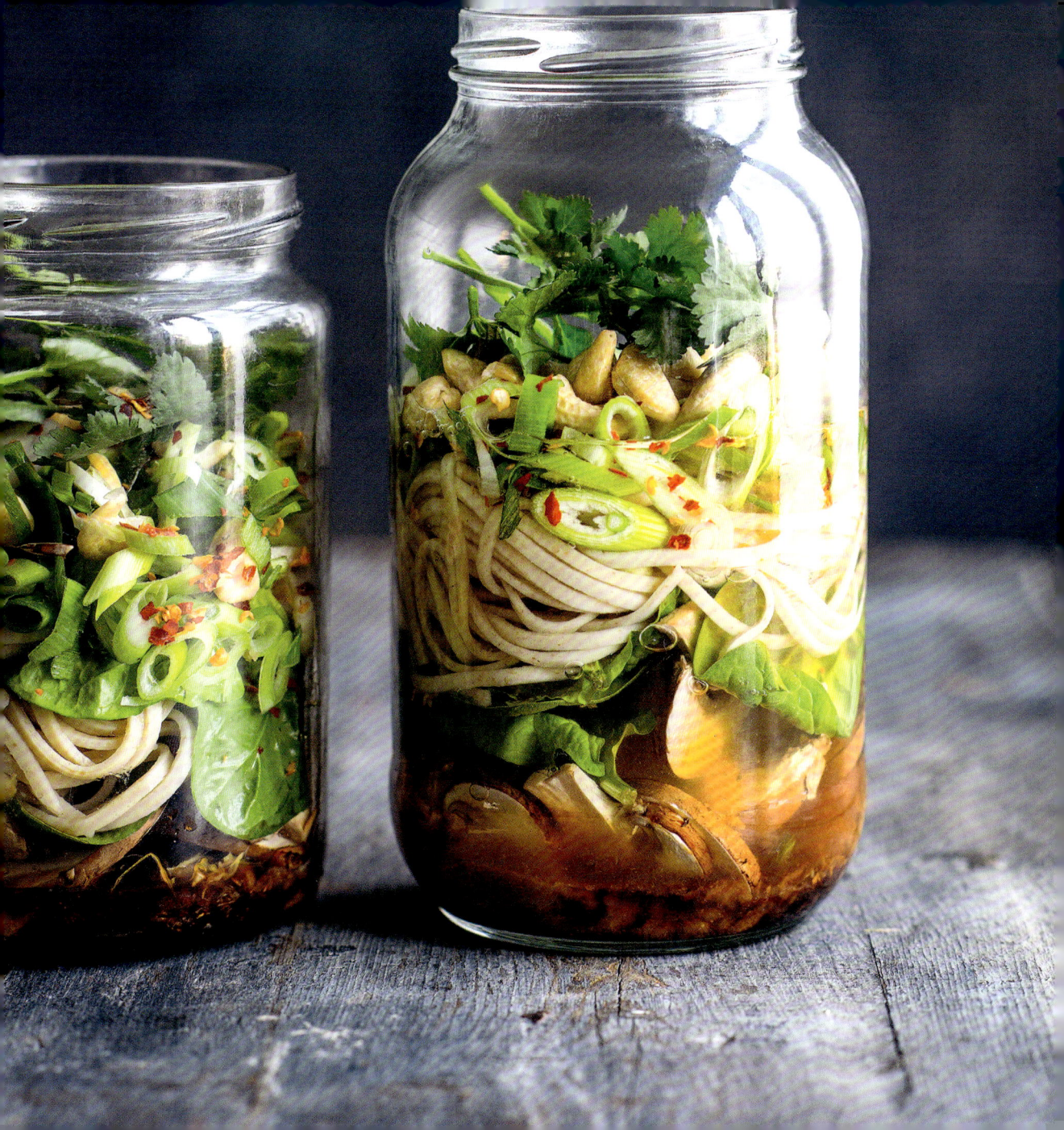

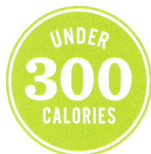

PER SERVING | **249cals** | PROTEIN **7g** | CARBS **18.5g**

Bean Soup with Kale and Pesto

SERVES | **PREP** | **COOK**
4 | **10** mins | **20** mins

2 tbsp olive oil
1 onion, roughly chopped
1 celery stick, cut into
roughly 1cm chunks
2 carrots, trimmed and
cut into roughly
1cm chunks
1 courgette, trimmed, halved
lengthways and cut into
roughly 1cm slices
1 × 400g can cannellini
beans, drained
1 × 400g can borlotti
or kidney beans, drained
1 vegetable or chicken
stock cube
75g kale or dark green cabbage,
thickly sliced and tough
stalks discarded
60g fresh basil pesto

NON-FAST DAYS
Serve with a drizzle of olive
oil and toasted wholegrain
sourdough bread. Add some
diced fried halloumi or bacon.

COOK'S TIP
You'll find tubs of fresh basil
pesto in the chilled department
of the supermarket, usually
with the fresh pasta, but you
could also use the jarred kind.

Super-quick and easy, this tastes fabulous topped
with the fresh basil pesto. You can use any of your
favourite beans – just keep the quantities the same.

1. Heat the oil in a large saucepan over a medium heat.
Add the onion, celery, carrots and courgette, and fry
gently for 10 minutes, stirring occasionally.

2. Tip the beans into the pan, add the stock cube and
1.2 litres water and stir to dissolve. Add the kale or cabbage
and bring to a simmer. Cook for 5–7 minutes, stirring
occasionally, until the vegetables are tender.

3. Season with salt and freshly ground black pepper
to taste, then ladle into warmed bowls and top with
the pesto.

VEGGIE · GLUTEN FREE · NUT FREE · DAIRY FREE

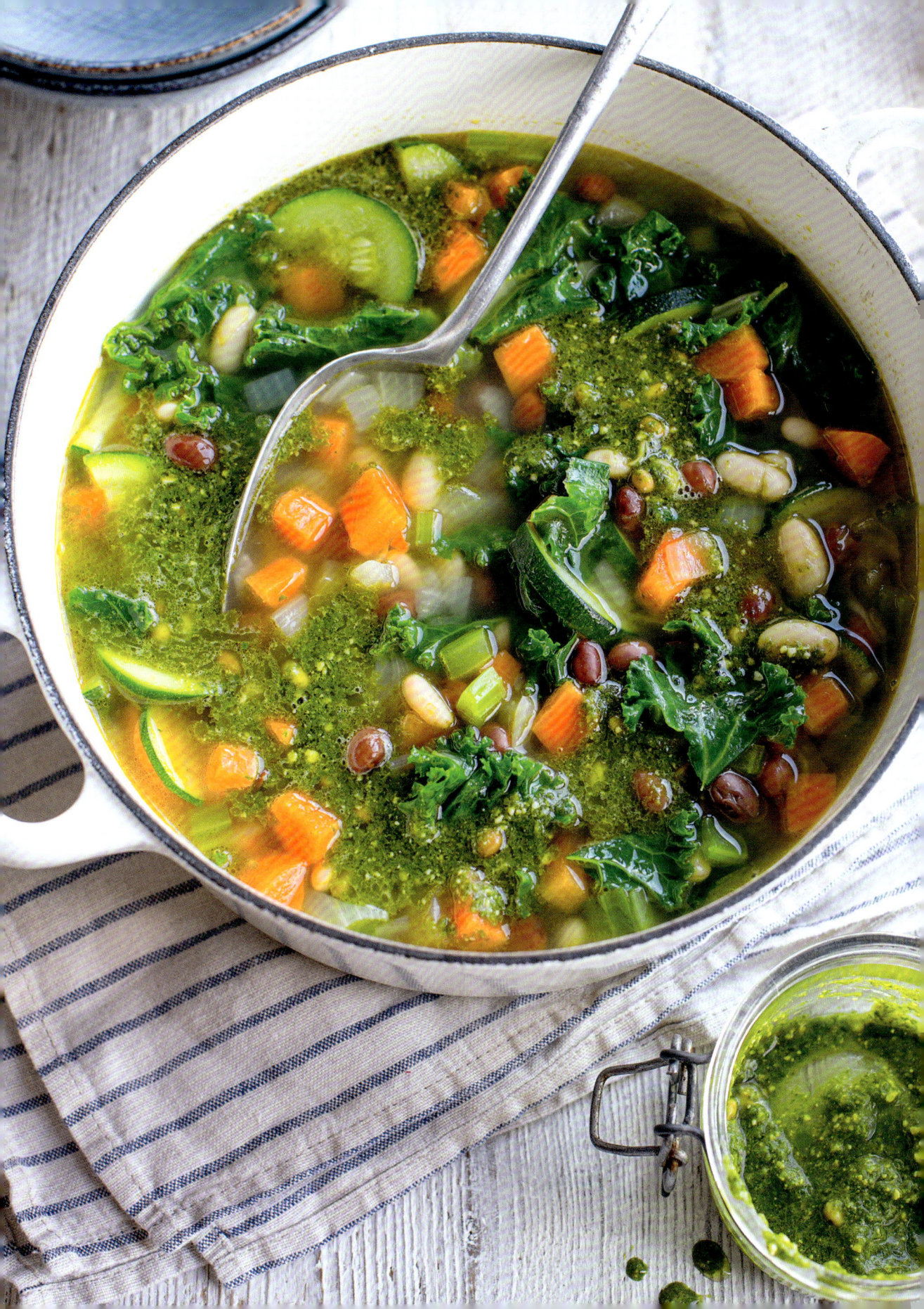

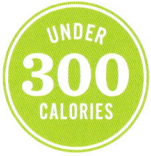

Creamy Broccoli, Ginger and Coriander Soup

SERVES	PREP	COOK
4	**5** mins	**20** mins

1 small onion, roughly chopped

40g fresh root ginger, roughly chopped (no need to peel)

1½ tbsp olive oil

1 head broccoli, roughly chopped

1 × 400ml can full-fat coconut milk

1 vegetable stock cube

15g fresh coriander, plus extra leaves to garnish

40g toasted flaked almonds, to garnish

COOK'S TIP

Add a protein top-up, if you like (see page 271). Fried diced bacon or feta cheese would work well.

A light soup with the warming qualities of coconut, ginger and coriander running through it. The recipe makes enough for four, but it keeps well in the fridge or freezer.

1. Place the onion, ginger and 1 tablespoon of the olive oil in a large saucepan over a medium heat and sauté for 3–4 minutes, until softened.

2. Add the broccoli, coconut milk, stock cube and 800ml water (simply refill the empty coconut milk can twice). Bring to the boil, reduce the heat and simmer for 10 minutes.

3. Remove from the heat, add the coriander and blitz with a stick blender until completely smooth. Season with salt and freshly ground black pepper, and serve topped with flaked almonds and coriander leaves, and drizzled with the remaining oil.

VEGAN · GLUTEN FREE · DAIRY FREE

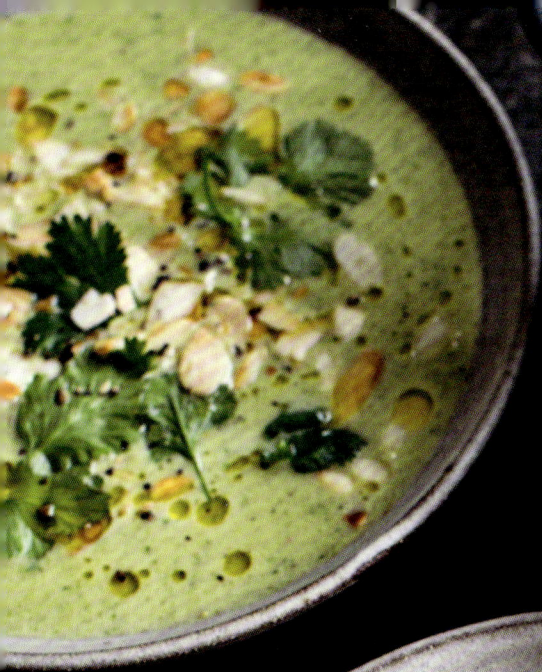

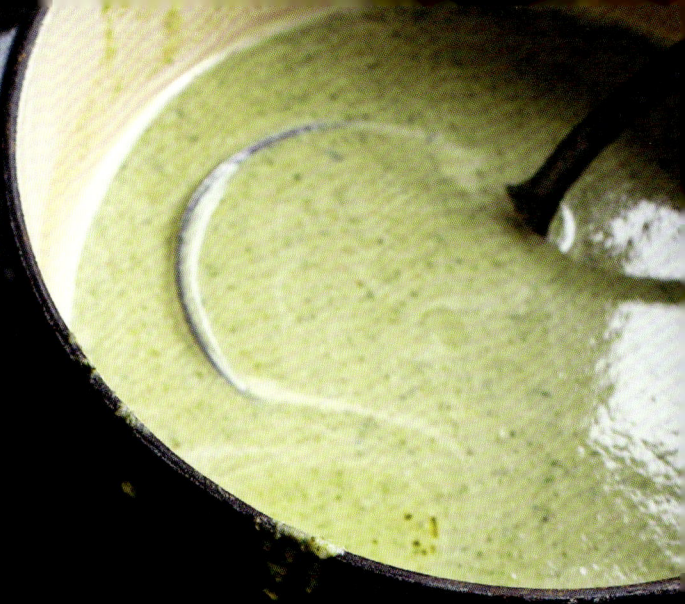

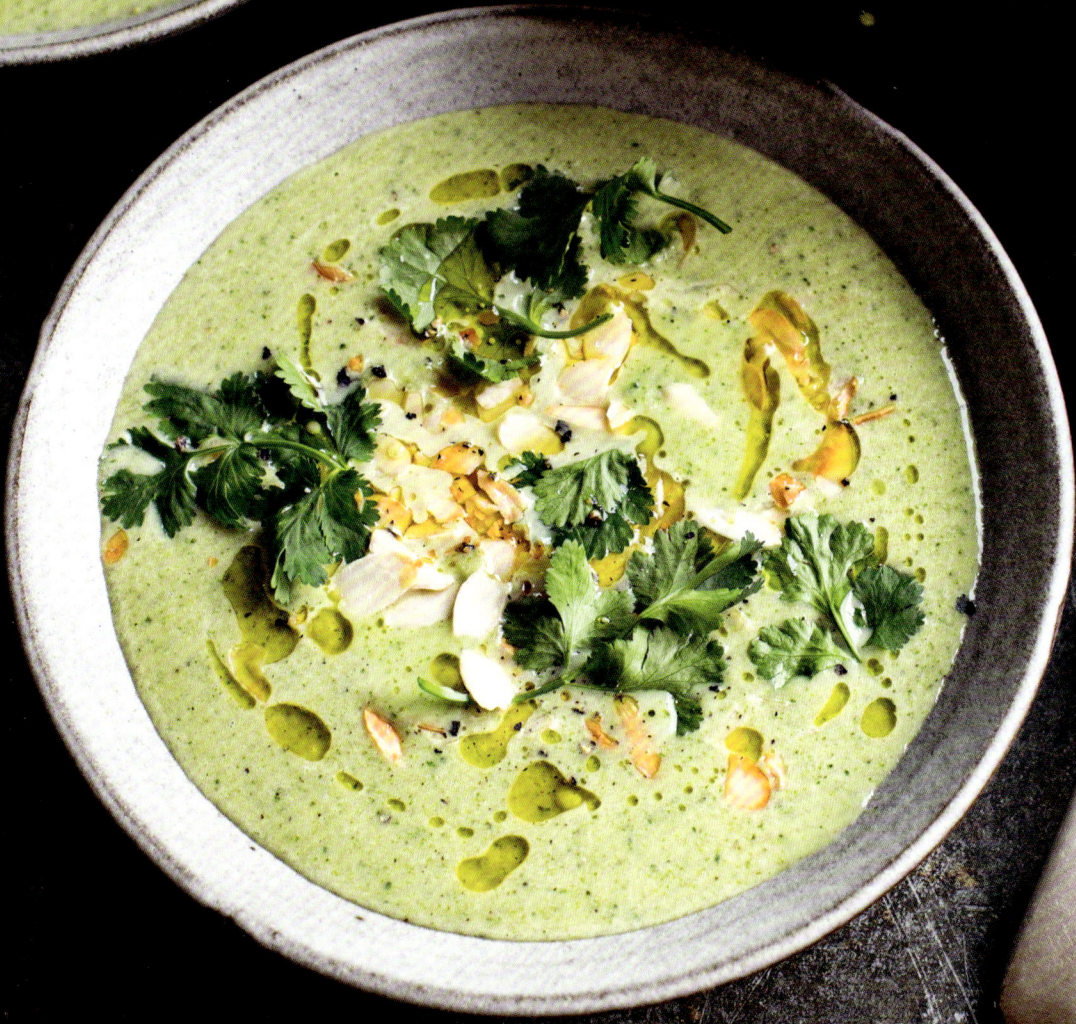

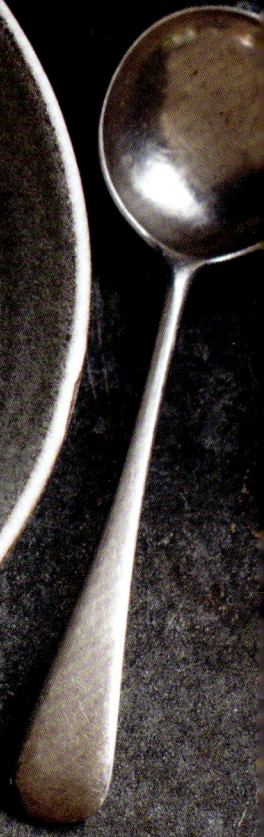

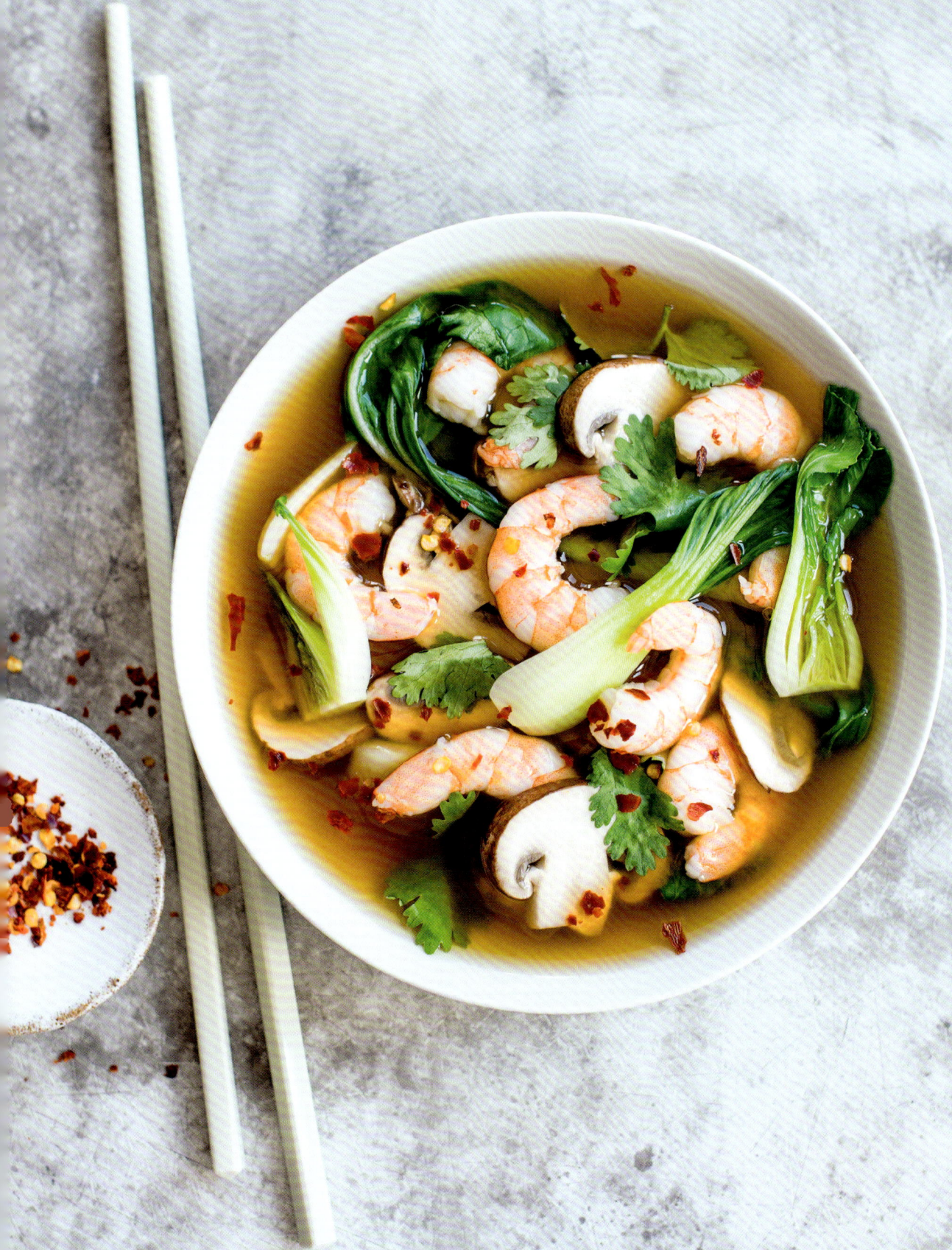

Miso Soup with Mushroom and Prawns

SERVES 1 | **PREP** 5 mins | **COOK** 5 mins

½ pak choi, leaves separated, washed and sliced

3 level tsp miso paste (around 15g)

1 closed cup mushroom, finely sliced

50g large cooked and peeled prawns, defrosted if frozen

small pinch crushed dried chilli flakes (optional)

small handful roughly chopped fresh coriander leaves, to serve (optional)

COOK'S TIP

For a vegan alternative, substitute tofu for the prawns.

Almost instant and very low-calorie, this is a fast-day life-saver. It was one of the recipes I demonstrated in our Channel 4 series *Lose a Stone in 21 Days*. Miso paste has a deliciously sweet, salty, slightly tangy flavour. The prawns add a good boost of protein and omega-3, along with other nutrients, including selenium (which most of us are lacking and is important for the immune system). You can add a handful of young spinach leaves or cooked greens as well. Simply add at the same time as the prawns. Having grown up in Hong Kong, Michael loved this exotic dish, rich in protein and fibre. Miso soup kept Michael going in his early 5:2 fast days.

1. Place the pak choi in a small saucepan with 250ml water.

2. Stir in the miso paste, add the sliced mushroom and bring to a simmer. Cook for 3–4 minutes, or until the pak choi is beginning to soften.

3. Add the prawns and cook for a further minute, or until the prawns are hot.

4. Remove from the heat, stir in the chilli and coriander, if using, and ladle into a deep bowl or large mug to serve.

GLUTEN FREE · NUT FREE · DAIRY FREE

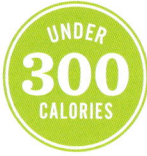

Harissa Lentil and Chickpea Soup with Spinach

SERVES **4** | PREP **5** mins | COOK **20** mins

2 tbsp olive or rapeseed oil
1 large onion, finely chopped
1 heaped tbsp harissa paste
1–2 tsp ground turmeric
   (optional)
1 × 400g can chopped tomatoes
1 × 250g sachet ready-cooked
   puy lentils (or use canned)
1 × 400g can chickpeas, drained
150g young spinach leaves
   or 3 balls frozen spinach
small handful coriander
   leaves, to serve (optional)

The lentils and chickpeas provide an excellent plant-based source of protein in this fragrant North African-flavoured soup. It is enhanced by a dollop of full-fat live Greek yoghurt – add 20cals for each 15ml tablespoon of yoghurt you use.

1. Heat the oil in a large saucepan over a low heat. Add the onion and gently fry for 5 minutes, or until softened, stirring regularly.

2. Add the harissa paste and turmeric, if using, and cook for a further minute, stirring.

3. Add the tomatoes, lentils, chickpeas and 600ml cold water. Bring to a simmer and cook for 10 minutes, stirring occasionally.

4. Stir in the spinach and cook for a further 1–2 minutes, or until well softened.

5. Season with salt and freshly ground black pepper, and ladle into warmed bowls. Sprinkle with coriander, if using, to serve.

VEGAN | GLUTEN FREE | NUT FREE | DAIRY FREE

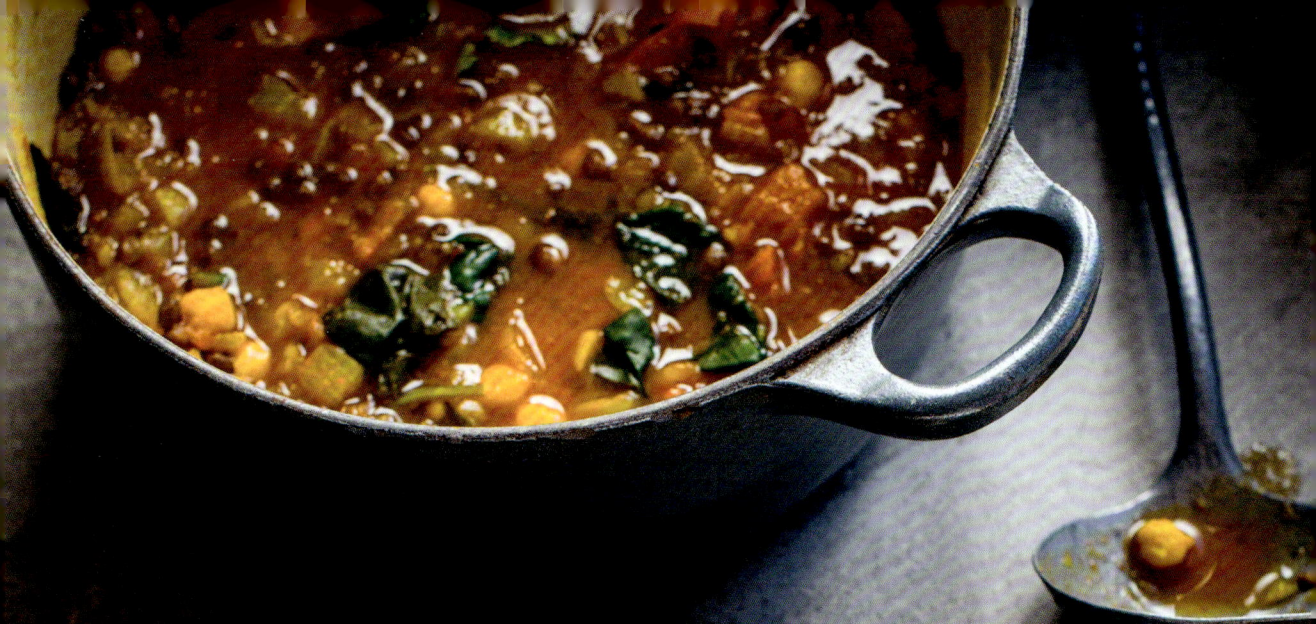

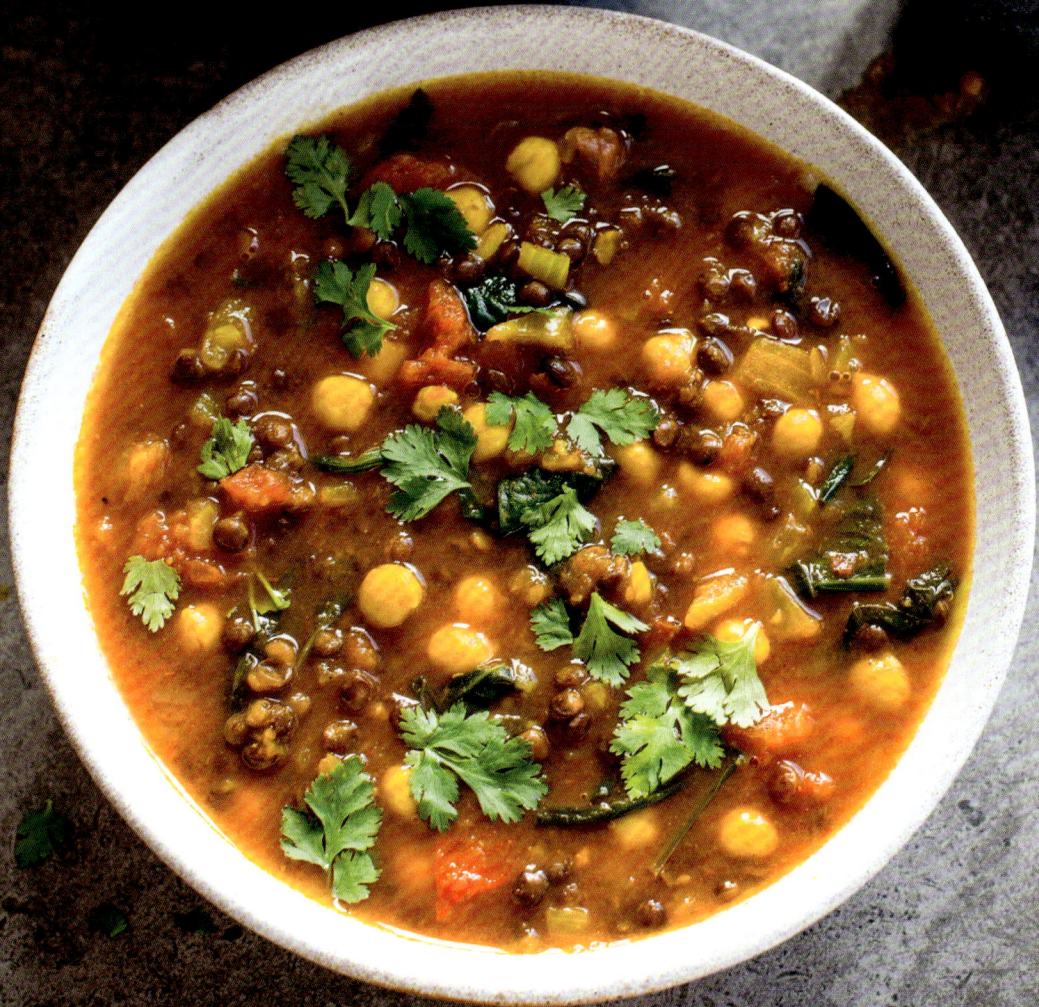

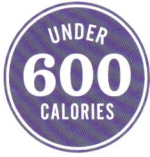

| PER SERVING | **542cals** | PROTEIN **33g** | CARBS **20g**

Salmon Salad Bowl

SERVES	PREP	COOK
2	**5** mins	**20** mins

25g wholegrain brown rice, or brown and wild rice mix
75g frozen edamame beans
2 × 120g salmon fillets
1 tsp sesame seeds
pinch crushed dried chilli flakes (optional)
2 large handfuls young spinach leaves or mixed baby salad leaves
½ avocado, peeled, stoned and chopped
1 carrot, trimmed and coarsely grated
2 spring onions, trimmed and finely sliced
4 radishes, trimmed and sliced
lime wedges, to serve

For the dressing
2 tbsp dark soy sauce
1 tbsp sesame oil
1 tsp fresh lime juice
1 tsp runny honey

NON-FAST DAYS
Choose larger fillets – you will need to cook them a few minutes longer – and increase the quantity of rice.

COOK'S TIP
Make the full amount, even if you only need one serving, as the rest will keep well in the fridge for the next day.

Serve the salad warm as a delicious lunch or supper, or take it to work in a lidded container for a nutritious and filling packed lunch. The dressing contains 39cals per tablespoon without the honey. Feel free to add it to another salad but don't forget to add the extra calories.

1. Preheat the oven to 200°C/Fan 180°C/Gas 6 and line a small baking tray with foil.

2. To make the dressing, combine the soy sauce, sesame oil, lime juice and honey in a small bowl and whisk well.

3. Half fill a small saucepan with water and bring to the boil. Add the rice and cook for about 20 minutes, or until tender. Add the edamame beans and return to the boil, stirring. Drain immediately.

4. Meanwhile, place the salmon, skin-side down, on the prepared tray and drizzle with 2 teaspoons of the dressing. Sprinkle with the sesame seeds and chilli flakes, if using. Bake for 10–12 minutes, or until just cooked. (It is ready when the salmon flakes into large pieces easily when prodded with a fork.)

5. Divide the leaves, rice and beans between two bowls. Arrange the avocado, carrot, spring onions and radishes alongside. Flake the salmon into the bowl (leaving behind the skin), drizzle with the remaining dressing and serve with lime wedges for squeezing over.

AIR-FRYER TIP
To cook the salmon in an air fryer: preheat the air fryer to 180°C, if needed. Prepare the salmon as Step 4, and air fry for 8 minutes, or until just cooked.

NUT FREE • DAIRY FREE

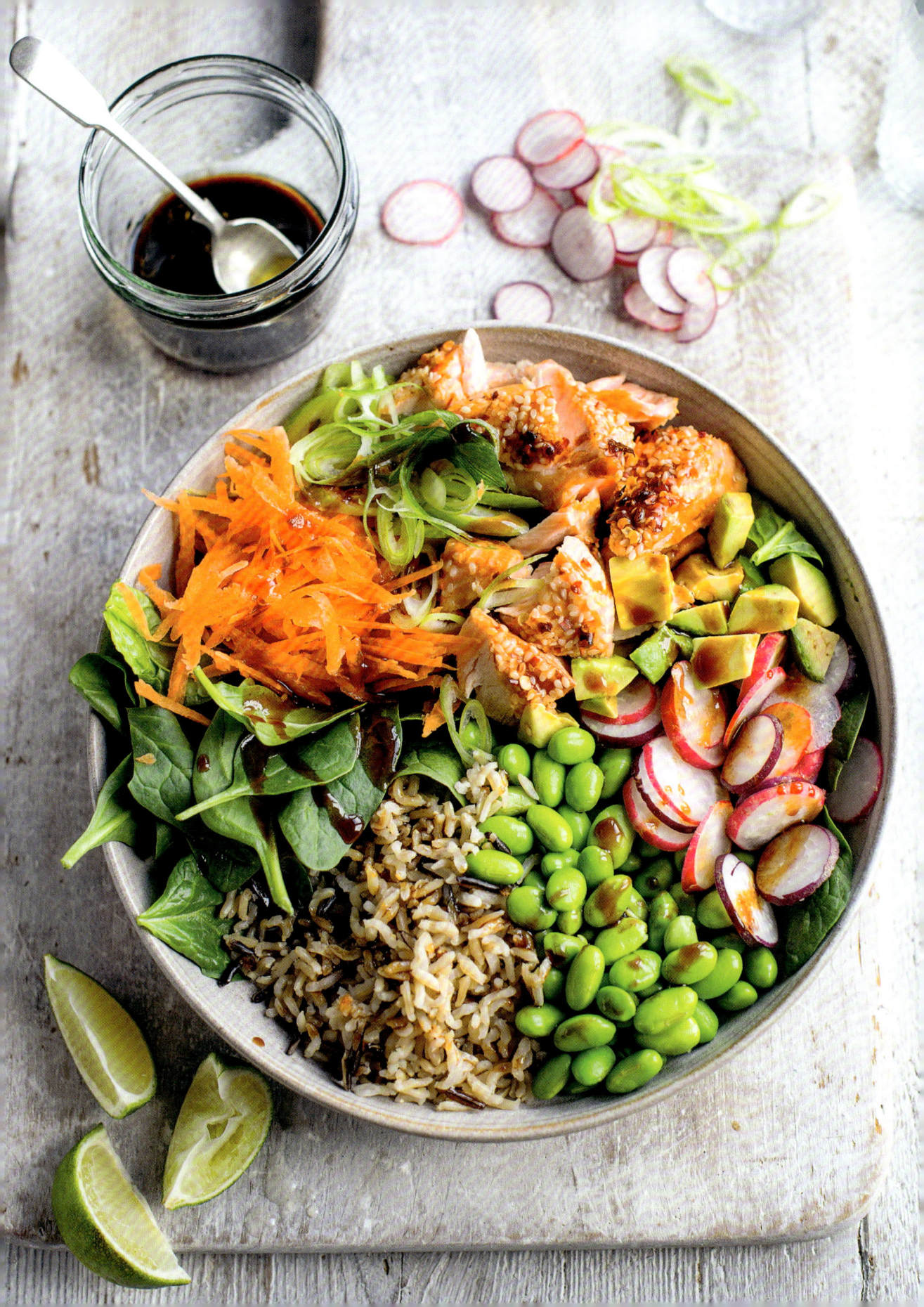

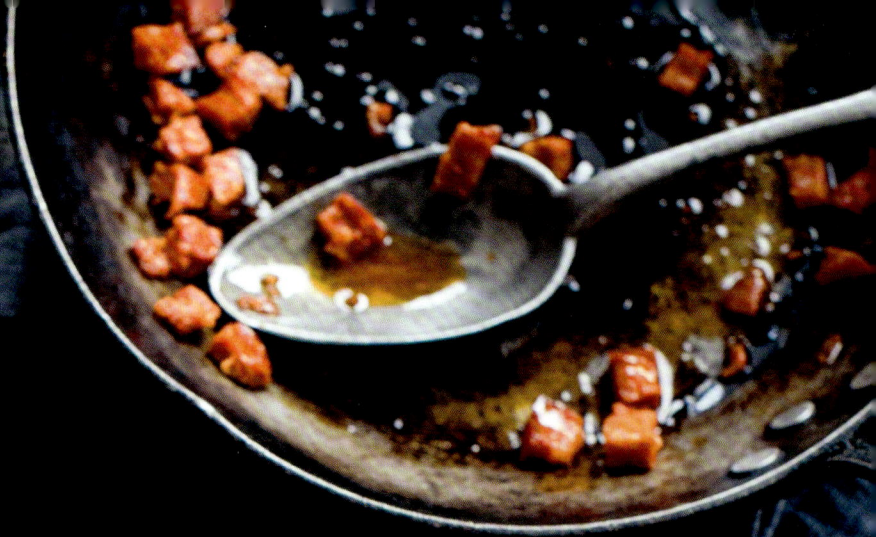

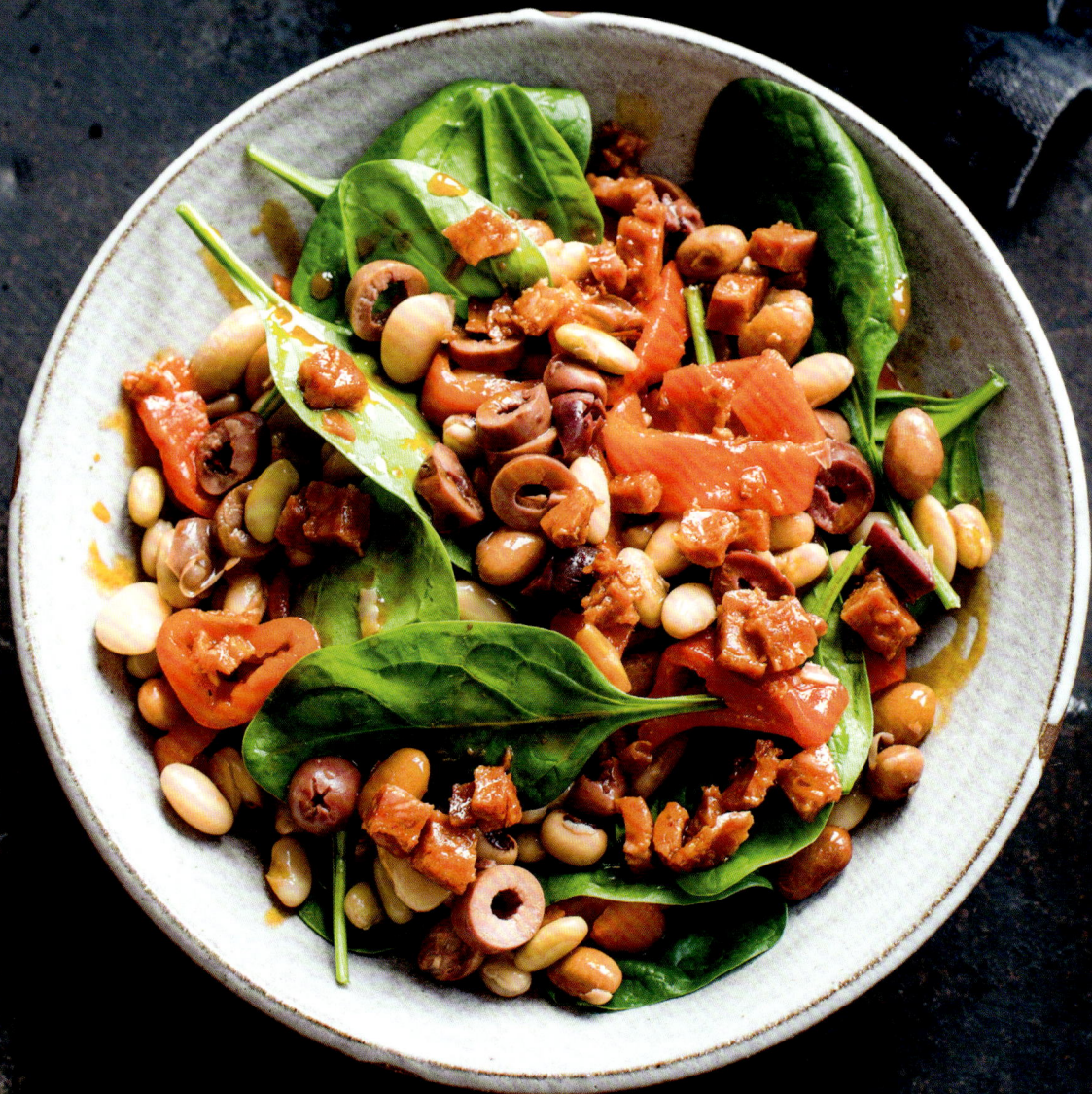

Chorizo and Bean Salad

SERVES **2** | **PREP** **10** mins | **COOK** **2** mins

25g chorizo, roughly chopped
2 tbsp extra-virgin olive oil
1 × 400g can mixed beans in
    water, drained and rinsed
100g roasted red peppers from
    a jar, drained and sliced
25g pitted olives, sliced
50g young spinach leaves
1 tbsp apple cider vinegar

COOK'S TIP
Roast your own peppers by
placing them on a baking tray
lined with foil and cooking
under a hot grill for about
10 minutes, or until the skins
are blistered and blackened,
turning regularly. Leave until
cool enough to handle, then
strip off the blackened skins
and cut the peppers into
strips, discarding the seeds.
Two smallish peppers will
give enough roasted pepper
for this recipe.

A high-protein, Mediterranean-style salad with
a boost of gut-friendly fibre. Choose the hard,
cured chorizo, rather than the soft, cooking kind.
Any beans or chickpeas work well; just make sure
they are canned in water.

1. Place the chorizo in a small frying pan with 1 tablespoon
of the oil over a medium heat. Cook for 2 minutes, or
until it begins to release its fat and turn lightly brown,
stirring regularly.

2. Meanwhile, mix the beans, peppers, olives and spinach
leaves in a large bowl.

3. Remove the pan from the heat and stir in the remaining
oil and the cider vinegar. Leave to sizzle for a few seconds,
then scatter the chorizo and warm dressing over the salad
and toss lightly.

4. Divide the salad between two shallow bowls or plates
and serve while still warm and before the leaves wilt.

GLUTEN FREE   NUT FREE   DAIRY FREE   ✓

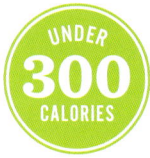

Chicken Caesar-ish Salad

SERVES | PREP
2 | **5**
mins

2 Little Gem lettuces,
 leaves separated
12 cherry tomatoes, halved
200g cooked chicken breast,
 cut or shred into small pieces
10g mixed seeds
20g Parmesan, grated

For the yoghurt dressing
75g full-fat live Greek yoghurt
½ small garlic clove,
 peeled and crushed
pinch dried mixed herbs
1 tbsp extra-virgin olive oil

NON-FAST DAYS
Increase the portion size
and add extra seeds.

COOK'S TIP
If taking as a packed lunch,
put the dressing in a small
lidded pot and drizzle over
the salad just before serving.
Keep the salad and dressing
chilled until needed.

The mixed seeds add the crunch usually provided by croutons and are far more nutritious. The dressing contains 34cals per tablespoon. Feel free to add it to another salad but don't forget to add the extra calories. For Michael, this ticked the box of an easy-to-make, flavourful lunch packed with protein.

1. To make the dressing, combine the yoghurt, garlic, herbs, oil and 2 tablespoons cold water in a bowl and mix well. Season with a pinch of salt and lots of freshly ground black pepper.

2. Divide the lettuce leaves between two shallow bowls or lidded containers and scatter with the tomatoes.

3. Place the chicken on top, then sprinkle with the mixed seeds and Parmesan. Drizzle with the dressing and season with ground black pepper to serve.

GLUTEN FREE | NUT FREE

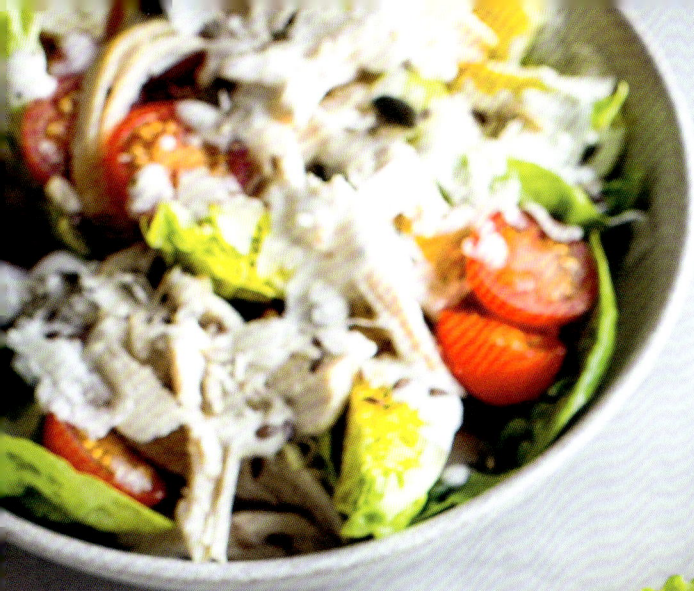

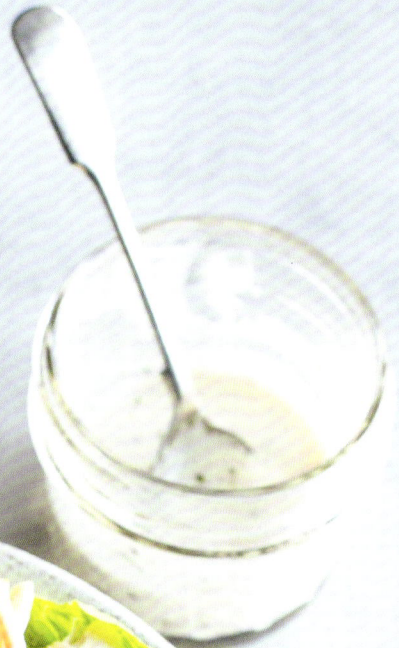

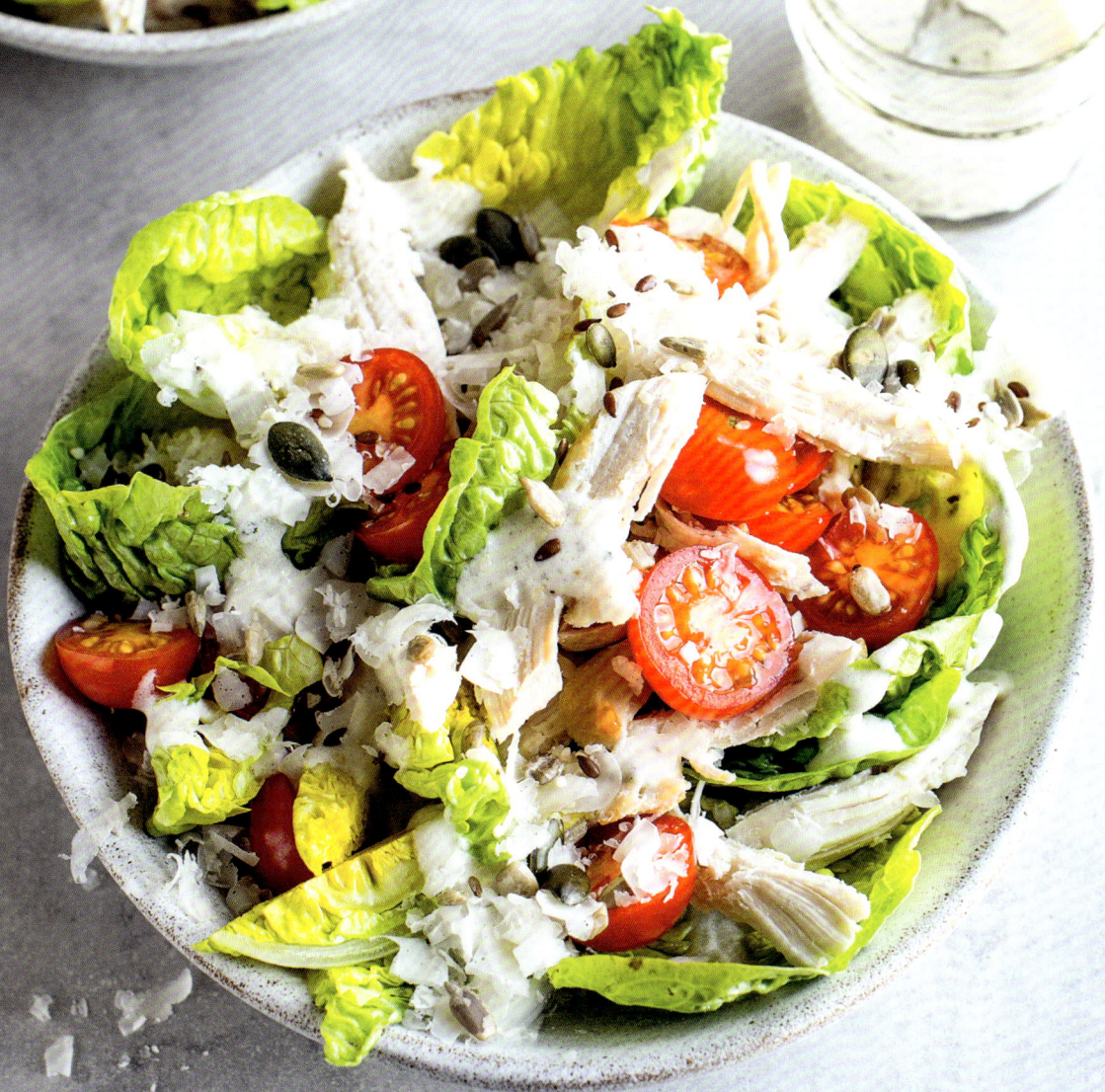

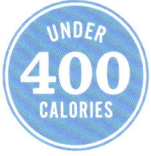

Black Bean and Mango Slaw

SERVES | PREP
2 | **20** mins

½ × 400g can black beans, drained and rinsed (around 120g drained weight)

1 red pepper, deseeded and cut into 1cm pieces

¼ small red cabbage, core removed and finely sliced

2–3 spring onions, trimmed and finely sliced

30g pine nuts

½ mango, diced (around 150g prepared weight)

2 generous handfuls rocket or watercress

1 small red chilli, finely sliced (deseeded, if preferred, for less heat)

small handful coriander, roughly chopped (optional)

For the dressing
1 tbsp fresh lime juice
2 tbsp full-fat live Greek yoghurt
1 tbsp full-fat mayonnaise

COOK'S TIP
You can use two halves of apricot or one peach from a can (around 100g) instead of mango, if you wish.

Although the beans and mango make this salad slightly higher in carbs than other slaws, these ingredients really make the salad sing! The beans also offer vital extra fibre to help feed your gut microbiome – which in turn supports your immunity, reduces inflammation, boosts mood and may even help with weight loss.

1. Mix the black beans, red pepper, red cabbage and spring onions together in a large bowl.

2. Toast the pine nuts in a dry frying pan over a medium heat for about 2 minutes, until they start to turn golden. Be careful they don't burn.

3. To make the dressing, place half the mango in a jug with the lime juice, yoghurt and mayo and blitz with a stick blender. Season with salt and freshly ground black pepper.

4. Stir the dressing into the beans and veg, then gently toss in the leaves. Divide between two plates and top with the remaining mango. Garnish with the pine nuts, chilli and coriander, if using, to serve.

VEGGIE   GLUTEN FREE   NUT FREE

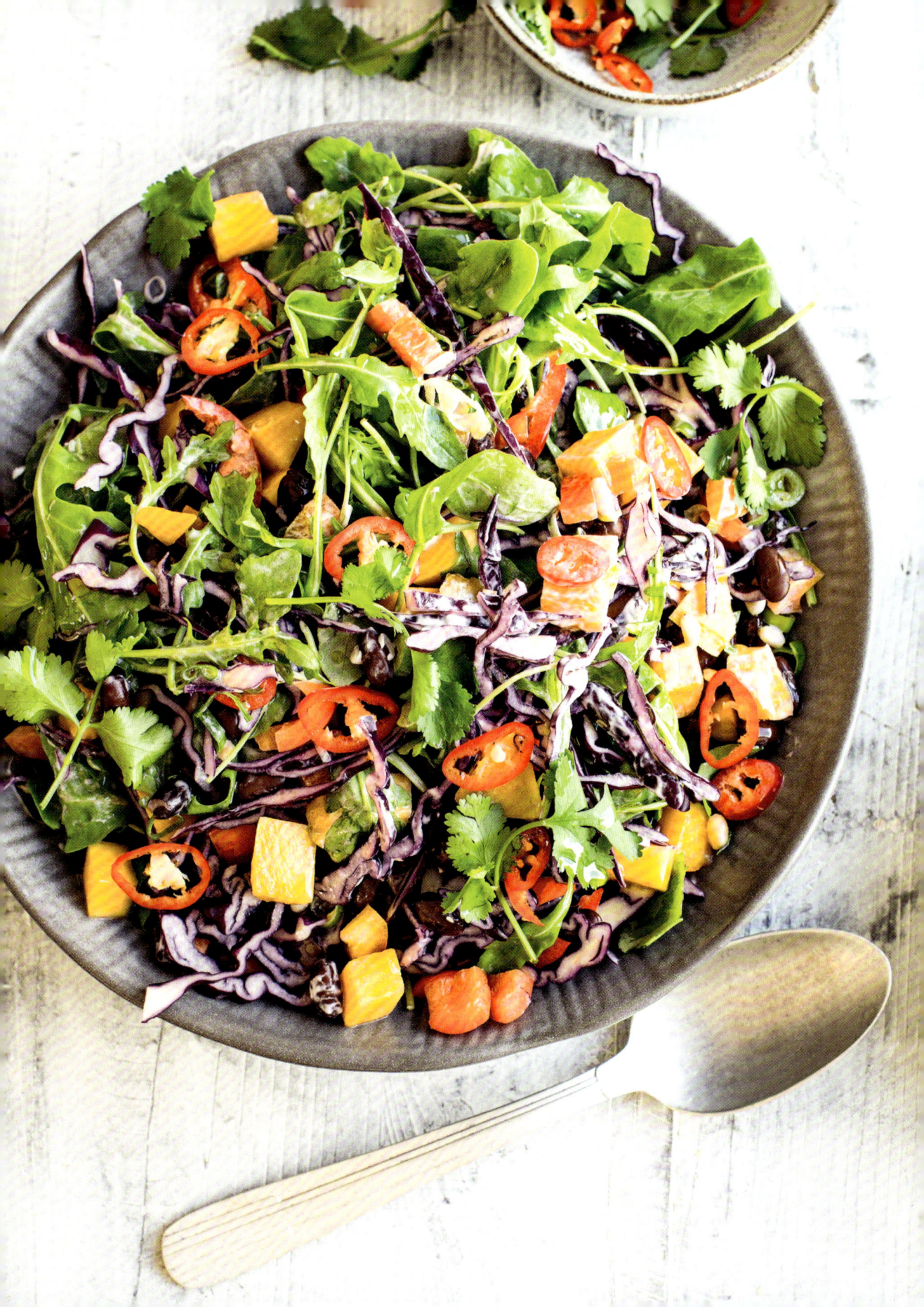

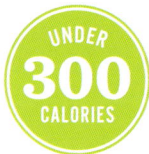

Warm Crispy Kale Salad with Mushrooms, Bacon and Goat's Cheese

SERVES **2** | PREP **8** mins | COOK **5** mins

125g curly kale, tough stalks
    stripped out and leaves
    roughly chopped
2 tbsp olive oil
½–1 tsp crushed dried
    chilli flakes
2 large Portobello mushrooms,
    finely sliced
4 rashers smoked streaky
    bacon, snipped into pieces
50g soft goat's cheese

NON-FAST DAY
Have an extra half portion,
and serve on toasted wholemeal
bread or seeded sourdough.

COOK'S TIP
Keep a close eye on the kale
to make sure it doesn't burn.

**Kale cooked in the oven becomes irresistibly crispy.
Eat this salad in a wide bowl.**

1. Preheat the oven to 200°C/Fan 180°C/Gas 6.

2. Tip the kale into a roasting dish, drizzle with 1 tablespoon of the olive oil, sprinkle over the chilli flakes and season with salt and freshly ground black pepper. Using both hands, massage the oil into the leaves so they are thoroughly coated. Roast in the oven for 5 minutes.

3. Meanwhile, place the mushrooms, bacon and remaining oil in a pan over a medium heat and sauté for about 5 minutes, until starting to brown and crisp. Remove from the heat.

4. To assemble, divide the kale, bacon and mushrooms between two bowls. Dot the goat's cheese all over and serve.

AIR-FRYER TIP
To crisp the kale in an air fryer: preheat the air fryer to 160°C, if needed. Prepare the kale as Step 2, using only 1½ teaspoons of oil with the chilli flakes and seasoning. Place the kale in the air fryer in an even layer (you may need to cook it in batches), and air fry for 3–4 minutes, or until crisp, turning halfway through.

GLUTEN FREE | NUT FREE

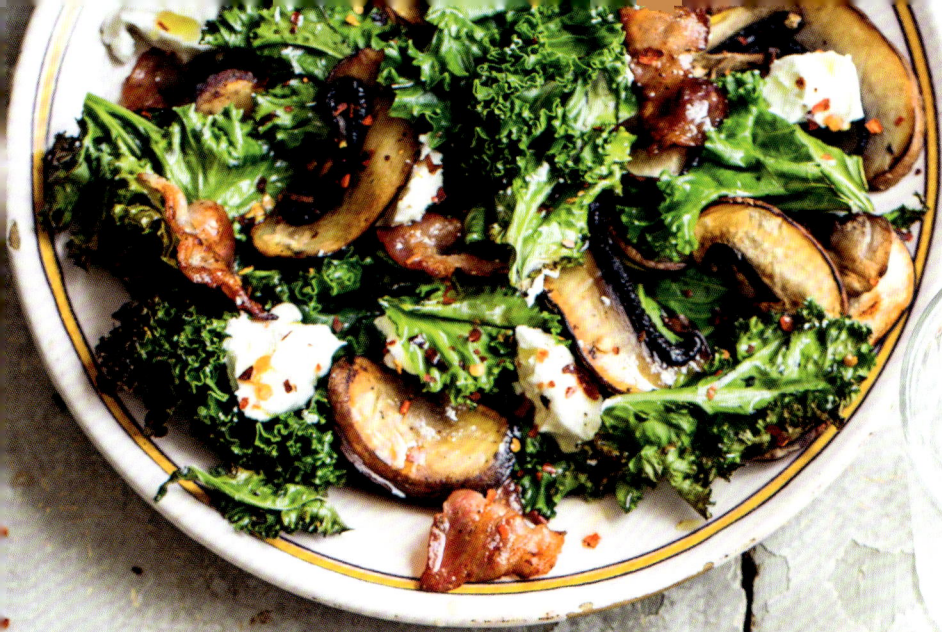

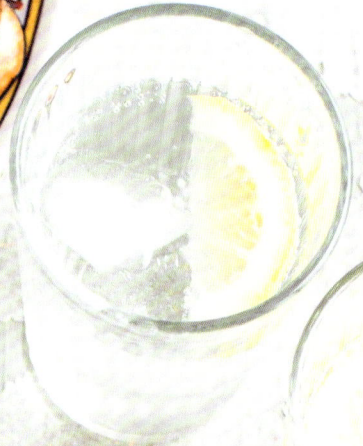

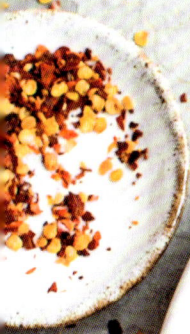

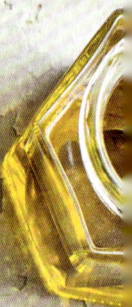

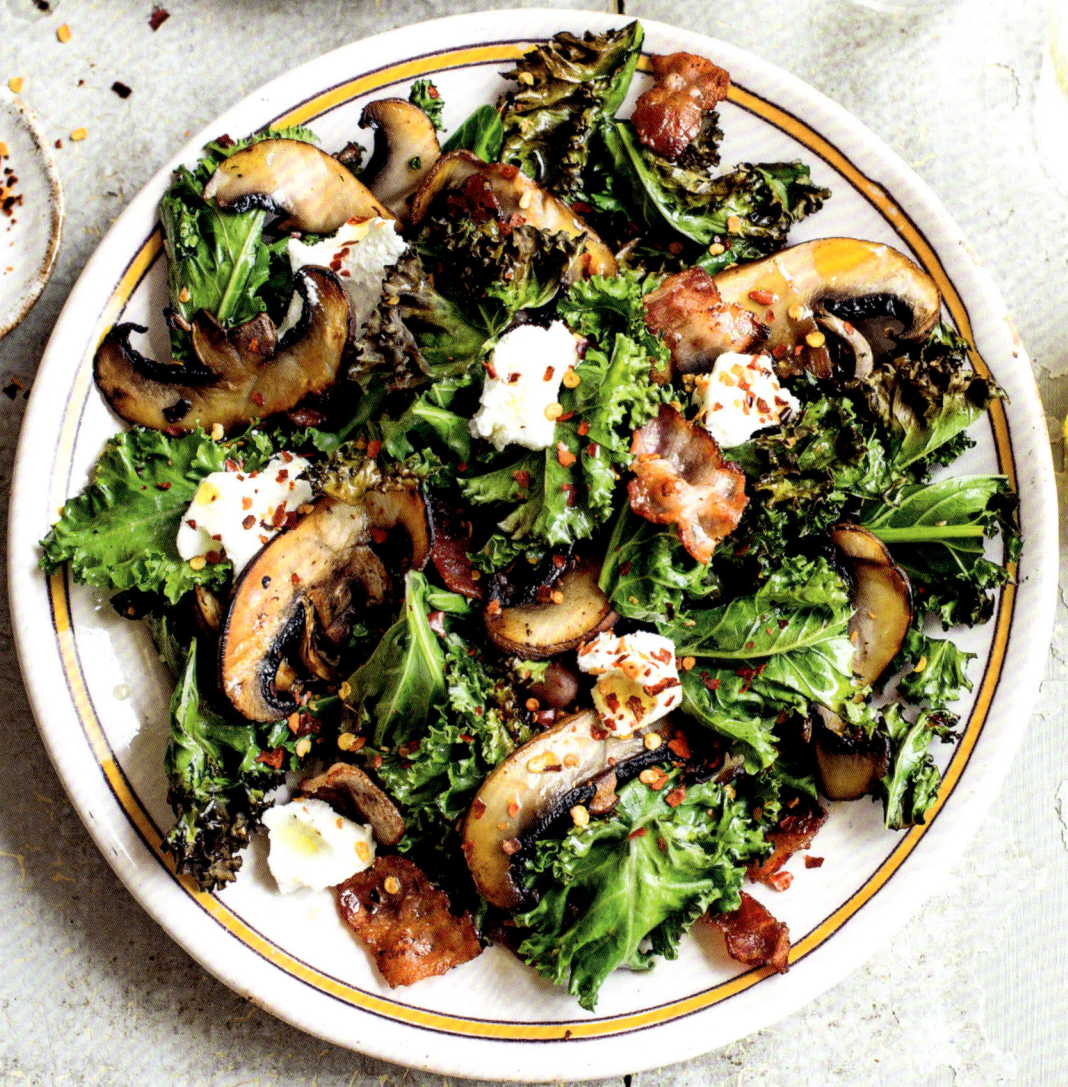

No-count Dressings

UNDER 100 CALORIES

PER SERVING | **75cals** | PROTEIN **1.5g** | CARBS **3.2g**

Sriracha Yoghurt Dressing

Sriracha has to be one of our favourite seasonings, adding a burst of sweet chilli and garlic. It's available in most big supermarkets.

SERVES **2** | PREP **2** mins

2 tbsp full-fat live Greek yoghurt
1 tbsp full-fat mayonnaise
1½ tbsp sriracha

1. Mix all the ingredients together in a small bowl, jug or jar.

COOK'S TIP
The dressing will keep in the fridge for up to a week. A squeeze of lime juice is a nice addition – 1 teaspoon will suffice.

UNDER 100 CALORIES

PER SERVING | **67cals** | PROTEIN **1.5g** | CARBS **0.8g**

Ranch Dressing

Our version of an American classic.

SERVES **2** | PREP **5** mins

2 tbsp full-fat live Greek yoghurt
1 tbsp full-fat mayonnaise
½ tsp garlic granules
1 tsp fresh lemon juice
5g fresh flat-leaf parsley, finely chopped

1. Place all the ingredients in a small bowl and mix together. Season with salt and lots of freshly ground black pepper.

PER SERVING | **73cals** | PROTEIN **1.7g** | CARBS **1.4g**

Curried Yoghurt Dressing

With its mild curry flavour, this goes with almost anything!

SERVES **2** | PREP **5** mins

2 tbsp full-fat live Greek yoghurt
1 tbsp full-fat mayonnaise
1 tsp curry powder
small handful coriander, leaves
   finely chopped (optional)

1. Place all the ingredients in a small bowl and mix together. Season to taste with salt and freshly ground black pepper.

PER SERVING | **79cals** | PROTEIN **0.4g** | CARBS **3.4g**

Ginger and Sesame Dressing

Bring your salad to life with this dressing – it works well in coleslaws, crunchy salads or drizzled on fish or tofu.

SERVES **2** | PREP **5** mins

1 tbsp rapeseed or olive oil
1 tbsp apple cider vinegar
1 tbsp light soy sauce
1 tbsp finely grated fresh root ginger
1 tsp sesame oil
½ tsp honey (optional)

1. Place all the ingredients in a small bowl, jug or jar and mix well. Season with a pinch of salt and a generous grinding of black pepper.

COOK'S TIP
The dressing will keep in the fridge for up to a week.

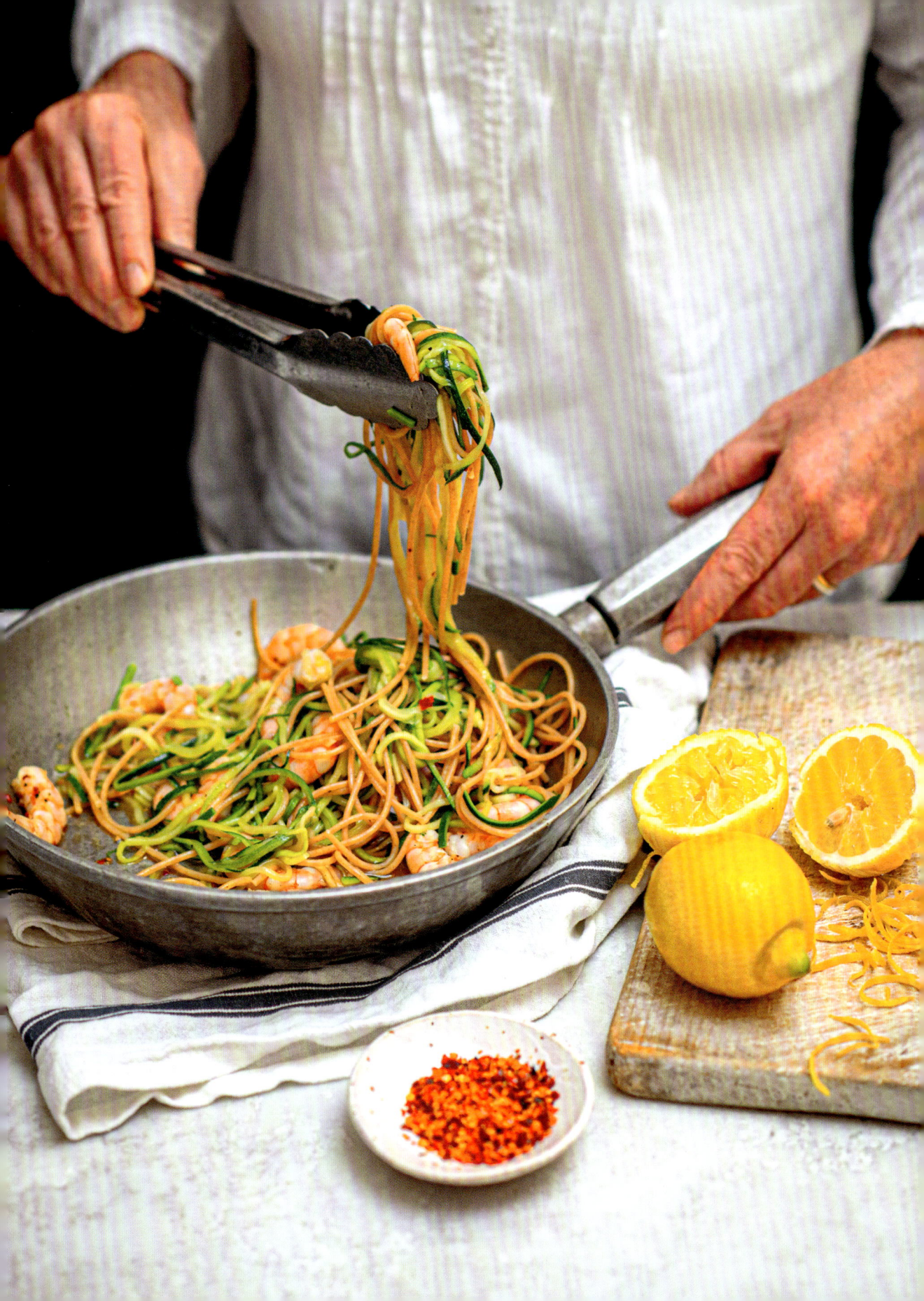

Fish and Seafood

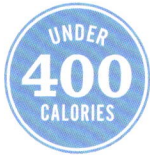

Pan-fried Fish with Lemon and Parsley

SERVES | PREP | COOK
1 | **2** mins | **5** mins

1 plaice fillet (around 175g),
   or other white fish fillet,
   defrosted if frozen
15g butter
1 tbsp extra-virgin olive oil
1 tbsp fresh lemon juice
small bunch parsley,
   leaves finely chopped
   (around 2 tbsp)

NON-FAST DAYS
Serve with a portion of warm white beans or some roasted vegetables. Add a knob of butter to your cooked greens or a generous splash of dressing to your salad. A serving of celeriac chips (see page 168) would also go well.

COOK'S TIP
Capers are a delicious addition to this dish. Simply add 1 tablespoon drained miniature capers at the same time as the lemon juice and parsley.

This is the ideal meal for one, but can easily be doubled up. Cook your vegetables or prepare a salad before you start frying the fish, as it takes less than 5 minutes. If you don't fancy plaice, sea bass or sea bream make good alternatives. If you want the dish to be dairy free, omit the butter and reduce by 28cals per serving. This classic fish dish was one of Michael's father's favourite meals, and Michael's too, served with plenty of steamed greens.

1. Season the fish on the skinless side with salt and freshly ground black pepper.

2. Melt the butter with the oil in a large frying pan over a medium heat. Add the plaice, skin-side down, and cook for 3 minutes. Carefully turn over and cook on the other side for a further 1–2 minutes, depending on the thickness of your fillet. (You can peel off the skin carefully at this point, if you like.)

3. Lift the plaice on to a warmed plate with a fish slice or spatula, turning on to the skin side. Return the pan to the heat, add the lemon juice and parsley, and simmer for a few seconds, stirring constantly.

4. Pour the buttery juices over the fish and serve with lots of green veg.

GLUTEN FREE | NUT FREE

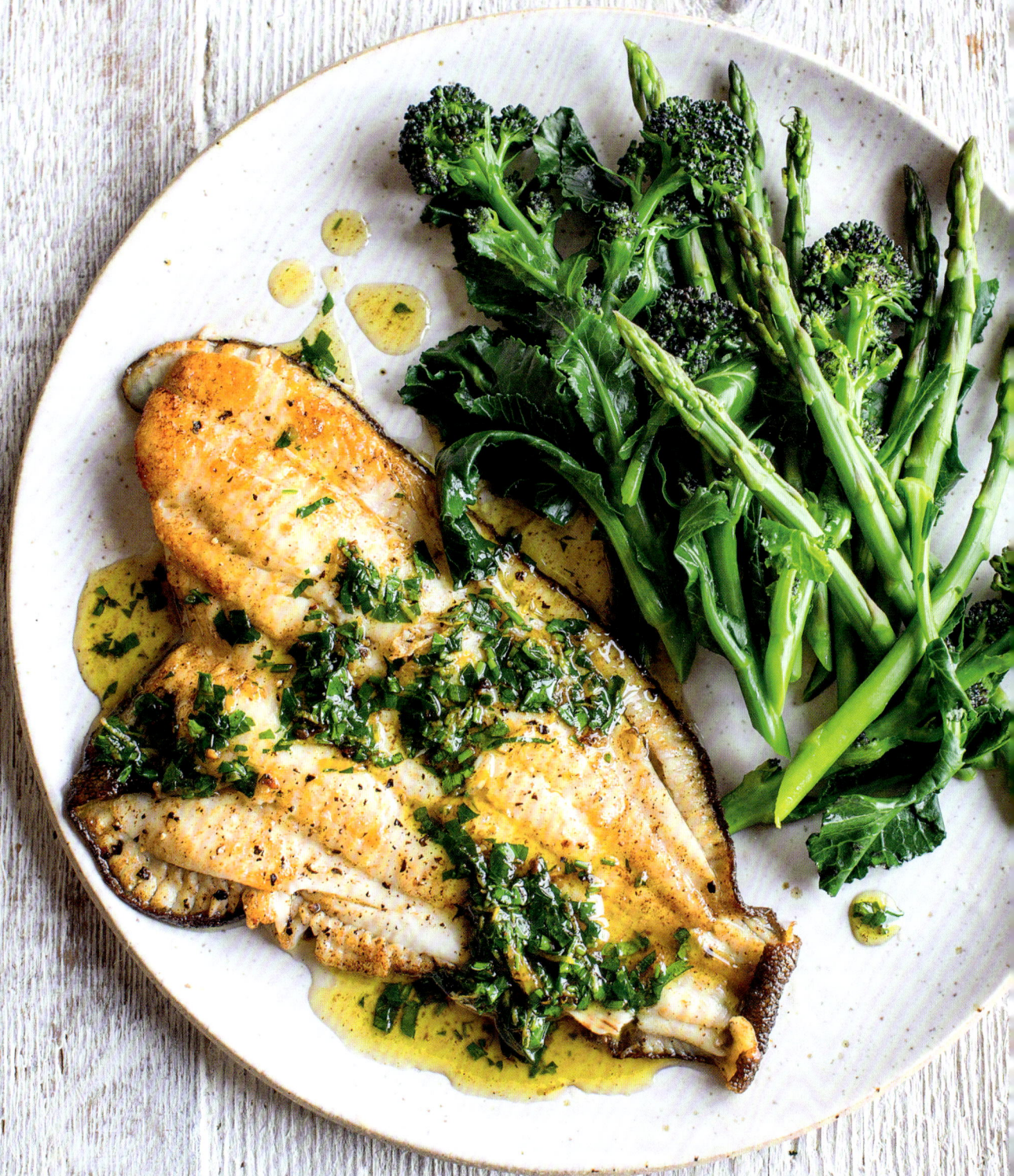

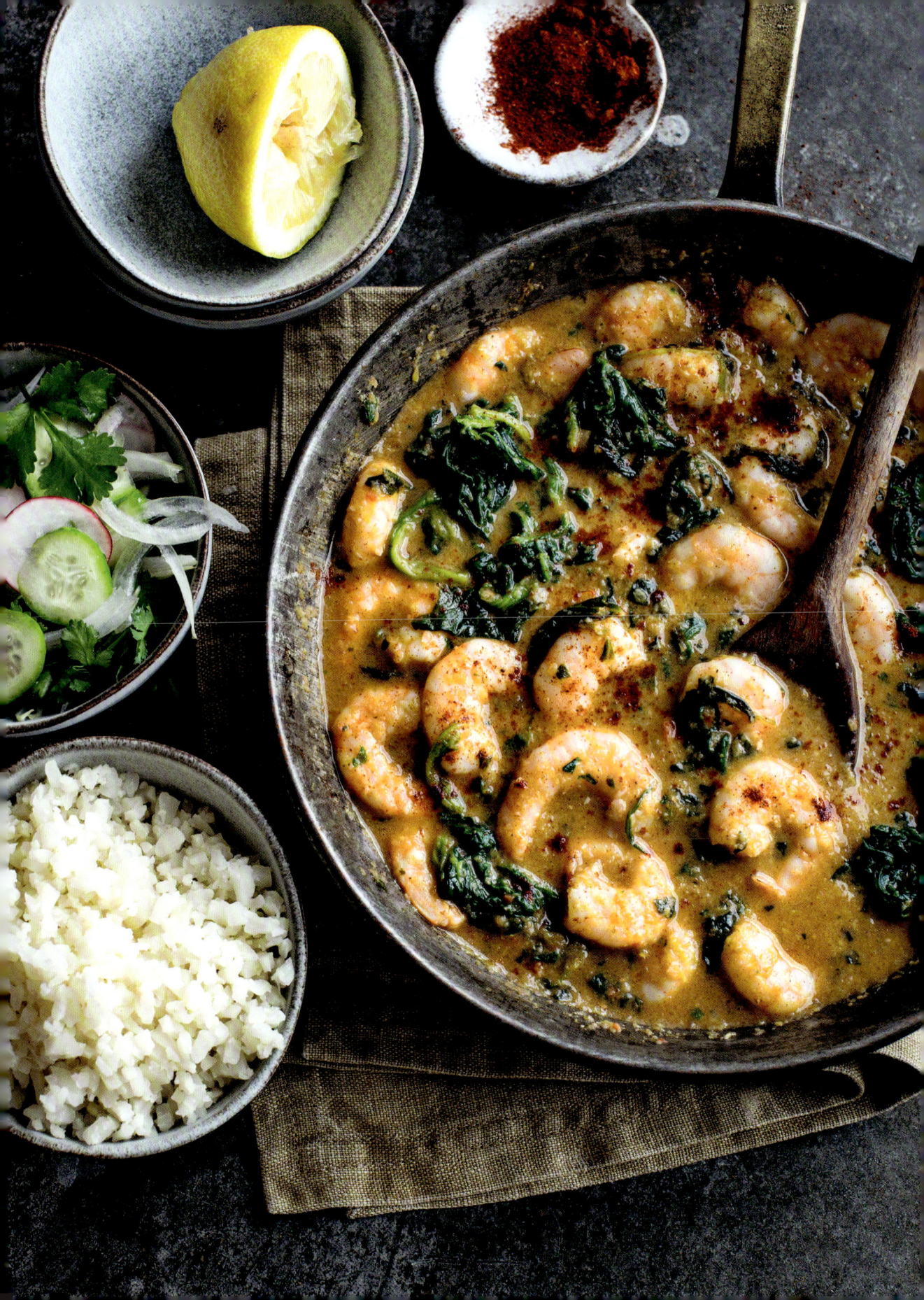

Made-in-minutes Goan Prawn Curry with Spinach

SERVES	PREP	COOK
4	**5** mins	**10** mins

1 small leek, trimmed
   and roughly chopped
3 garlic cloves, peeled
20g fresh root ginger
   (no need to peel)
2 tsp ground cumin
1 tsp ground coriander
1 tsp paprika
1 tsp garam masala
1 vegetable stock cube
1 small tomato, quartered
1 tbsp olive oil
1 × 400ml can full-fat
   coconut milk
100g frozen spinach
400g raw, peeled, frozen
   king prawns, defrosted
juice of ½ lemon (optional)

NON-FAST DAY
Serve a double portion and/or
serve with 2–3 tablespoons
cooked brown rice.

COOK'S TIP
Get ahead with this recipe
by creating the curry base
up to the point the coconut
milk is added. It will keep
in the fridge for up to 4 days.

This luscious dish has the feel of a curry that has been laboured over for hours. The flavour is condensed into a paste, creating the most fabulous, creamy, coconut base for the spinach and prawns. Although it has quite a few ingredients, most are found in the cupboard or freezer. Serve with steamed leafy greens. A big fan of curried prawns, Michael sometimes used a curry paste from the supermarket to make this, instead of adding individual spices.

1. Place all the ingredients up to and including the tomato in a food processor or blender and blitz until smooth.

2. Tip the paste into a saucepan, add the oil and fry over a medium heat, stirring from time to time, for 3–4 minutes.

3. Pour in the coconut milk and add the frozen spinach. Simmer for 3–4 minutes to allow the flavours to mingle and the spinach to defrost.

4. Finally, add the defrosted prawns and cook for no more than 2 minutes, until they have just turned pink.

5. Stir in the lemon juice, if using, and serve.

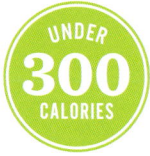

Salmon, Ginger and Coriander Fish Cakes with Soy and Lime

SERVES	PREP	COOK
2	**15** mins	**4** mins

150g salmon fillet,
   skin removed
10g fresh root ginger,
   peeled and finely grated
5g fresh coriander,
   finely chopped
1 level tbsp ground almonds
1 tbsp olive oil
2 tbsp light soy sauce
Juice of ½ lime (around 1 tbsp)

NON-FAST DAY
Increase the portion
size and/or serve with
wholegrain noodles
or 2–3 tablespoons
cooked wholegrain rice.

Fresh and clean in flavour – without a starchy coating – these fish cakes need little more than some lettuce leaves on the side (peppery rocket works well) to make a great lunch. A generous plate of steamed greens will make them into a delicious dinner.

1. Place the salmon on a clean work surface and chop finely, using a very sharp knife. The salmon should be slightly paste-like, but still have small chunks.

2. Transfer the salmon to a bowl and add the ginger, coriander and ground almonds. Season generously with salt and freshly ground black pepper, and mix until thoroughly combined.

3. Shape into four small patties, squeezing each one between the palm of your hands to make sure it is tightly packed together.

4. Heat the olive oil in a frying pan over a medium heat. Add the fish cakes and fry for 2 minutes on each side. Transfer to a sheet of kitchen paper to mop up the excess oil.

5. Meanwhile, mix the soy sauce and lime juice together in a dipping bowl and serve alongside the fish cakes.

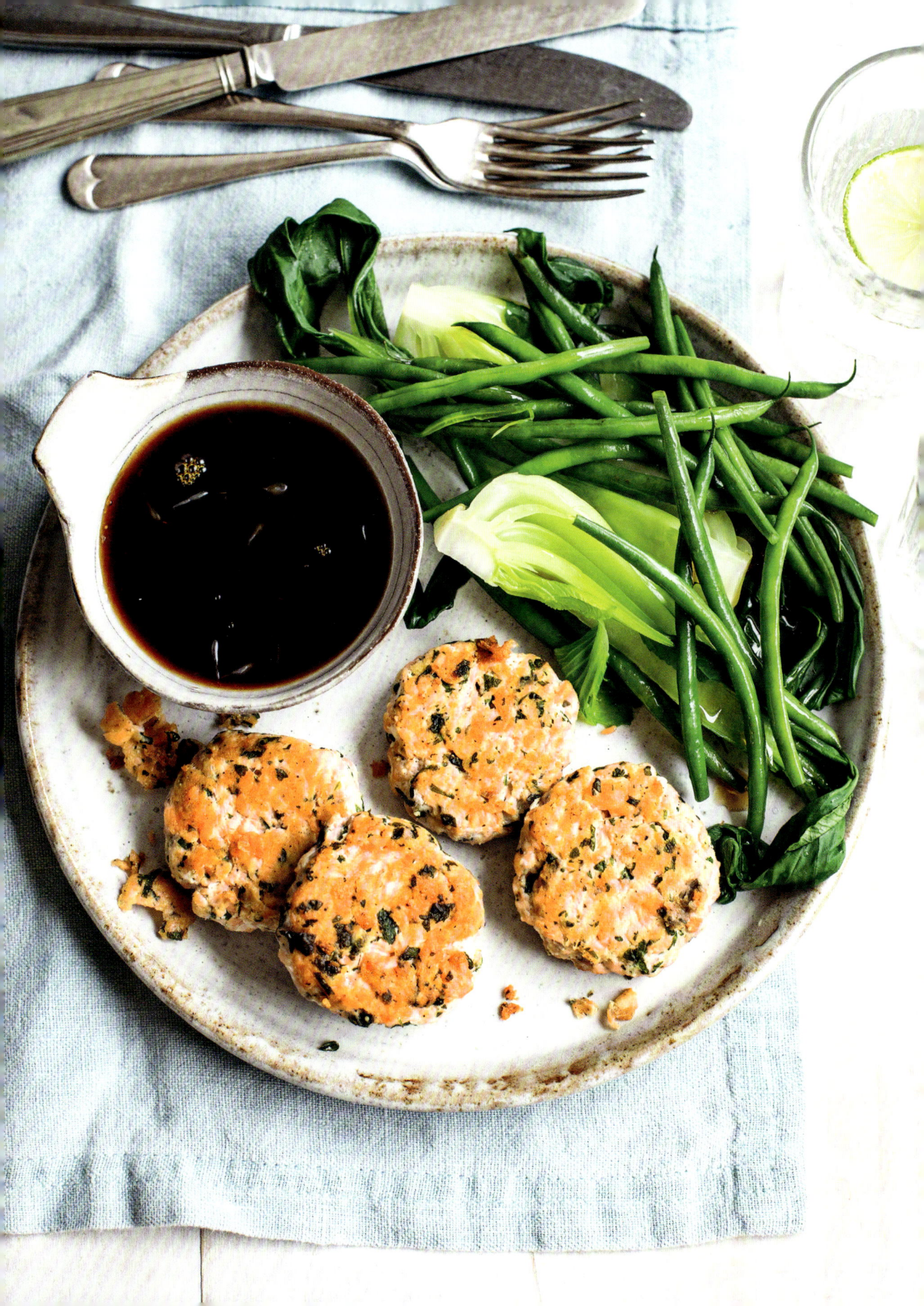

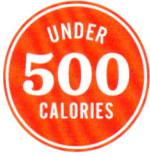

Scallops with a Mushroom and Sun-dried Tomato Sauce

SERVES	PREP	COOK
2	**5** mins	**6** mins

240g frozen scallops, defrosted
1 tbsp olive oil
2 sun-dried tomatoes from a jar, finely chopped, plus 1 tbsp of the oil
100g chestnut mushrooms, finely sliced
1 large garlic clove (or 2 small cloves), peeled and finely chopped
100ml crème fraîche
5g fresh dill, roughly chopped

NON-FAST DAY
Have a larger portion and add some cooked peas or beans.

This recipe is super quick to make and results in a truly restaurant-level meal. I use frozen scallops as they are cheaper and readily available in supermarkets. Serve with a generous plate of greens.

1. Season the scallops with a pinch of salt and freshly ground black pepper.

2. Place the oil in a frying pan over a high heat. When it is really hot, add the scallops and fry on one side for 2 minutes, until they have a golden crust. Turn and fry on the other side for 1 minute, then remove from the pan and keep warm.

3. Add the sun-dried tomato oil to the pan with the mushrooms and sauté for 1 minute.

4. Stir in the garlic and sun-dried tomatoes, and fry for 30 seconds.

5. Add the crème fraîche, dill and 1 tablespoon of water to loosen the sauce. Stir to heat through and return the scallops to the pan for a final 30 seconds. Check the seasoning and serve.

GLUTEN FREE NUT FREE

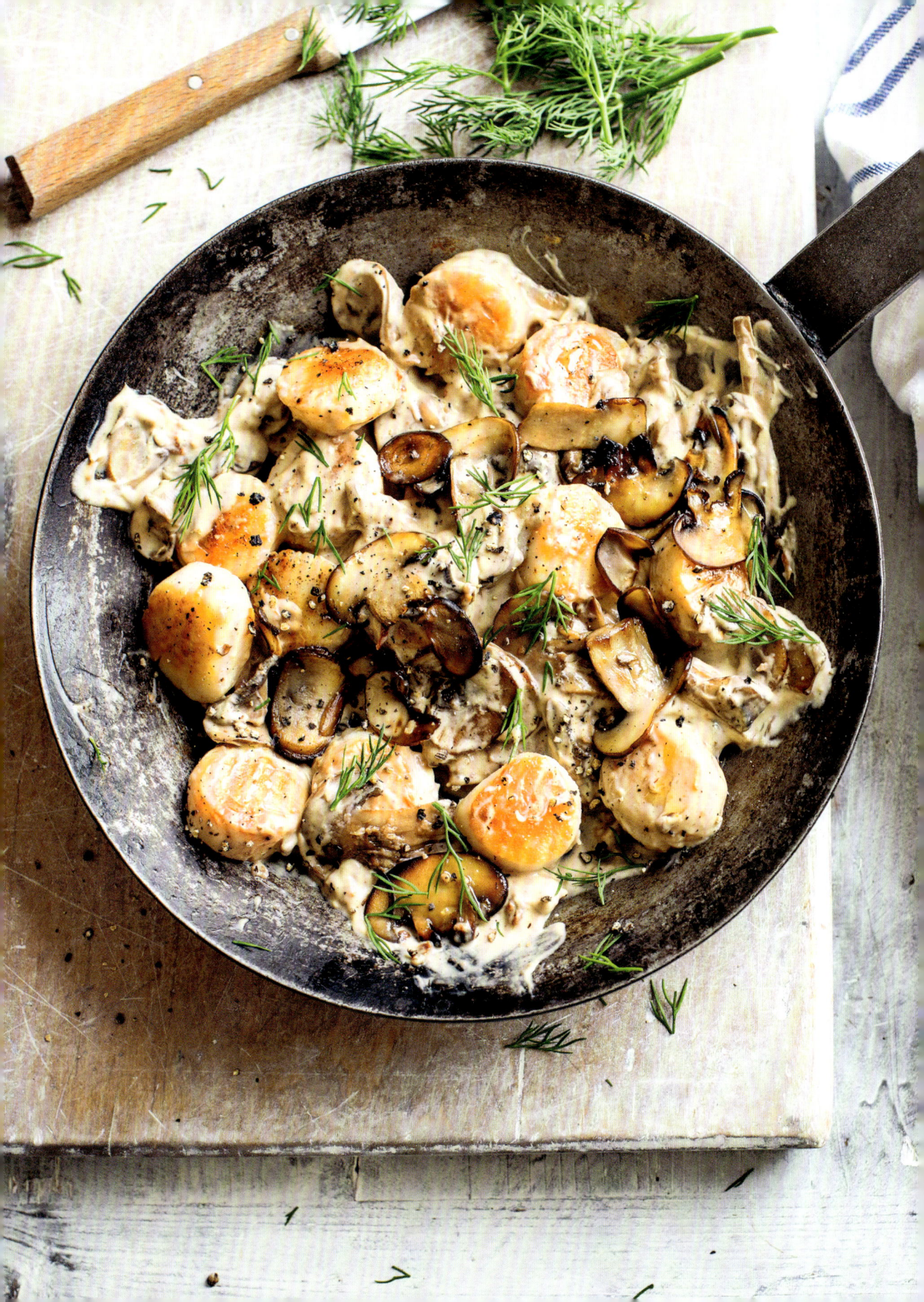

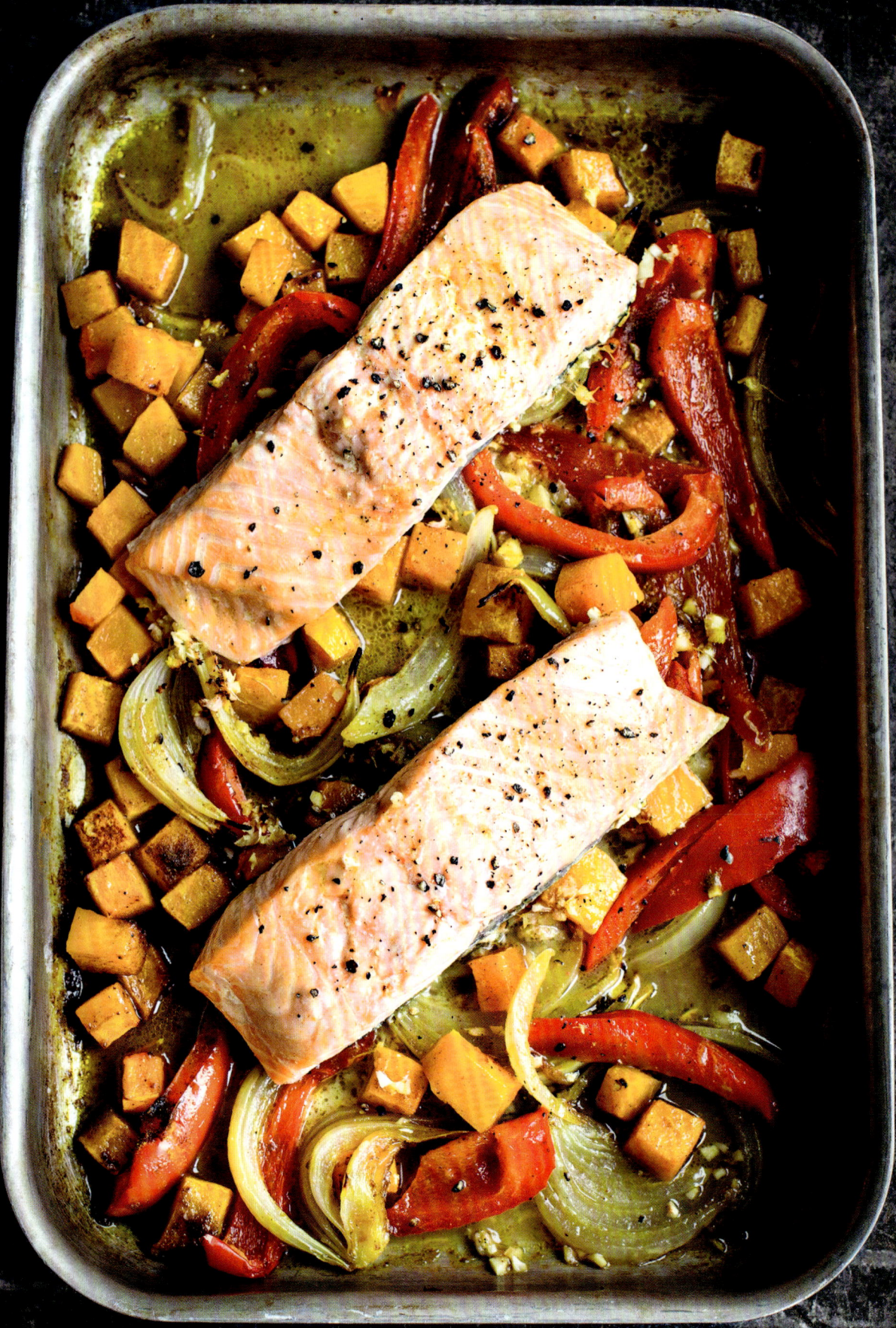

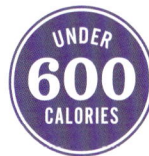

Spicy Salmon and Butternut Squash Traybake

SERVES 2 | **PREP** **20** mins | **COOK** **25** mins

½ onion, sliced into wedges about 1cm thick

200g butternut squash, peeled and cut into 1cm dice

1 red pepper, deseeded and sliced

1 tsp medium curry powder

1 tbsp olive oil

¼ × 400ml can full-fat coconut milk

1 large garlic clove, finely chopped

1 tsp finely chopped fresh root ginger

2 salmon fillets (around 130g each)

2 tsp Thai fish sauce

NON-FAST DAY
Enjoy a larger portion and/or serve with 2–3 tablespoons cooked wholegrain rice.

We all love traybakes – throw in the ingredients, let the oven do its bit, and hey presto! Here the mildly curried veg contrasts with the salmon in its creamy, spiced coconut sauce. This fabulous traybake includes many of Michael's favourite ingredients, as well as having lots of protein.

1. Preheat the oven to 200°C/Fan 180°C/Gas 6.

2. Place the onion, squash and red pepper in a baking dish or roasting tin and sprinkle the curry powder over the top. Drizzle with the olive oil and toss to coat. Roast the veg in the oven for 15 minutes.

3. Remove the tray from the oven and gently stir in the coconut milk, garlic and ginger. Place the salmon fillets on top, drizzle with the fish sauce and season with salt and freshly ground black pepper. Return to the oven for 10 minutes, or until the salmon is cooked through.

AIR-FRYER TIP

Preheat the air fryer to 180°C, if needed. Prepare the vegetables as Step 2. Place the vegetables in the air fryer in an even layer and cook for 15 minutes. Remove the air fryer basket and gently stir in the coconut milk, garlic and ginger. Place the salmon on top, drizzle with the fish sauce and season. Air fry for another 8 minutes until the salmon is cooked through.

GLUTEN FREE — NUT FREE — DAIRY FREE

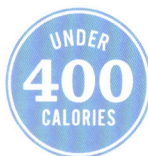

PER SERVING | **304cals** | PROTEIN **25g** | CARBS **3g**

Salmon Burgers

SERVES	PREP	COOK
2	**15** mins	**8** mins

2 × 120g skinless salmon fillets,
   cut into large chunks
15g bunch coriander,
   leaves roughly chopped,
   plus extra to serve
1 garlic clove, finely grated
15g fresh root ginger,
   peeled and finely grated
2 tsp dark soy sauce or
   1 tsp Thai fish sauce
2 spring onions, trimmed
   and finely sliced
1 red chilli, finely chopped,
   or ½–1 tsp crushed
   dried chilli flakes
2 tsp olive, coconut
   or rapeseed oil
lime wedges, to serve

A simple fish burger that can be knocked up in very little time. Serve with some finely diced red chilli, if you like a bit more heat.

1. Put the salmon in a food processor with the coriander, garlic, ginger and soy or fish sauce. Season with lots of ground black pepper and blitz on the pulse setting until it comes together as a thick, slightly chunky paste. Don't allow it to become too smooth.

2. Remove the blade and stir the spring onions and chilli into the mixture. Form into two balls and flatten into burger shapes.

3. Heat the oil in a frying pan over a moderate heat. Add the burgers and fry for 3–4 minutes on each side, or until golden brown and cooked through.

4. Serve with lime wedges and a mixed salad.

GLUTEN FREE · NUT FREE · DAIRY FREE

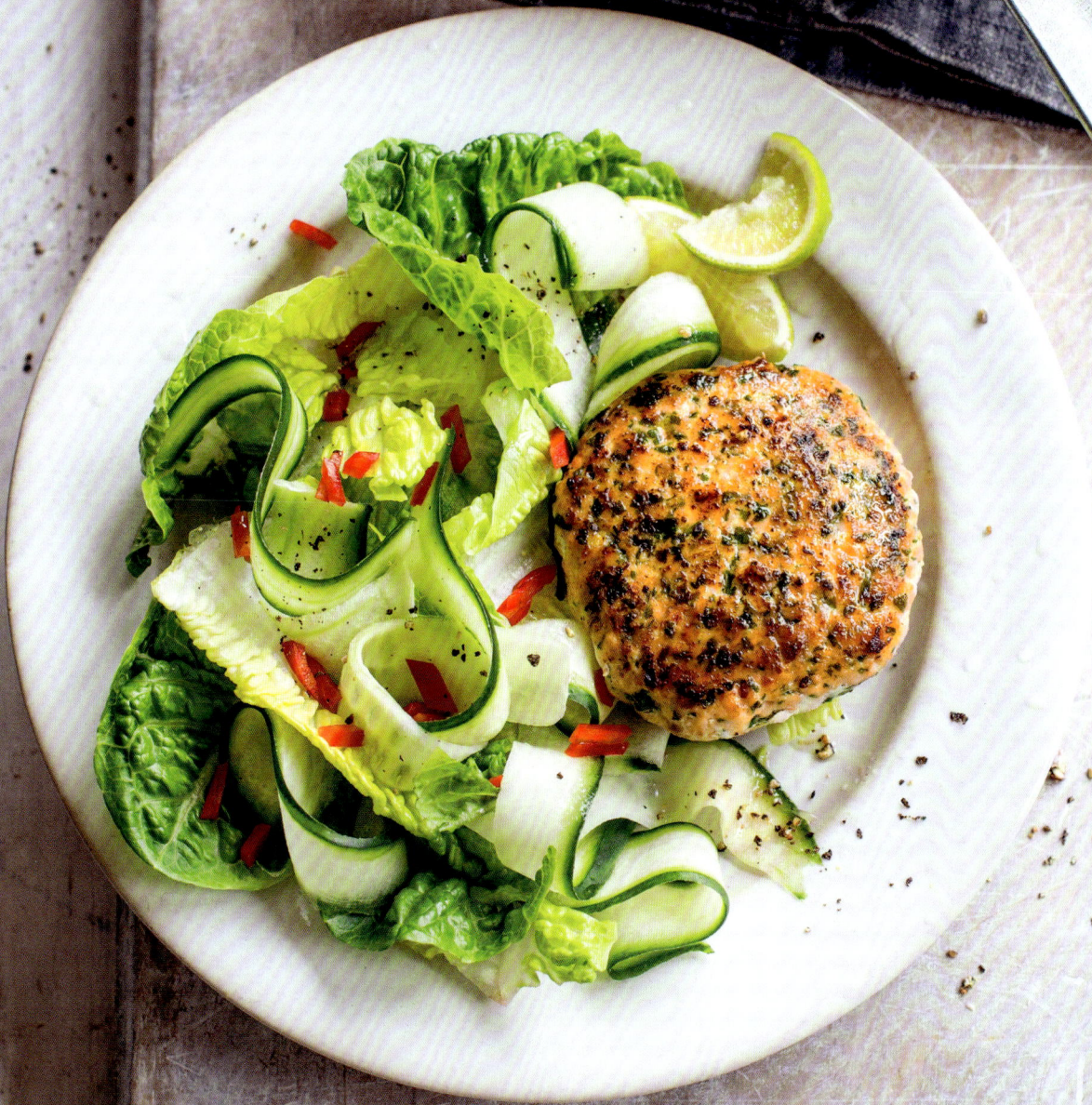

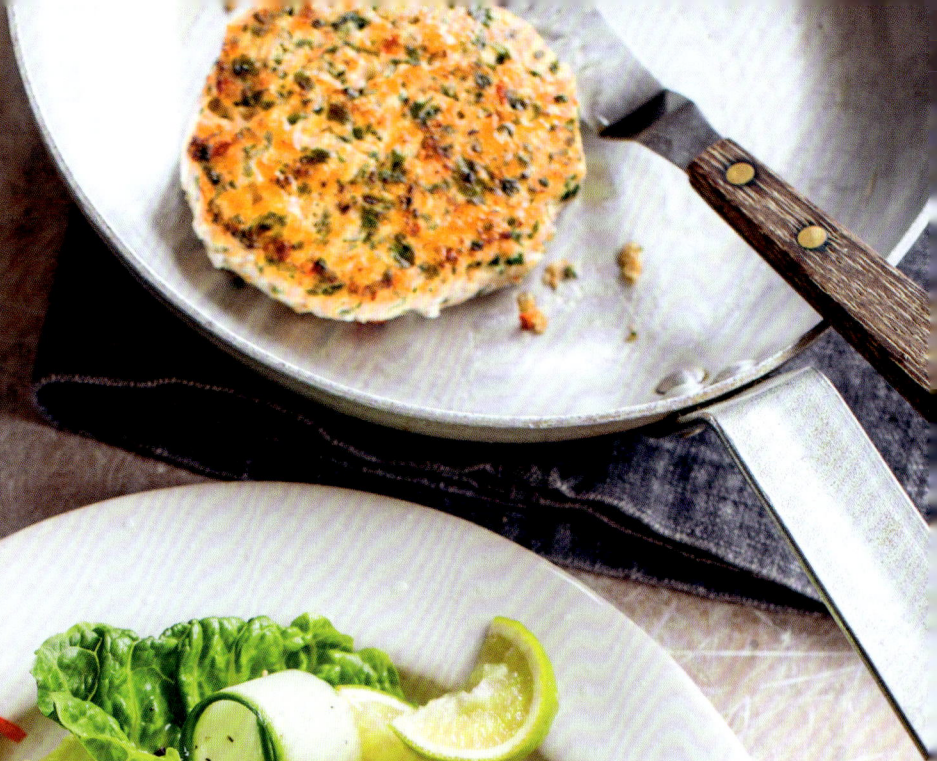

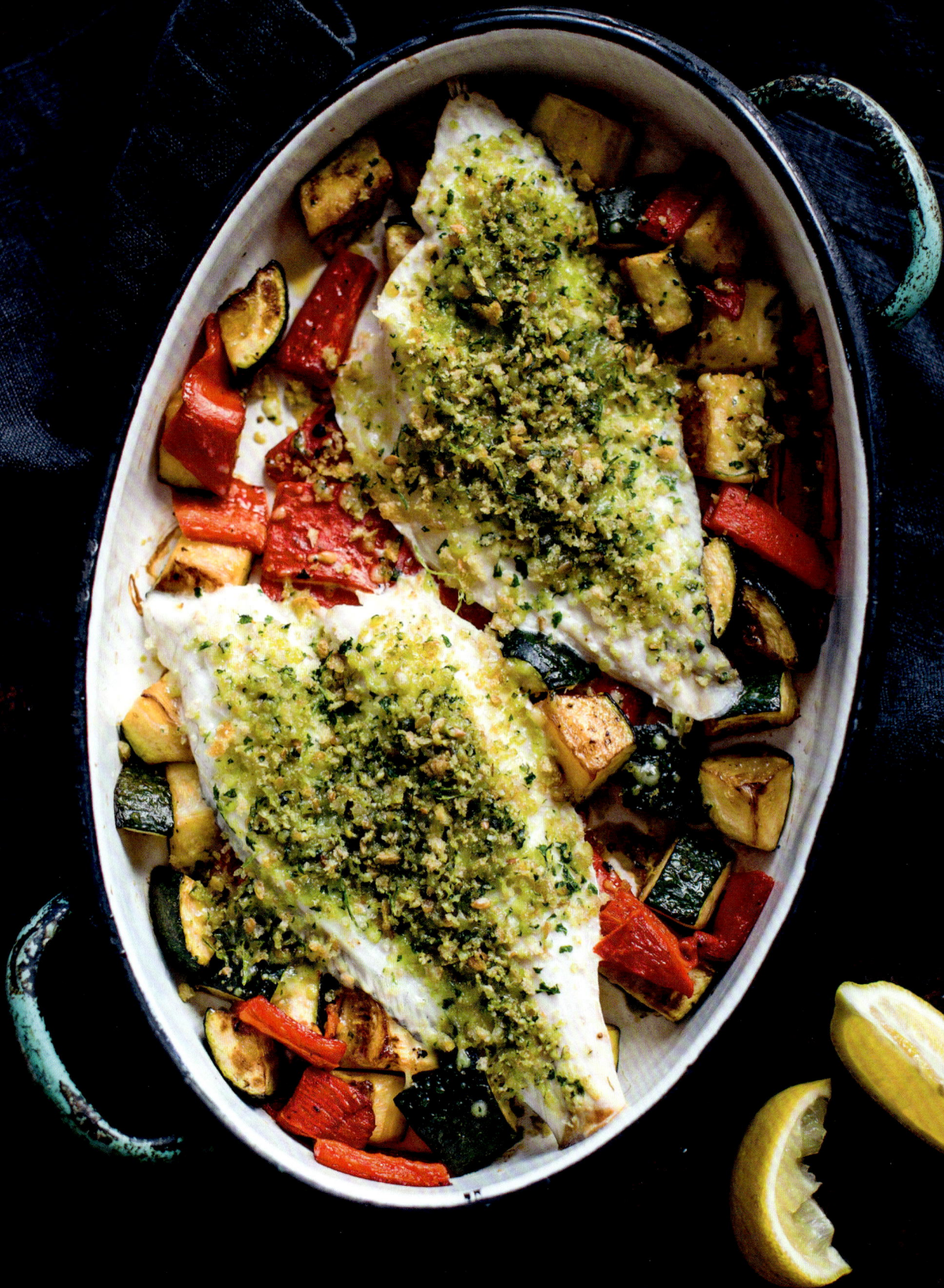

Roasted Fish with a Cheese and Parsley Crumb

SERVES 2

PREP 10 mins

COOK 27 mins

1 courgette, trimmed and cut into roughly 1.5cm chunks

120g roasted red peppers from a jar, drained and roughly sliced

2 tsp extra-virgin olive oil

20g wholegrain sourdough bread, blitzed into breadcrumbs

20g mature Cheddar, coarsely grated

few parsley sprigs, leaves finely chopped

finely grated zest of ¼ lemon, plus extra lemon wedges, to serve

2 sea bream or sea bass fillets (each around 90g)

COOK'S TIP
We keep sliced sourdough in the freezer, so we can turn it into toast or crumbs any time.

This is a simple way to cook fish and an easy introduction if it's not something you prepare often. If you don't have fresh parsley, use frozen, or finely sliced spring onions instead.

1. Preheat the oven to 200°C/Fan 180°C/Gas 6.

2. Place the courgette and roasted pepper in a small baking tray, drizzle over the oil, season with freshly ground black pepper and toss together lightly. Roast for 15 minutes.

3. Meanwhile, mix the breadcrumbs, cheese, parsley and lemon zest together in a small bowl to make the topping. Season with a little salt and lots of black pepper.

4. Remove the tray from the oven and turn the courgette and pepper pieces. Place the fish fillets on the vegetables, skin-side down, and sprinkle the breadcrumb mixture on top of the fish. Bake for about 12 minutes, or until the fish is cooked and the crumbs are lightly browned.

5. Serve with lots of green vegetables or a large mixed salad and extra lemon wedges for squeezing over.

AIR-FRYER TIP
Preheat the air fryer to 180°C, if needed. Prepare the vegetables and breadcrumb mixture as above. Air fry the vegetables for 12–14 minutes, then remove the air fryer basket, turn the roasted vegetables and place the fish on top. Sprinkle the breadcrumb mixture over the fish, and air fry for another 7–8 minutes until the fish is cooked and the crumbs are lightly browned.

NUT FREE

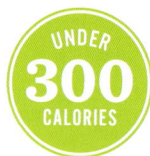

Prawn Courgetti and Spaghetti with Chilli and Lemon

SERVES	PREP	COOK
2	**10** mins	**12** mins

40g dried wholewheat
   spaghetti
1 large courgette, trimmed
   and spiralized or peeled
   into ribbons, or use a pack
   of courgetti
2 tbsp extra-virgin olive oil
200g cooked peeled prawns,
   defrosted if frozen
2 garlic cloves, crushed
   or finely grated
1–1½ tsp crushed dried
   chilli flakes
finely grated zest and juice
   of 1 small lemon

COOK'S TIP
You can use raw prawns
but you will need to cook them
for 1–2 minutes before adding
the chilli and garlic. They should
be hot and pink throughout
before tossing with the
spaghetti and courgetti.

Prawns, lemon and chilli are a winning combination. Here we have swapped in some courgetti, so you get the luxurious feel of pasta but with far fewer calories. Michael liked his spaghetti mixed with courgetti to add fibre, and he always served it with plenty of protein.

1. Half fill a large pan with water and bring to the boil. Add the pasta and cook according to the packet instructions. Stir in the courgetti for the last 15–20 seconds of the cooking time. Drain the pasta and courgetti in a colander and set aside.

2. Meanwhile, heat the oil in a large pan, add the prawns, garlic and chilli and fry over a medium heat for about 2 minutes, or until heated through, stirring regularly. Don't overcook the prawns or they will toughen.

3. Add the spaghetti and courgetti, lemon zest and juice to the pan, and toss together well. Season with salt and plenty of ground black pepper and serve in warmed bowls.

NUT FREE · DAIRY FREE

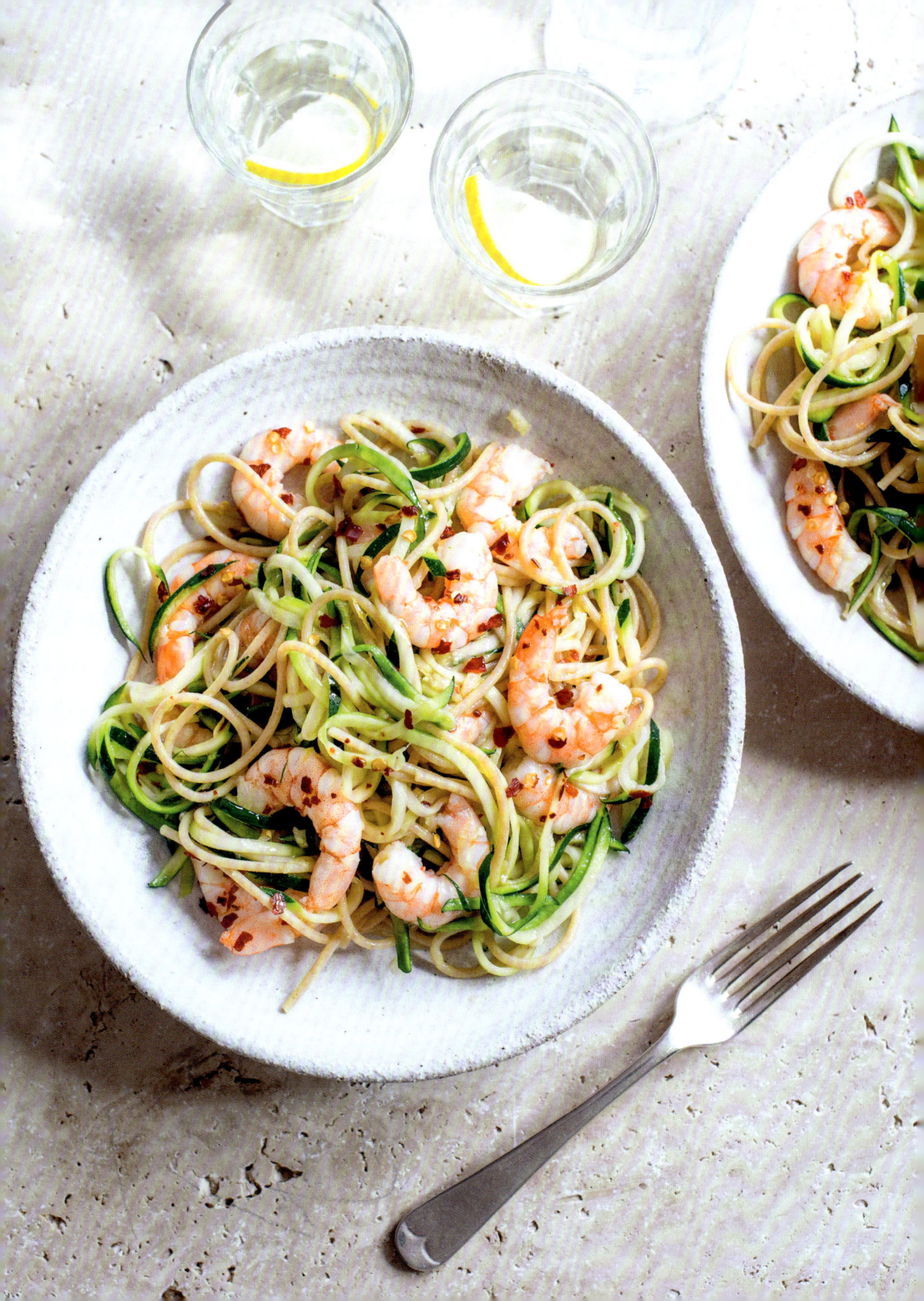

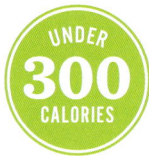

Tuna Provençal

SERVES **2** | PREP **5** mins | COOK **5** mins

2 tsp extra-virgin olive oil,
    plus 1 tbsp
2 × 115g fresh tuna steaks,
    defrosted if frozen
40g slow-roasted tomatoes
    (semi-dried) from a jar
    or tub, drained and
    roughly chopped
10 pitted black olives
    (around 30g), ideally
    kalamata, halved
1 tbsp fresh lemon juice
small handful roughly
    chopped parsley leaves,
    to serve (optional)

Fresh tuna steak is surprisingly filling and packed with protein. Here, we pan-fry it and serve it alongside a punchy tomato and olive sauce. Anyone not following the Fast 800 can add a small portion of new potatoes.

1. Heat the 2 teaspoons of oil in a frying pan over a medium heat. Season the tuna steaks on both sides with a little salt and plenty of freshly ground black pepper. Add them to the pan and cook for 2 minutes.

2. Turn the tuna and add the tomatoes, olives, the tablespoon of oil and the lemon juice to the pan. Cook for a further 1–2 minutes, or until the tuna is cooked to taste, crushing the tomatoes and olives together to make a loose sauce.

3. Divide the tuna between two plates and spoon the tomato and olive sauce over the top. Sprinkle with the parsley, if using, and serve with salad or freshly cooked green beans.

GLUTEN FREE | NUT FREE | DAIRY FREE

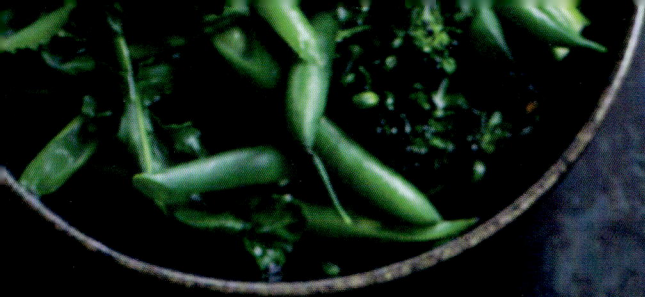

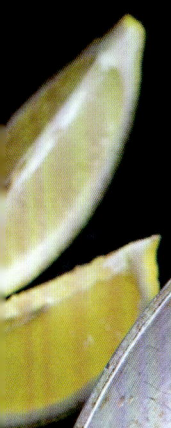

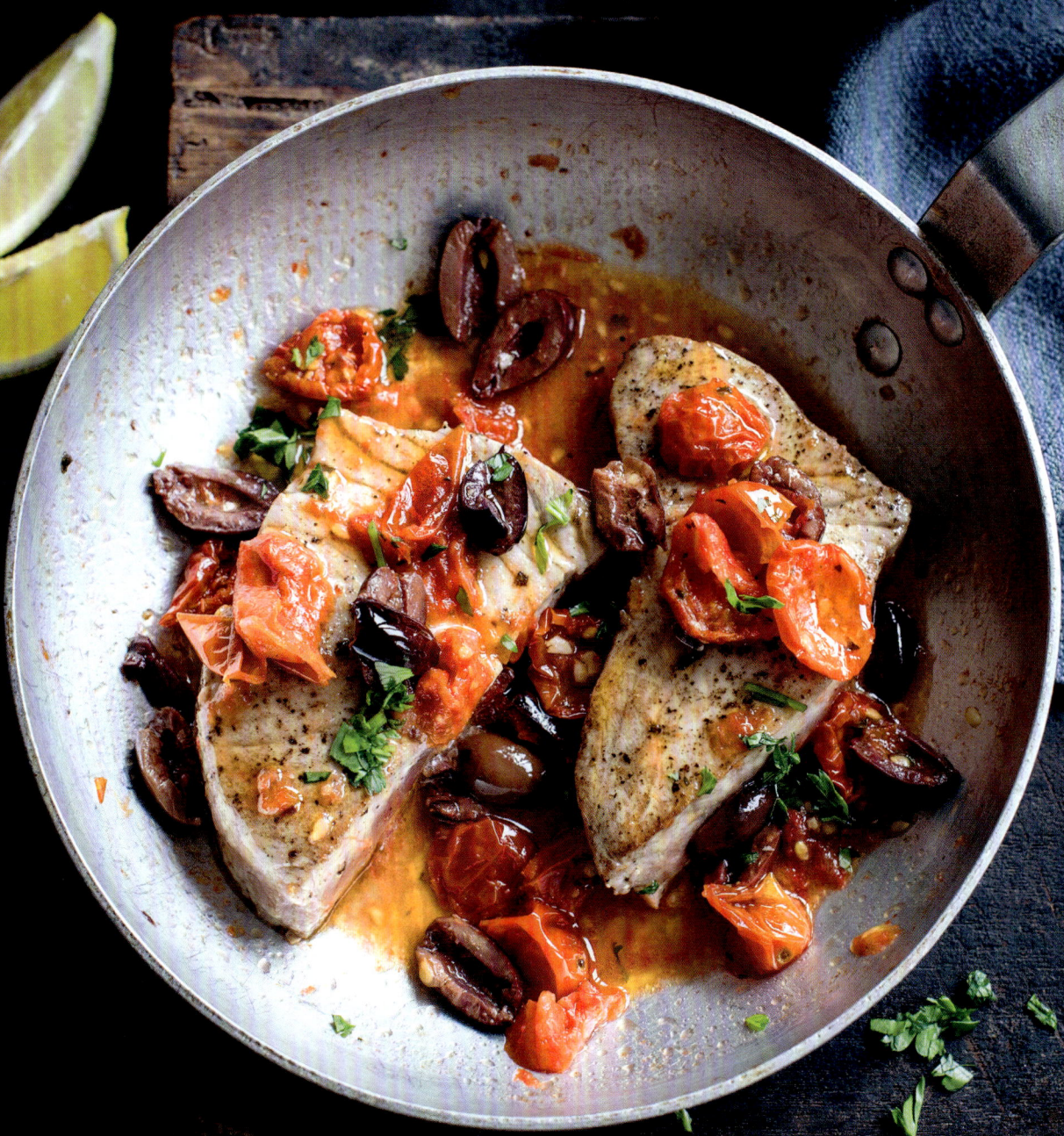

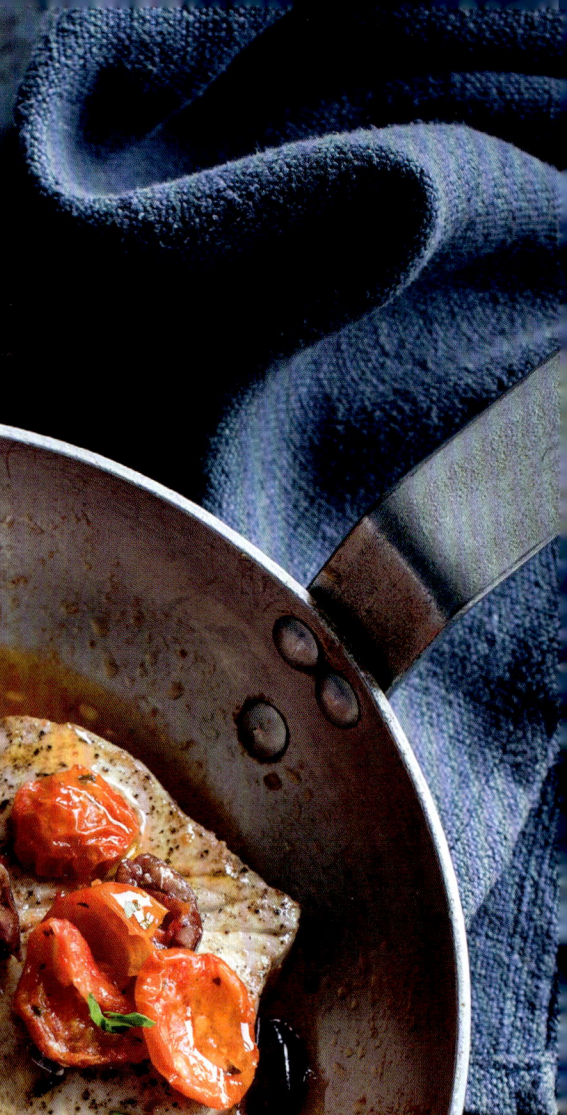

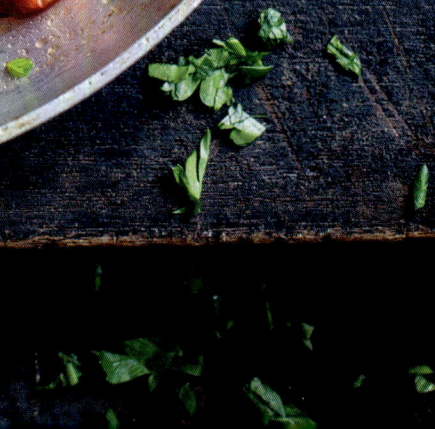

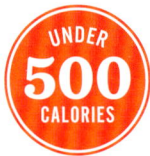

PER SERVING | **434cals** | PROTEIN **42g** | CARBS **29g**

Smoked Haddock with Lentils

SERVES | PREP | COOK
2 | **10** mins | **16** mins

2 tbsp olive oil
½ onion, finely chopped
1 celery stick, trimmed
   and finely sliced
1 carrot, trimmed, halved
   lengthways and sliced
   diagonally
1 rosemary sprig or
   ¼ tsp dried rosemary
1 garlic clove, very finely sliced
1 × 250g sachet ready-cooked
   puy lentils (or use canned)
200ml vegetable stock
   (made with ½ stock cube)
2 × 140g smoked haddock
   or cod fillets, skinned
   (see below)
small handful roughly
   chopped parsley
   leaves (optional)

NON-FAST DAYS
Top the fish with a poached egg
for an extra 78cals per serving,
or add 1–2 tablespoons of cooked
quinoa to the lentils just before
the end of the cooking time.

COOK'S TIP
To skin the fillet, place the
fish on a board, skin-side
down, and carefully work a
knife horizontally between
the skin and the fish using
a gentle sawing motion
until separated.

A simple one-pan dish where the slightly smoky,
salty flavour of the fish holds its own and enhances
the earthiness of the lentils. Serve with a large
portion of cooked leafy greens.

1. Heat the oil in a non-stick frying pan or wide-based
saucepan over a low heat. Add the onion, celery and carrot
and gently fry for 5 minutes, or until soft but not browned.

2. Add the rosemary and garlic and cook for a few seconds
more, stirring. Tip the lentils into the pan and add the stock.
Bring to a gentle simmer then place the fish fillets on top.
Season well with ground black pepper and sprinkle with
chopped parsley, if using.

3. Cover the pan with a lid (or a heatproof plate) and cook
the fish for about 8 minutes, or until just beginning to flake
when prodded with a knife.

4. Divide the lentils between two warmed plates or bowls,
and top with the fish.

GLUTEN FREE   NUT FREE   DAIRY FREE

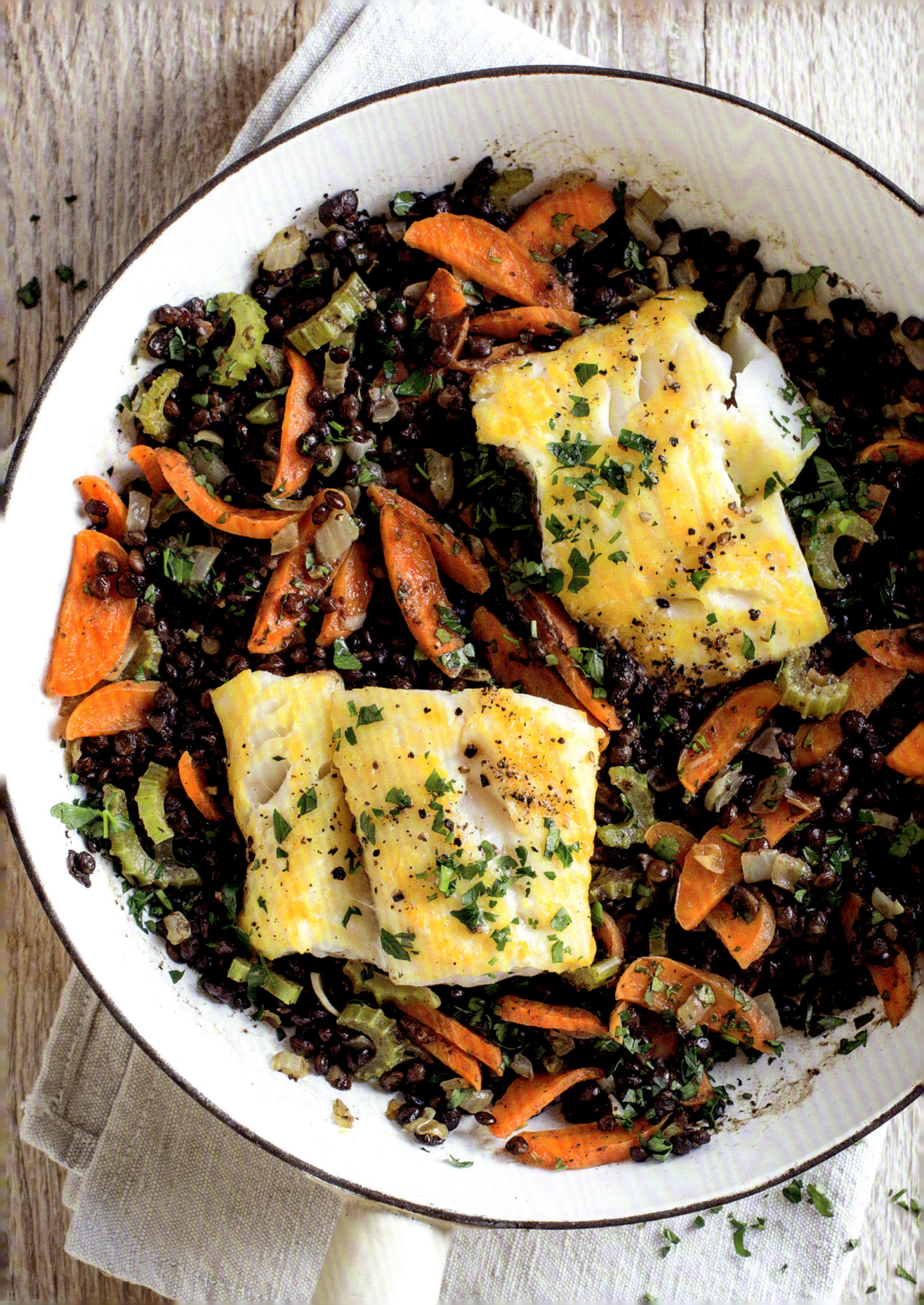

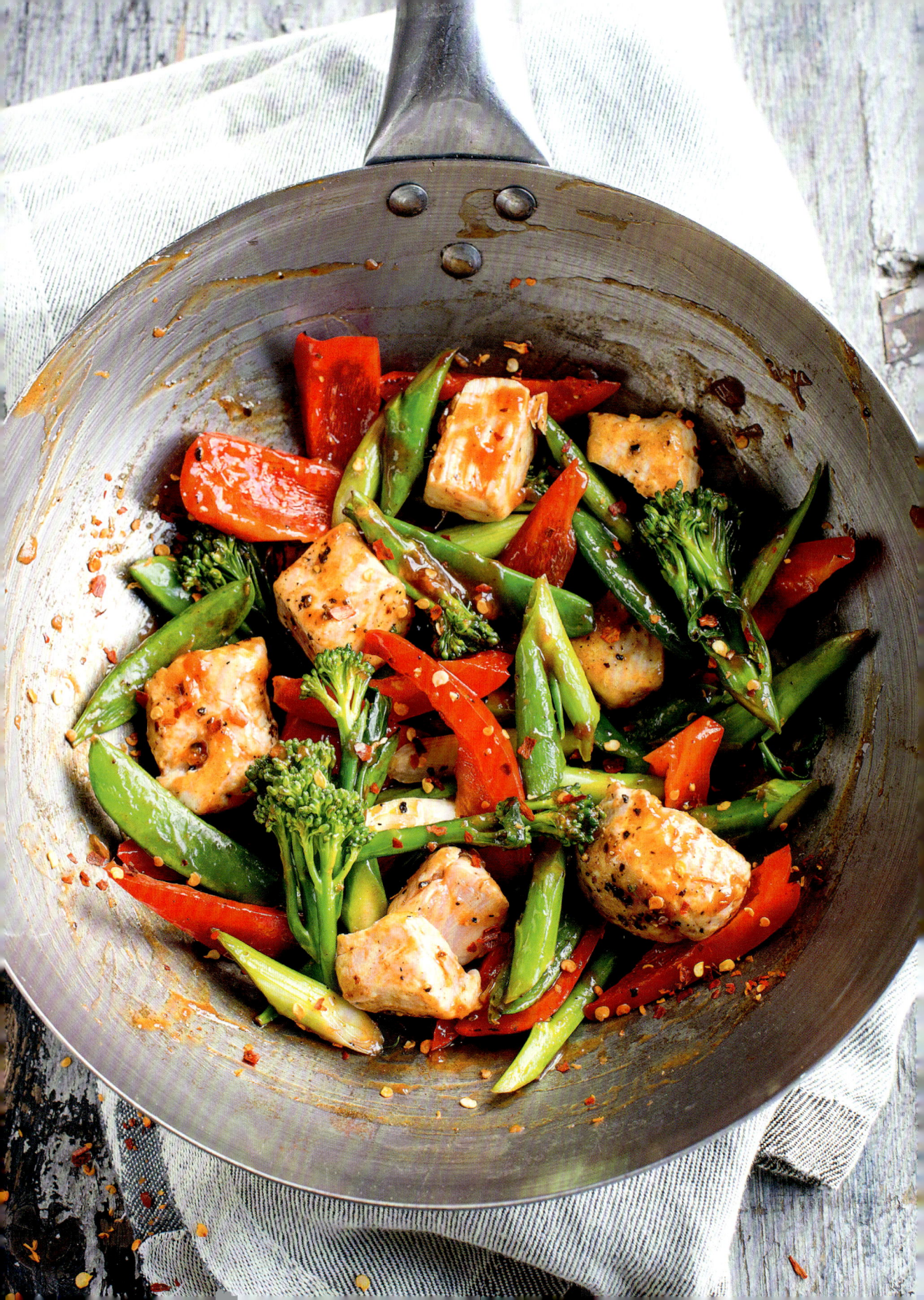

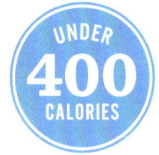

Stir-fry Tuna with Hoisin Sauce

SERVES | PREP | COOK
1 | **1** min | **5** mins

1 × 110g fresh tuna steak,
   cut into roughly 3cm chunks
1 tbsp coconut or rapeseed oil
1 × 300–350g pack stir-fry
   vegetables
2 tbsp hoisin sauce
pinch crushed dried chilli
   flakes (optional)

NON-FAST DAYS
Serve with a small portion of
wholewheat noodles or brown
rice. You could also add a few
tablespoons of defrosted
edamame beans at stage 2.

COOK'S TIP
Use any firm fish for this easy
dish – salmon and cod work
well. Prawns could be used,
as could thin strips of chicken
breast. You'll need to adjust
the calories if you make any
substitutions (tuna is 118cals).

This quick tuna dish is the perfect meal after a busy
day. Packs of ready-prepared stir-fry vegetables
save time and are easily available. Or make your
own combination with any fresh crispy vegetables.
And don't worry about the minor variations in the
calorie count of the stir-fried veg, just enjoy it!
Michael often made a good stir fry with plenty
of protein and extra chilli flakes.

1. Season the tuna with salt and freshly ground
black pepper.

2. Heat the oil in a large frying pan or wok over a
high heat. Add the tuna and vegetables and stir fry
for 3–4 minutes, or until the tuna is lightly browned.

3. Drizzle over the hoisin sauce and toss with the
fish and vegetables for 20–30 seconds.

4. Sprinkle with the chilli flakes, if using, and
serve immediately.

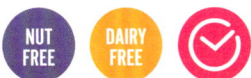

NUT FREE · DAIRY FREE

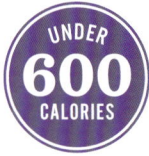

PER SERVING | **507cals** | PROTEIN **34.5g** | CARBS **2.5g**

Leek and Salmon Quiche in a Dish

SERVES
2

PREP
10
mins

COOK
30
mins

1 tbsp olive oil, plus
  extra for greasing
1 leek, trimmed and thinly
  sliced (around 100g
  prepared weight)
1 garlic clove, crushed
generous handful young
  spinach leaves
100g cooked salmon
  fillet, skinned
4 large free-range eggs
½ tbsp fresh thyme leaves
  or ½ tsp dried thyme
45g full-fat crème fraîche
15g Parmesan, grated

NON-FAST DAYS
Add a dressing to the salad,
if serving one alongside, and
serve with a few tablespoons
of cooked pearl barley or lentils.

COOK'S TIP
Use freshly snipped dill or
chopped parsley instead
of thyme, if you like.

Abandoning the pastry crust makes this quiche much lower in calories and carbs. Enjoy it warm with a large leaf salad or cold as a high-protein packed lunch.

1. Preheat the oven to 190°C/fan 170°C/Gas 5. Generously oil a small ovenproof baking dish, to hold around 900ml of liquid, or two small dishes (each around 450ml).

2. Heat the oil in a frying pan over a medium heat. Add the leek and fry gently for 3 minutes, or until softened but not browned, stirring. Add the garlic and spinach, and cook for about 2 minutes, or until the spinach has wilted and softened, stirring constantly.

3. Transfer the leeks and spinach to a sieve and press out any excess liquid with the back of a spoon. Tip the veg into the oiled dish or divide between the dishes.

4. Flake the salmon into chunky pieces and add to the leeks and spinach, spreading loosely over the base of the dish.

5. Whisk the eggs, thyme and crème fraîche in a small bowl. Add 2 tablespoons of the Parmesan, season with salt and freshly ground black pepper and stir well.

6. Pour the egg mixture gently over the salmon and veg. Sprinkle with the remaining Parmesan and bake for about 25 minutes (15–20 minutes, if using two dishes), or until slightly puffed up, golden brown and just set.

AIR-FRYER TIP
Preheat the air fryer to 170°C, if needed. Prepare the filling mixture as above, then pour into an oiled 18cm square baking dish (or 2 smaller dishes). Air fry for 18–20 minutes (13–16 minutes if using 2 dishes), or until golden and just set. Cover the dish with foil, if the quiche starts to brown too quickly.

GLUTEN FREE   NUT FREE

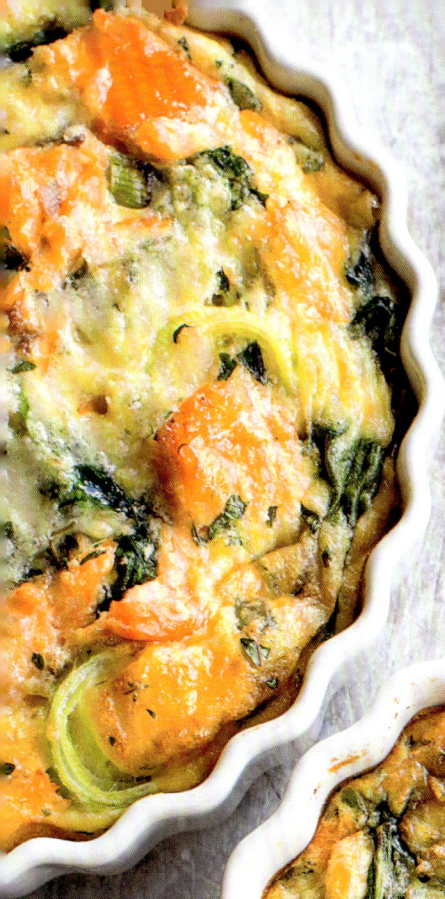

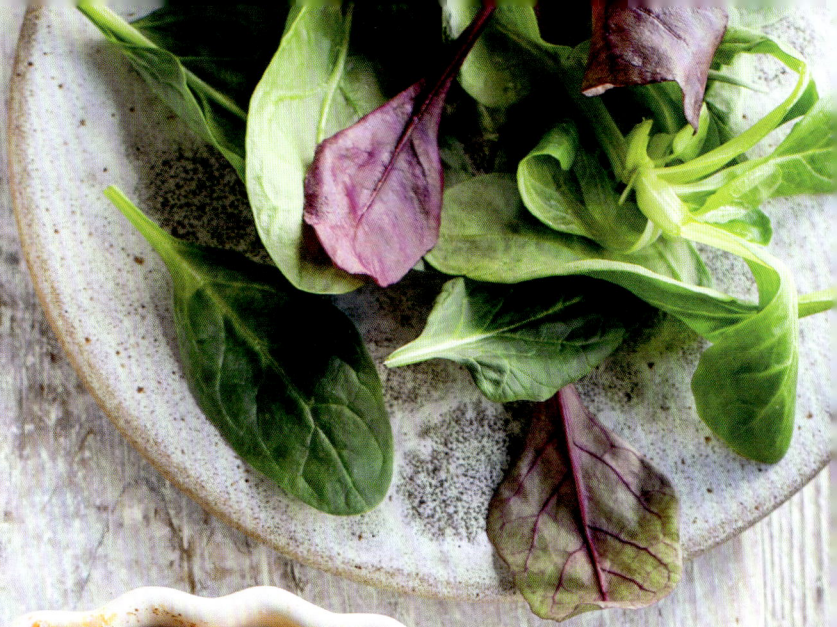

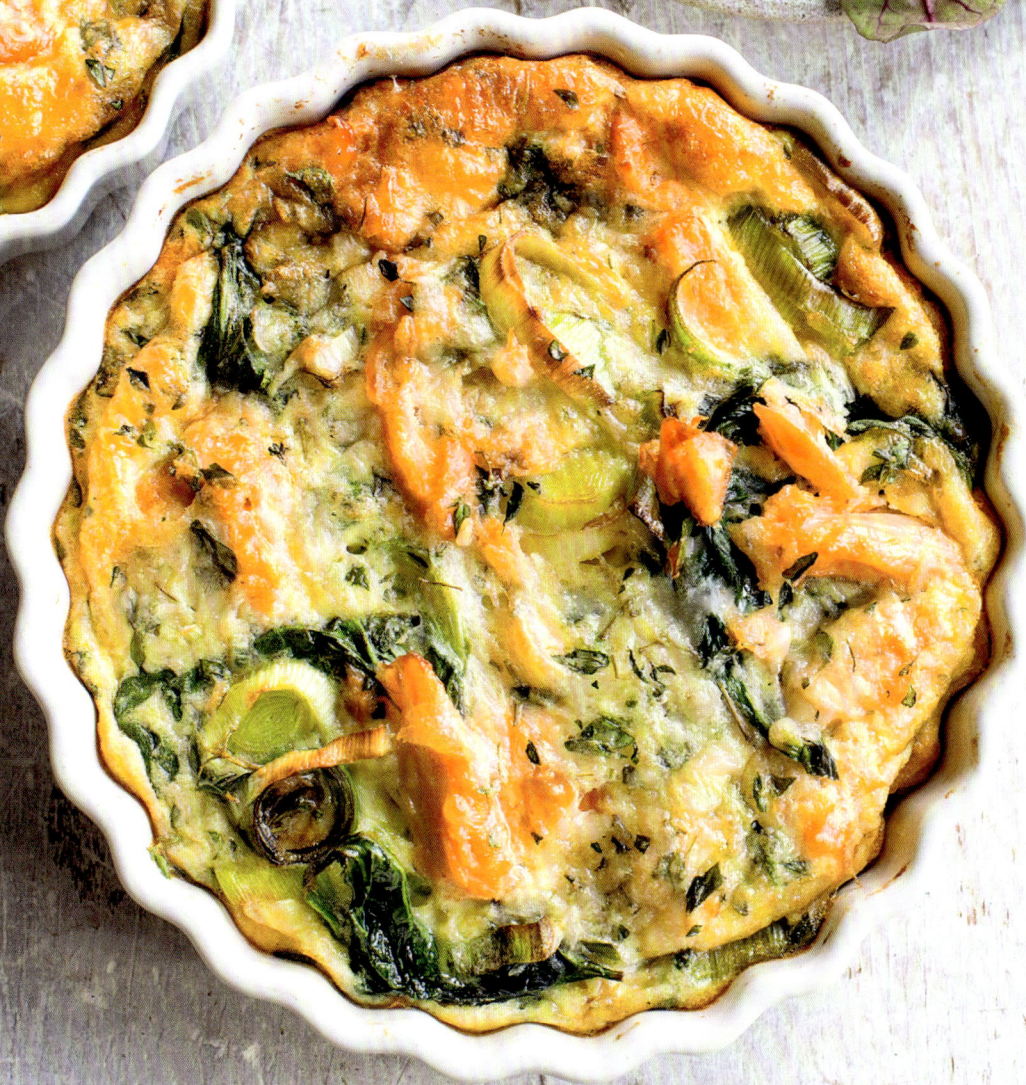

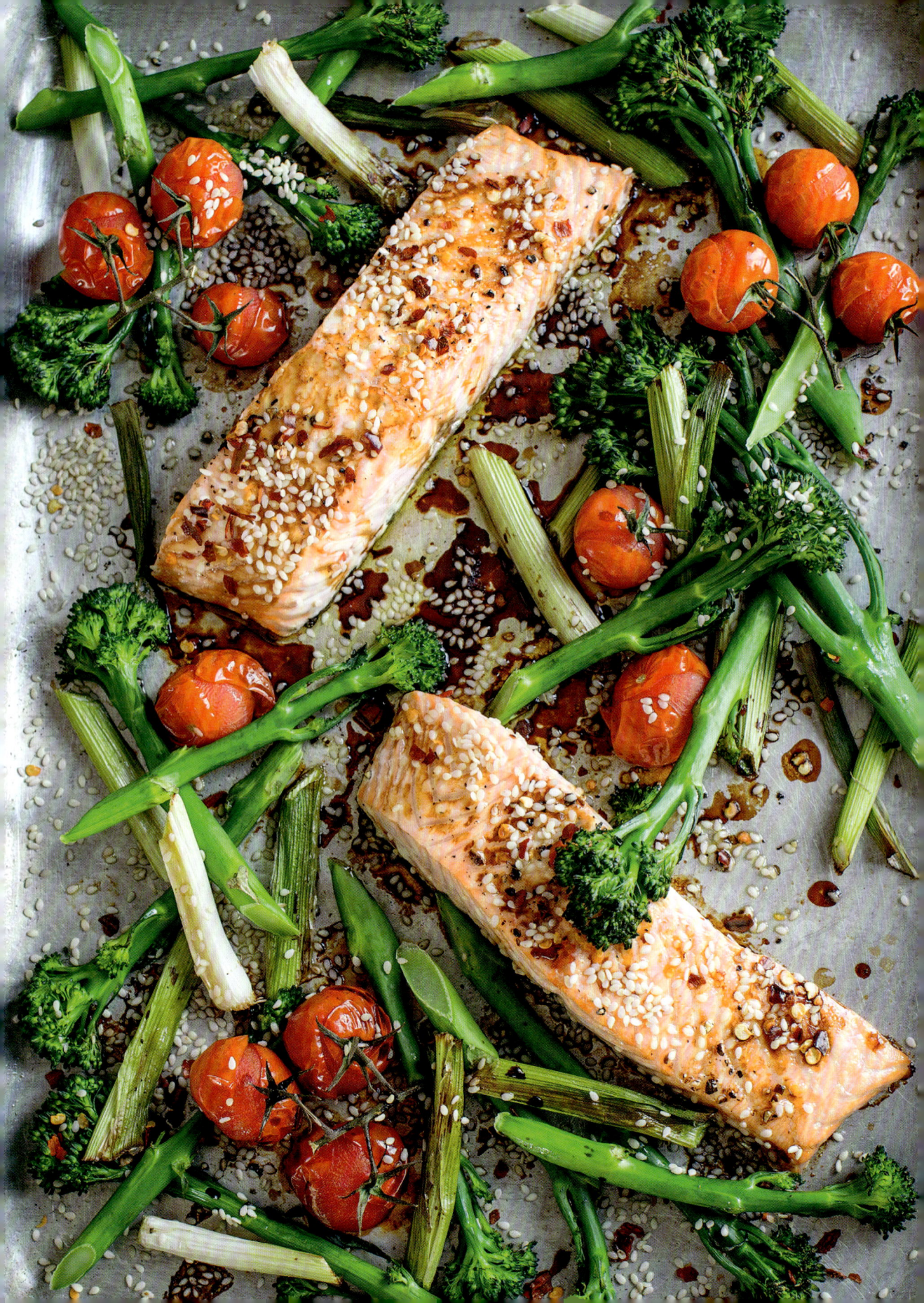

Sesame Salmon with Broccoli and Tomatoes

SERVES 2 | **PREP** 2 mins | **COOK** 12 mins

2 tsp olive or rapeseed oil
2 × 125g salmon fillets
6 spring onions, trimmed
    and each cut into 3 pieces
12 cherry tomatoes
200g long-stemmed
    broccoli, trimmed
1 tbsp dark soy sauce
1 tsp sesame oil
½ tsp crushed dried
    chilli flakes
1 tsp sesame seeds

NON-FAST DAYS
Serve with wholegrain noodles or brown rice. Or try pea, bean or lentil pasta for a delicious and gluten-free alternative. Soba noodles work well, too.

COOK'S TIP
You can see if the salmon is ready by prodding it with the side of a fork. It should flake into large pieces and look pale pink and opaque on the outside but slightly translucent in the middle.

This is wonderful served hot for supper or cold for lunch on the go. If you don't fancy salmon, any other chunky fish fillet will work well.

1. Preheat the oven to 200°C/Fan 180°C/Gas 6. Drizzle a baking tray with the oil.

2. Place the salmon fillets in the tray, skin-side down, add the spring onions and tomatoes and season with lots of freshly ground black pepper. Bake for 8 minutes.

3. Meanwhile, third fill a pan with water and bring to the boil. Add the broccoli and return to the boil. Cook for 4 minutes, then drain.

4. Remove the tray from the oven and add the broccoli. Drizzle the soy sauce and sesame oil over the fish. Sprinkle everything with the chilli flakes and sesame seeds, and return to the oven for a final 3–4 minutes, or until the salmon is just cooked.

5. Divide between two warmed plates and serve.

AIR-FRYER TIP

Preheat the air fryer to 180°C, if needed. Put the salmon and spring onions (not the tomatoes) on an oiled tray. Season with pepper and air fry for 6 minutes. Turn the spring onions, add the tomatoes and blanched broccoli as Step 4. Drizzle the soy sauce and sesame oil over the fish. Sprinkle everything with chilli flakes and sesame seeds and air fry for another 2 minutes, or until the salmon is just cooked.

GLUTEN FREE · NUT FREE · DAIRY FREE

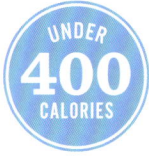

PER SERVING | **381cals** | PROTEIN **27g** | CARBS **4g**

Mussels with Creamy Tarragon Broth

SERVES	PREP	COOK
2	**20** mins	**12** mins

1kg fresh, live mussels
1 tbsp olive oil
1 leek, trimmed and thinly
  sliced (around 100g
  prepared weight)
2 garlic cloves, thinly sliced
100ml dry white wine
75g full-fat crème fraîche
3–4 sprigs of tarragon
  (around 5g), leaves
  roughly chopped,
  or 1 tsp dried tarragon

NON-FAST DAYS
Serve with celeriac chips
(see page 168) or a slice
of brown sourdough or
whole-grain bread.

COOK'S TIP
If you can't get hold
of tarragon, use freshly
chopped parsley or
dill instead.

Mussels make a fabulous, cheap, low-calorie yet high-protein meal. If you haven't cooked them before, don't be put off, they are incredibly easy and the quality of farmed mussels in the UK is superb. Keen on sustainability, Michael felt mussels were a juicy, affordable and flavourful option, delivering lots of protein.

1. Tip the mussels into the sink, scrub well under cold running water and remove the 'beards'. Discard any mussels with damaged shells or those that don't close immediately when tapped on the side of the sink. Put the good ones into a colander.

2. Heat the oil in a deep, lidded, wide-based saucepan or shallow flameproof casserole, over a low heat. Add the leek and garlic and fry very gently for 2–3 minutes, or until softened but not browned.

3. Add the white wine, crème fraîche and tarragon, and season generously with salt and freshly ground black pepper. Increase the heat under the pan and bring the wine to a simmer.

4. Stir in the mussels, cover tightly with a lid and cook for about 4 minutes, or until most of the mussels have steamed open. Stir well, then cover and cook for a further 1–2 minutes, or until the rest are open.

5. Divide the mussels between two bowls, removing any that haven't opened, and pour the tarragon broth over the top.

GLUTEN FREE   NUT FREE

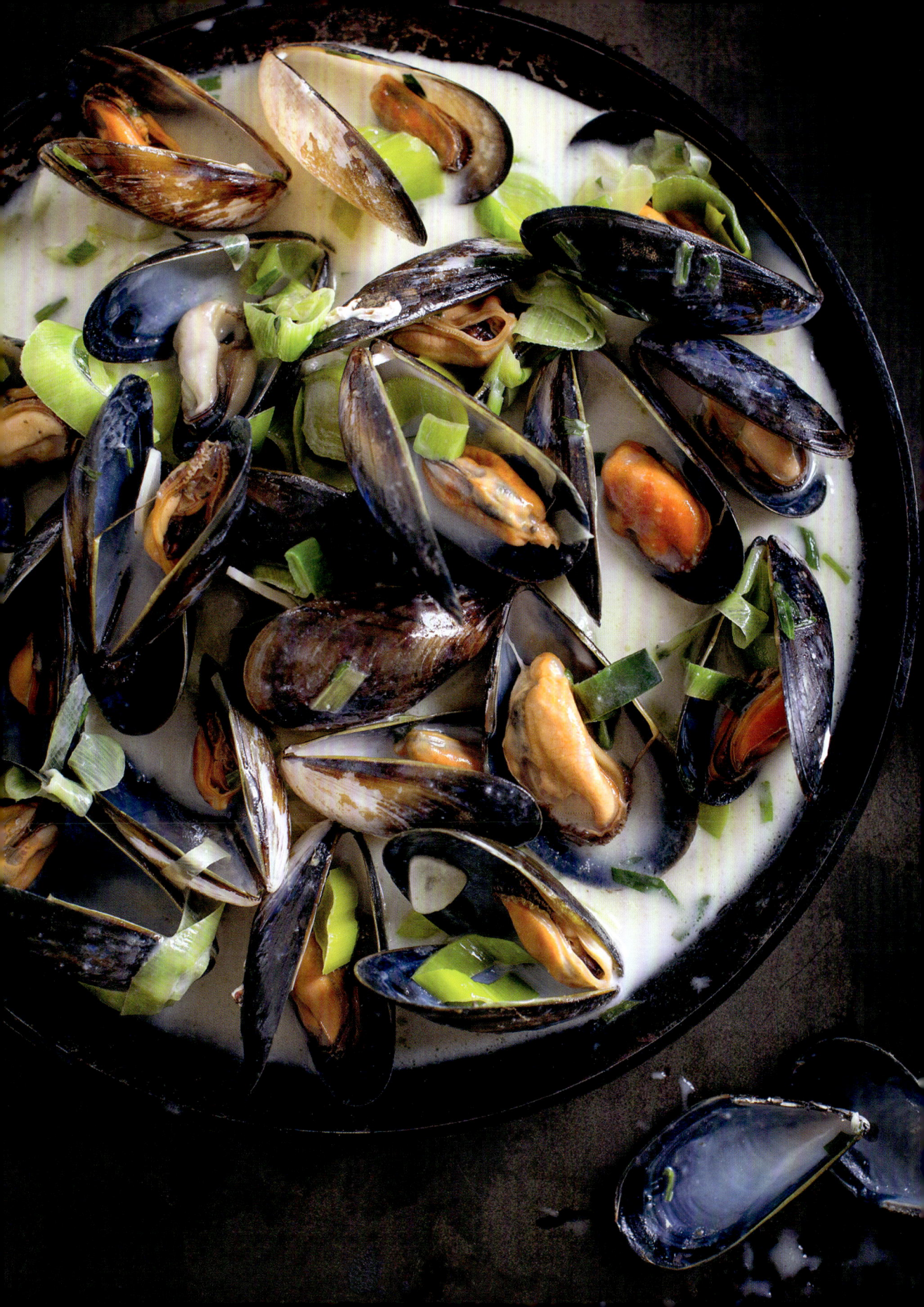

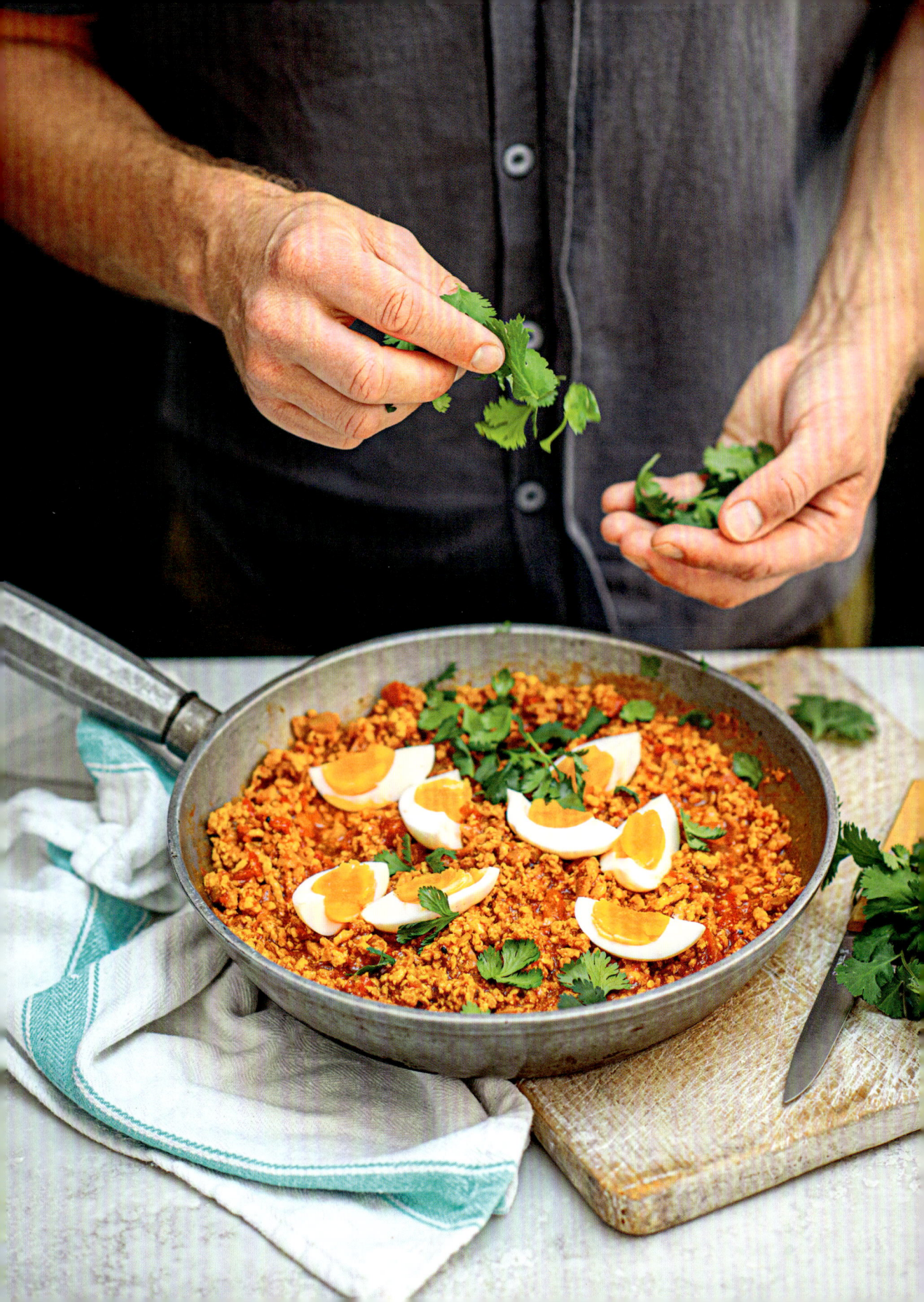

Chicken, Turkey
and Duck

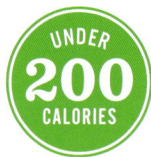

PER SERVING | **195cals** | PROTEIN **28g** | CARBS **7.5g**

Turkey Fajitas

SERVES	PREP	COOK
4	**10** mins	**8** mins

1 whole iceberg lettuce
1 tbsp olive or rapeseed oil
400g turkey breast steaks,
   cut into thin strips
1 red onion, cut into 12 wedges
2 peppers (1 red and 1 yellow),
   deseeded and thinly sliced
1 tsp hot smoked paprika
1 tsp ground cumin
1 tsp ground coriander
handful fresh coriander,
   leaves roughly chopped
100g full-fat live Greek yoghurt
lime wedges, to serve

NON-FAST DAYS
Top the turkey with guacamole
and grated cheese, and serve
in a small, good-quality
wholemeal wrap, if you like.

COOK'S TIP
Try to avoid the temptation
to use a fajita mix, as most
contain added sugars.

Turkey makes a fantastic alternative to chicken here and iceberg lettuce is the perfect carrier for this tasty Mexican-style filling. Let everyone help themselves at the table. When the family were around, Michael produced some scrumptious feasts.

1. Turn the lettuce over and cut around the stalk end with a small knife to separate the leaves. Carefully peel away at least eight leaves, wash and drain well. Place the leaves on a board or serving platter.

2. Heat the oil in a large frying pan over a medium heat. Add the turkey, onion and peppers and fry for 5–6 minutes, or until the turkey is cooked and the vegetables are softened and lightly browned, stirring regularly.

3. Add the spices and cook for 1–2 minutes, stirring. Season with salt and lots of freshly ground black pepper.

4. Take the pan to the table or transfer to a warmed dish and sprinkle with lots of coriander.

5. Pile the hot turkey into the leaves, top with yoghurt and serve with lime wedges for squeezing over.

GLUTEN FREE · NUT FREE

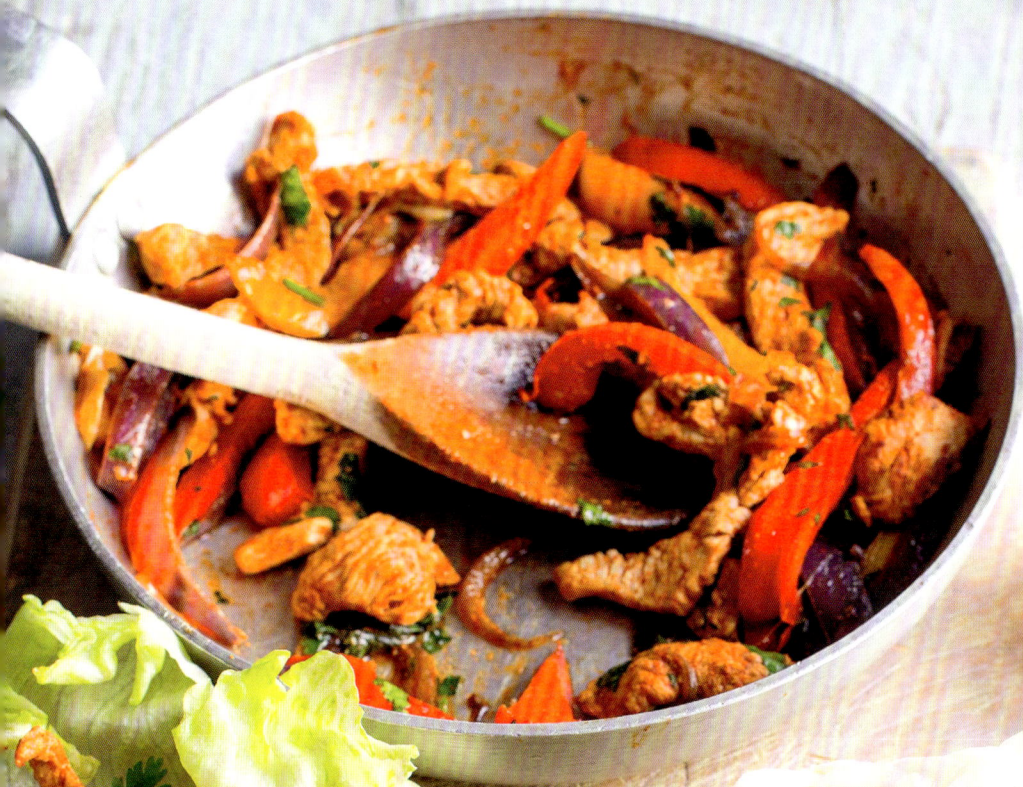

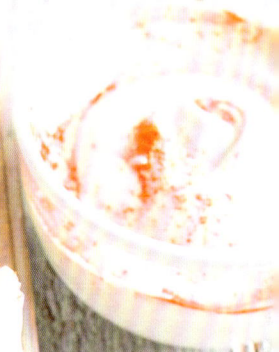

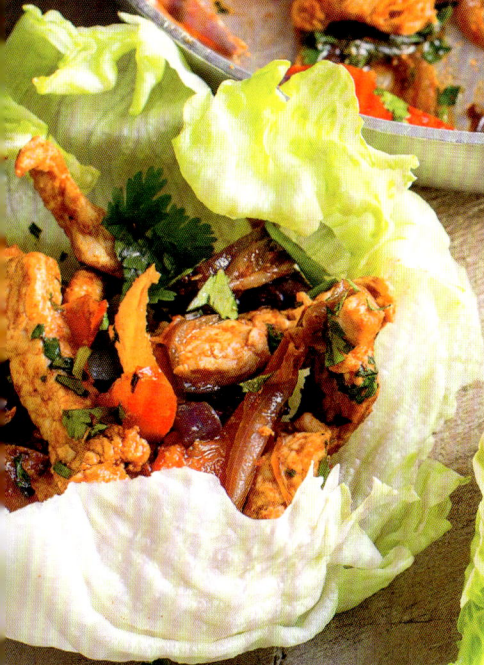

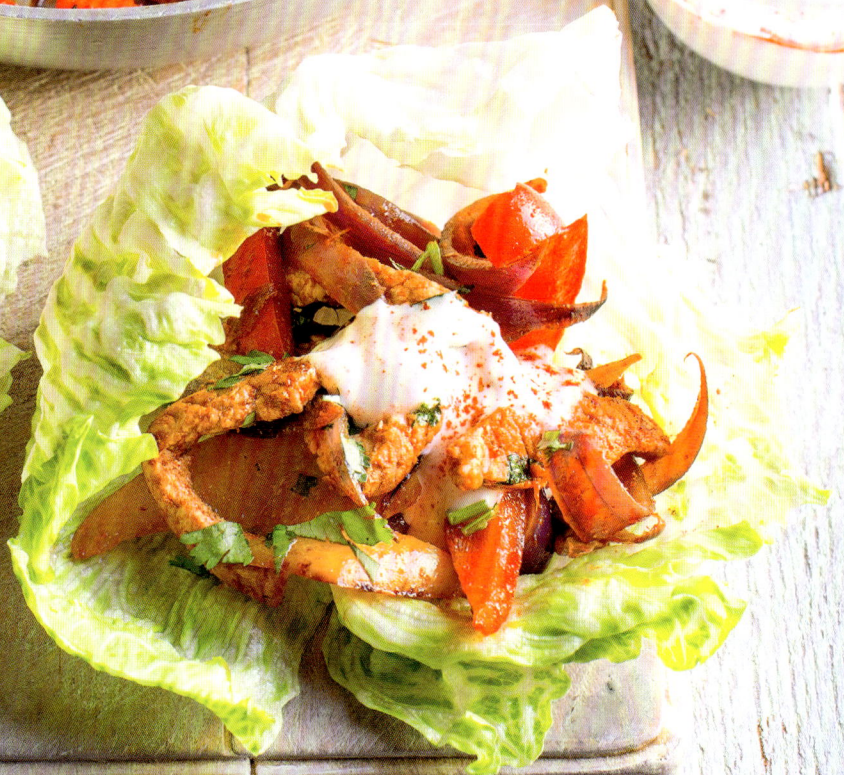

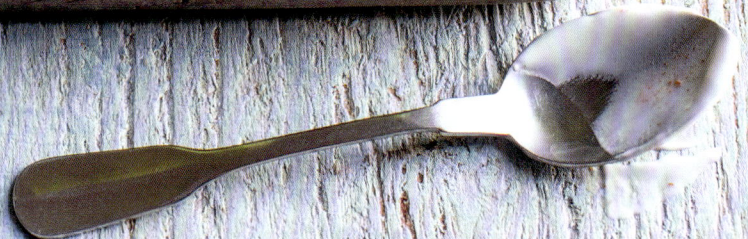

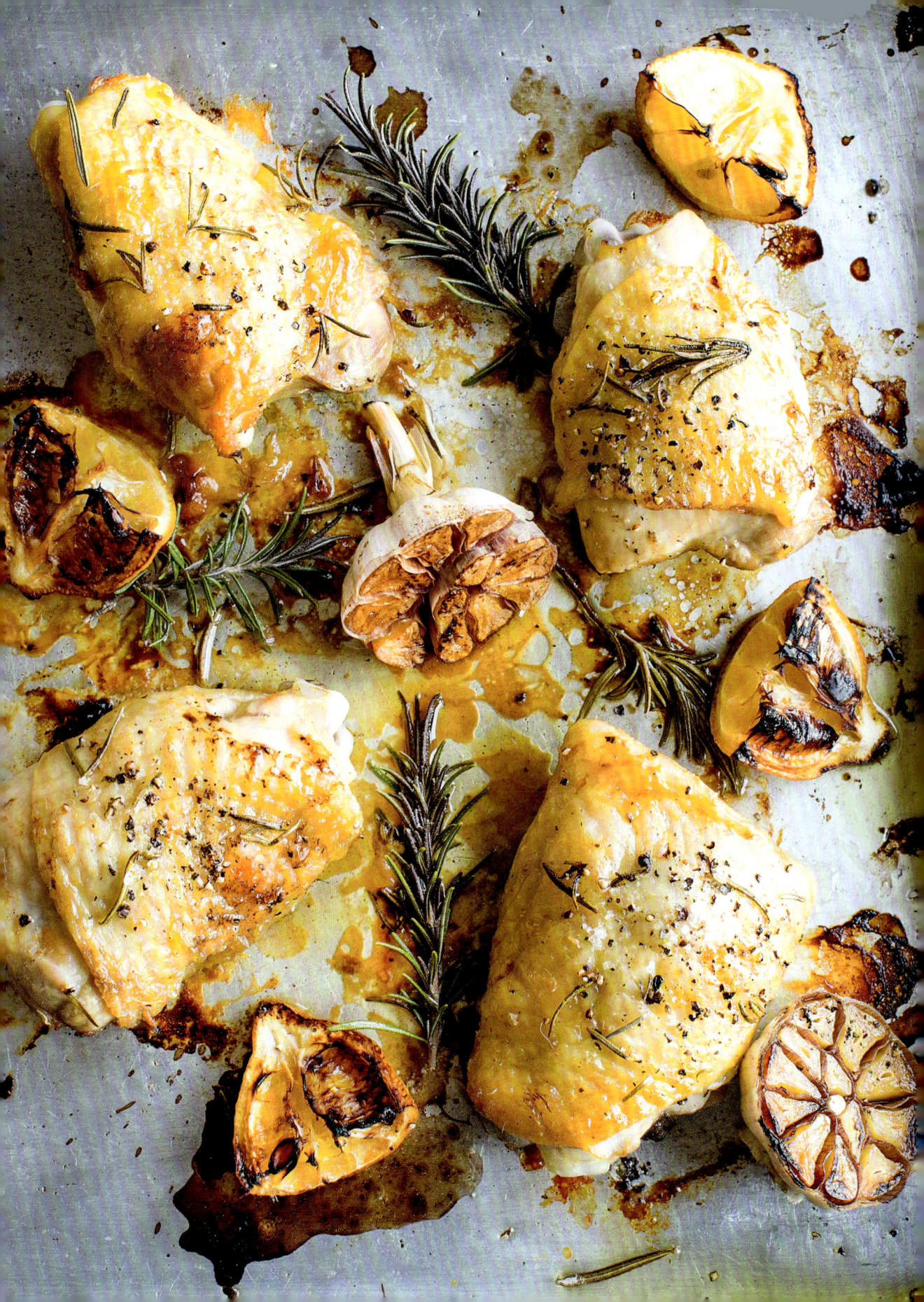

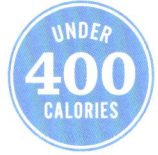

Roast Chicken Thighs with Lemon

SERVES **2** | **PREP** **5** mins | **COOK** **40** mins

4 bone-in chicken thighs
(each around 150g)
1–2 lemons, juice of 1
(around 2 tbsp), the other
quartered (optional)
1 tbsp olive oil
2 tbsp fresh thyme leaves
or 3–4 rosemary sprigs
(or use 1 tsp dried herbs)
1 bulb garlic, halved (optional)

NON-FAST DAYS
Serve with roasted butternut
squash and/or 3 tablespoons
of cooked quinoa or brown
or wild rice.

COOK'S TIP
If you remove the chicken
skin before eating, you will
save 25cals per serving.
Add extra herbs for garnish
about 10 minutes before
the end of the cooking
time, if you like.

This juicy, herb-infused chicken is perfect served
with a large green and coloured leaf salad, dressed
with a no-count dressing (see pages 88–9), or
a generous serving of freshly cooked vegetables.
It works brilliantly on the barbecue, too.

1. If cooking the chicken straight away, preheat the oven
to 200°C/Fan 180°C/Gas 6.

2. Put the chicken in a bowl with the lemon juice and oil.
Add the thyme or rosemary and season with salt and lots
of freshly ground black pepper. Toss well together. If you
have time, cover and leave to marinate in the fridge for
at least 1 hour and up to 4 hours.

3. Place the chicken, skin-side up, in a roasting tin
with the herbs and quartered lemon, if using, and bake
for 15 minutes. Remove the tin from the oven, add the
garlic, if using, and cook for a further 20–25 minutes,
or until the chicken is lightly browned, tender and
cooked all the way through.

AIR-FRYER TIP

Prepare the chicken thighs as above. When ready
to cook, preheat the air fryer to 180°C, if needed.
Put the chicken, skin-side down, in the air fryer with
the herbs and lemon quarters, if using, and cook for
12 minutes. Turn the chicken, add the garlic, brushing
the cut-side with the juices in the pan. Air fry for
another 18 minutes, or until the chicken is lightly
browned and cooked through.

GLUTEN FREE | NUT FREE | DAIRY FREE

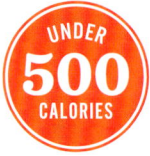

Easy Chicken Tagine

SERVES 2 | **PREP 5** mins | **COOK 54** mins

2 tbsp olive oil
1 onion, thinly sliced
3 boneless, skinless chicken thighs (around 300g), quartered
1½ tsp ground cumin
1½ tsp ground coriander
¼ tsp ground cinnamon
1 red pepper, deseeded and cut into roughly 3cm chunks
1 × 400g can chopped tomatoes
1 × 210g can chickpeas, drained (around 130g drained weight)
4 dried apricots (around 25g), roughly chopped
1 chicken stock cube
handful coriander or parsley leaves, to serve

NON-FAST DAYS
Increase the portion size and serve with 3 tablespoons of quinoa or bulgur wheat.

COOK'S TIP
For a more fiery taste, add 1 tablespoon harissa paste with the tomatoes. For a meat-free version, omit the chicken, which is 163cals per serving, use a veggie stock cube and add 200g cubed butternut squash instead.

A filling Moroccan-inspired casserole with lovely fibre-rich chickpeas. Don't be put off by the number of ingredients – once the chicken is browned, it's a throw-it-all-in-the-oven number. You could use a Moroccan-flavoured spice blend from the supermarket, or a paste from a jar for simplicity, if preferred. It was dishes such as this, where I discreetly slip in a tin of lentils, that helped Michael change his tastes and come to embrace beans and lentils – so full of much-needed fibre and protein.

1. Preheat the oven to 200°C/Fan 180°C/Gas 6.

2. Place the oil in a flameproof casserole over a medium heat. Add the onion and chicken and fry gently for 6–8 minutes, or until the onion is lightly browned, stirring regularly.

3. Sprinkle in all the spices and cook for a few seconds, stirring.

4. Add the pepper, tomatoes, chickpeas, apricots and crumbled stock cube. Pour in 250ml water, season with salt and plenty of freshly ground black pepper, and bring to a simmer. Cover with a lid and cook in the oven for 45 minutes, or until the chicken is tender and the sauce has thickened.

5. Sprinkle with coriander or parsley to serve with a large portion of green beans or a generous leafy salad.

GLUTEN FREE · NUT FREE · DAIRY FREE

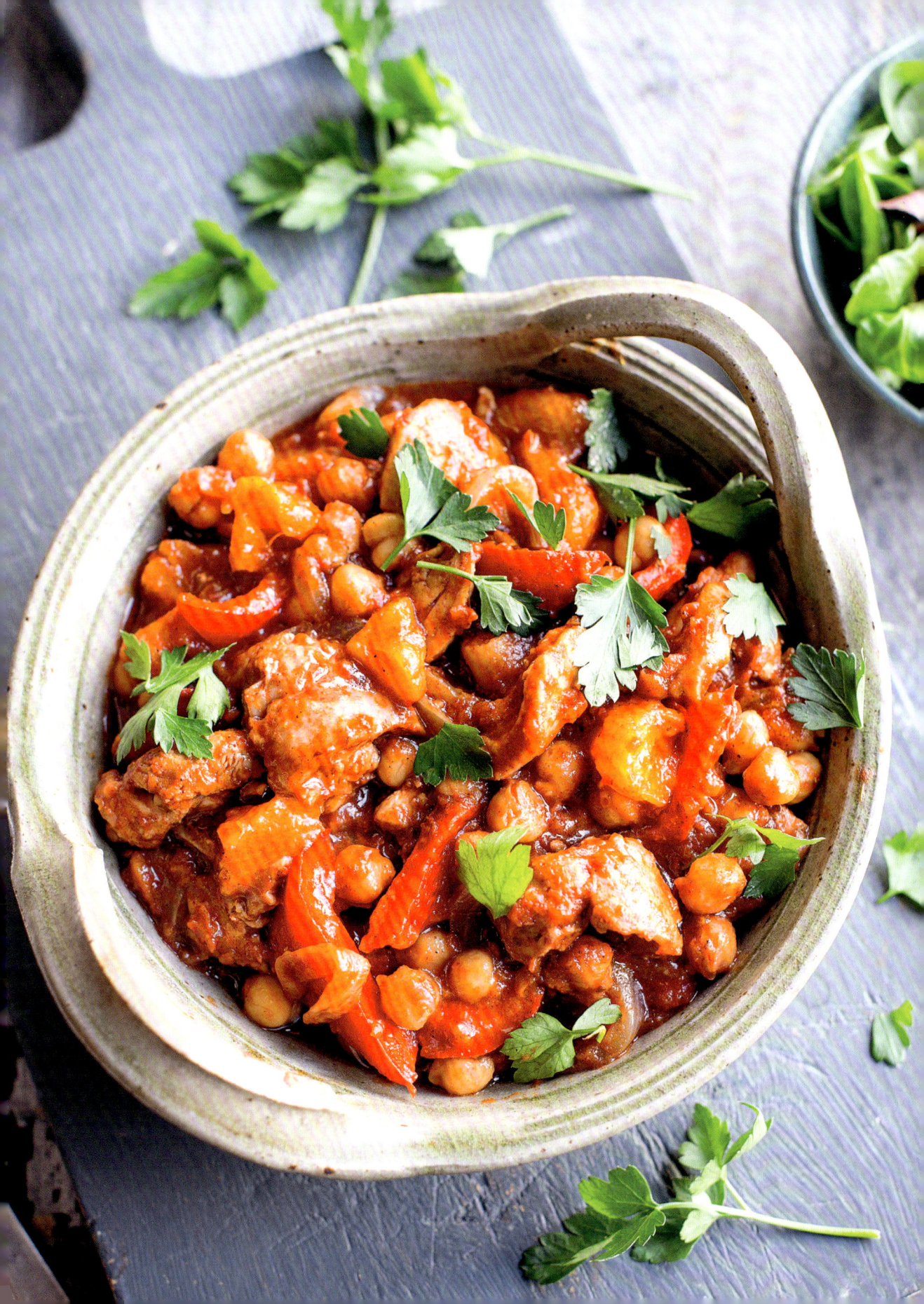

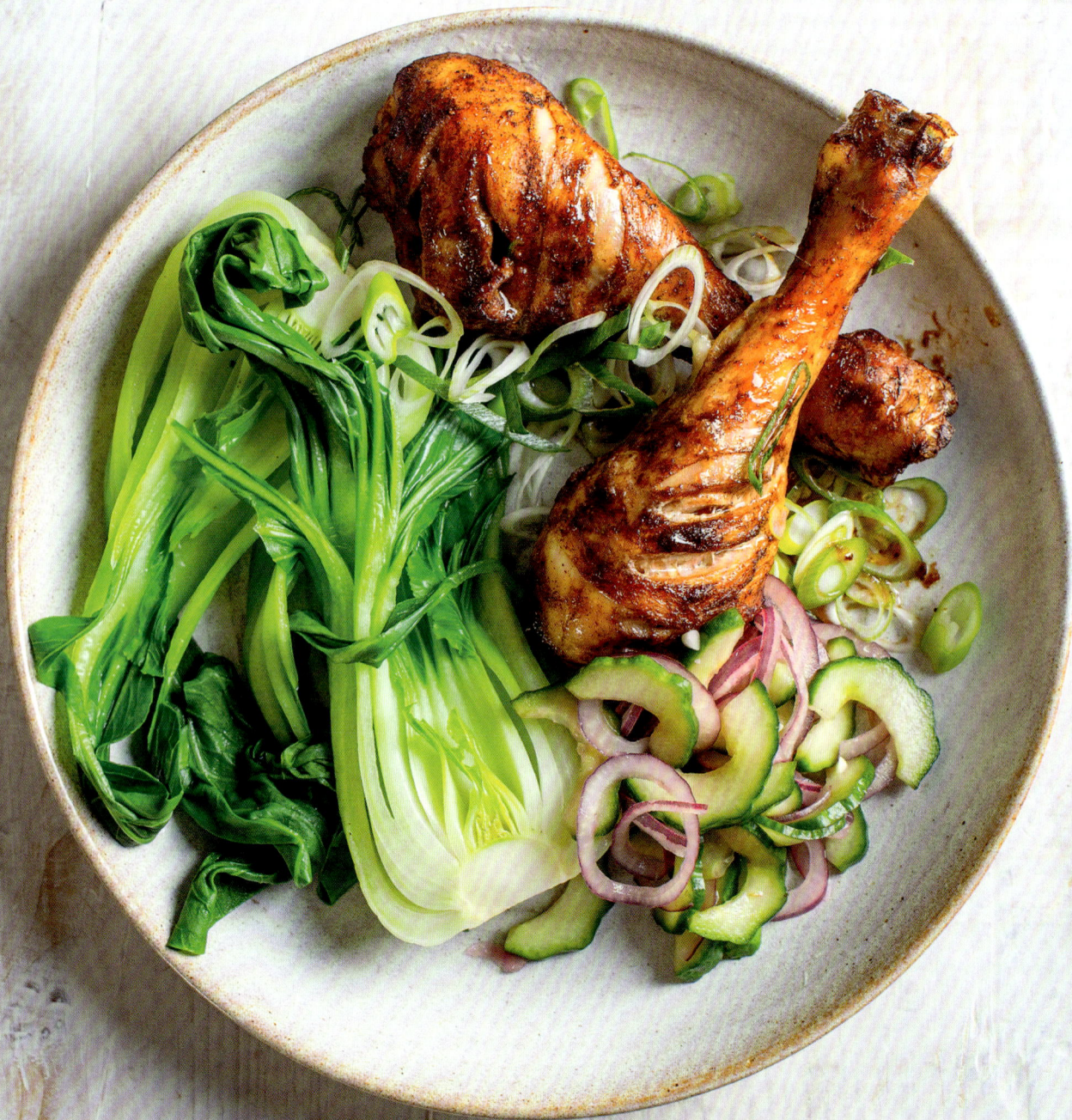

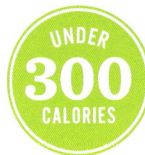

Chinese-style Drumsticks

SERVES
4

PREP
30
mins

COOK
35
mins

2 tsp Chinese five spice powder
4 tbsp dark soy sauce
2 tsp sesame oil
2 garlic cloves, finely grated
8 chicken drumsticks
2 spring onions, trimmed
    and finely sliced (optional)

NON-FAST DAYS
Enjoy with 3 tablespoons
of brown rice or quinoa.

COOK'S TIP
Make quick pickled cucumber
to serve with the drumsticks
by mixing half a very thinly
sliced small red onion with
half a deseeded and thinly
sliced cucumber. Top with
1½ tablespoons apple cider
vinegar and season with a
generous pinch of salt. Leave
to stand for 30 minutes.

These can be oven-baked but are great for cooking
on the barbecue, too. Serve with steamed pak choi
or spring greens, or a large mixed salad.

1. Put the five spice, soy sauce, sesame oil and garlic
in a large bowl and mix thoroughly. Slash each chicken
drumstick through the thickest part 2–3 times and add
to the marinade. Mix well, then cover and leave in the
fridge to marinate for at least 30 minutes, or ideally
several hours, turning occasionally.

2. Preheat the oven to 220°C/Fan 200°C/Gas 7.
Line a large baking tray with foil.

3. Place the drumsticks on the prepared tray, reserving
any marinade left in the bowl, and bake for 20 minutes.

4. Remove from the oven, brush the chicken generously
with the remaining marinade and return to the oven for
a further 10–15 minutes, or until the chicken is golden
and cooked through.

5. Garnish with spring onions, if using, to serve.

AIR-FRYER TIP
Prepare the spice mix and chicken as above. When ready
to cook, preheat the air fryer to 190°C, if needed. Put the
chicken in the air fryer, brushing it with some of the
marinade (you may need to cook it in batches). Air fry
for 15 minutes, then turn the chicken and brush with
more of the marinade. Air fry for another 8–10 minutes
until golden and cooked through.

NUT FREE

DAIRY FREE

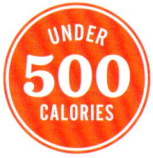

PER SERVING | **427cals** | PROTEIN **46g** | CARBS **11.5g**

Chicken Tikka Masala

SERVES	PREP	COOK
2	**65** mins	**20** mins

1 tbsp tikka curry paste
4 tbsp full-fat live
   Greek yoghurt
2 boneless, skinless chicken
   breasts (around 350g), cut
   into roughly 3cm chunks
1 tbsp coconut or rapeseed oil
handful coriander leaves,
   to serve (optional)
½ red chilli, sliced, to serve
   (optional)

For the masala sauce
1 tbsp coconut or rapeseed oil
1 onion, finely chopped
2 garlic cloves, finely grated
15g fresh root ginger,
   peeled and finely grated
2 tbsp tikka curry paste
1 tbsp tomato purée

NON-FAST DAYS
Serve with 2–3 heaped
tablespoons of brown
rice or a wholemeal roti.

COOK'S TIP
If you don't have a stick blender,
you can leave out the blitzing
but the sauce won't be as
smooth and creamy.

A healthy version of a favourite curry, which is much better than a take-away. Choose a good-quality tikka curry paste. Michael loved a good, protein-rich curry and often served it with steamed greens or cauli-rice (see page 232).

1. To prepare the chicken, combine the curry paste, yoghurt and 2 generous pinches of salt in a bowl. Add the chicken and mix until well coated. Cover and leave to marinate in the fridge for at least 1 hour, preferably longer or even overnight.

2. Fifteen minutes before you are ready to serve, make the sauce. Place the oil in a large non-stick saucepan over a medium heat. Add the onion and fry gently for 5 minutes, or until softened, then stir in the garlic, ginger and curry paste and cook for 1½ minutes more. Pour 300ml water into the pan, stir in the tomato purée and bring to a simmer. Cook for 5 minutes, then remove the pan from the heat and use a stick blender to blitz the sauce. Set aside.

3. Heat the oil for the chicken in a large frying pan over a medium–high heat. Add the marinated chicken and fry for 3 minutes, or until lightly browned, turning regularly.

4. Stir the prepared sauce into the pan and bring to a simmer. Cook for 3–4 minutes, or until the chicken is cooked, stirring constantly. Add a splash of water, if the sauce thickens too much.

5. Sprinkle with coriander and chilli, if using, to serve.

GLUTEN FREE · NUT FREE

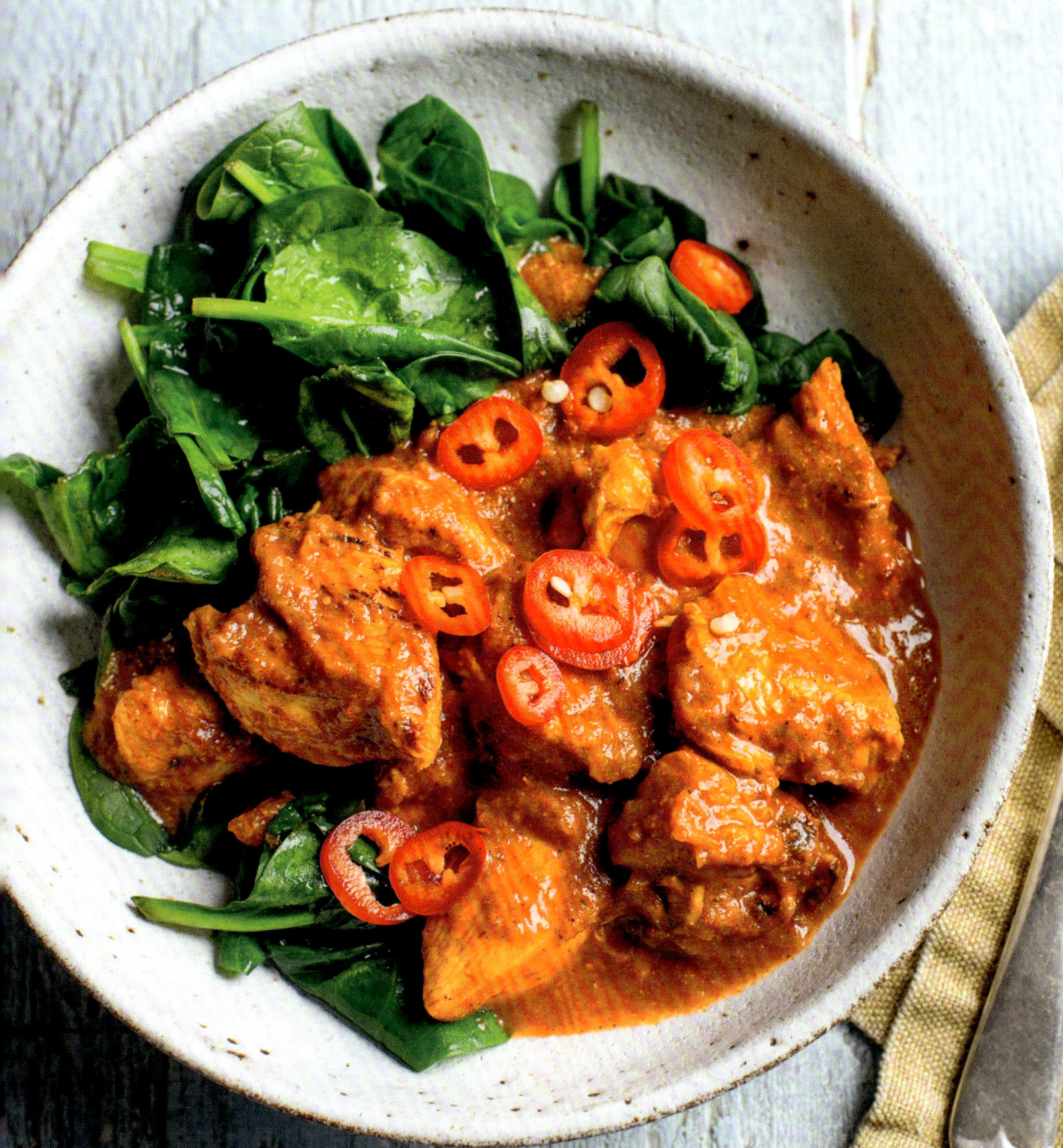

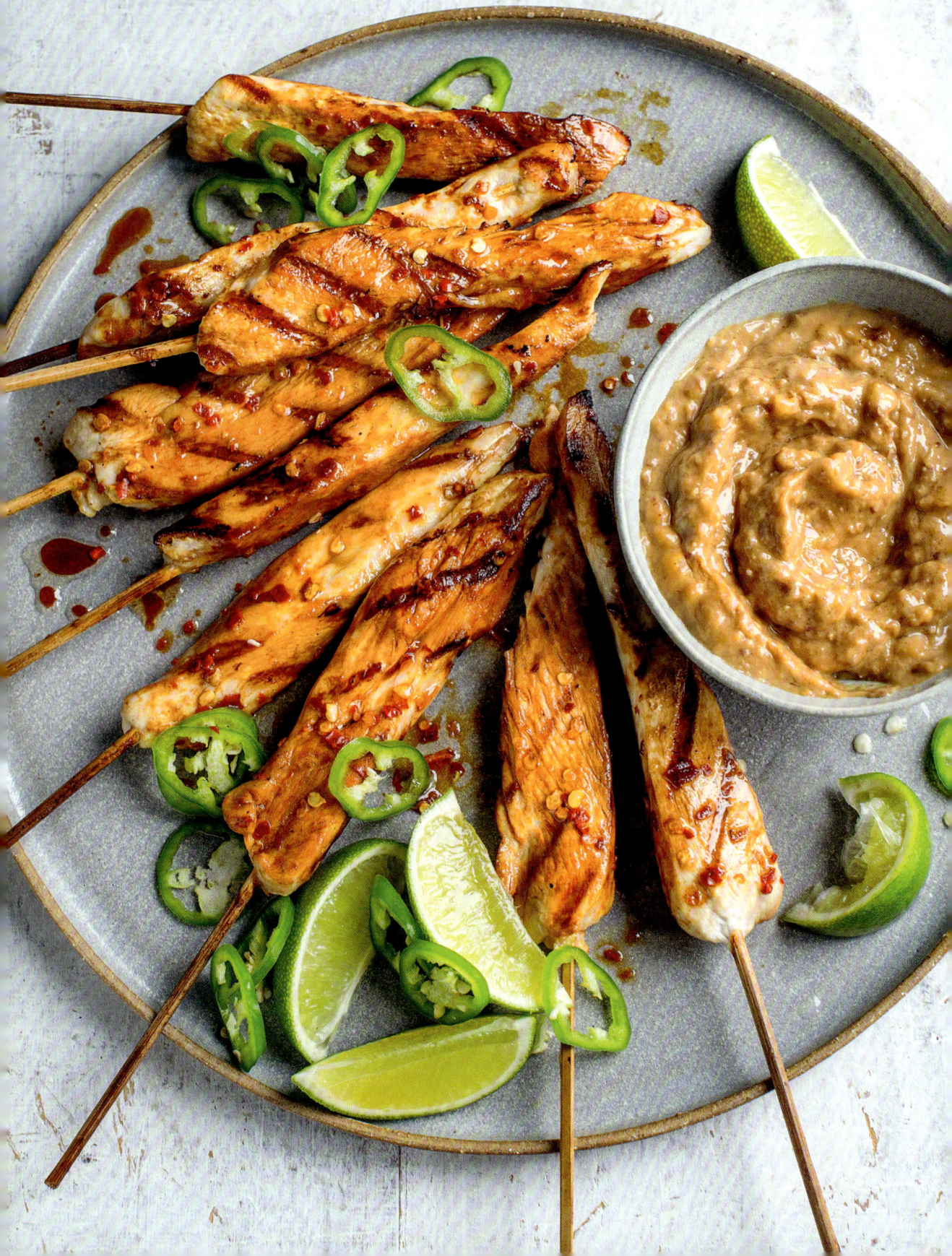

PER SERVING | **264cals** | PROTEIN **36g** | CARBS **3g**

UNDER 300 CALORIES

Satay Chicken

SERVES	PREP	COOK
4	**25** mins	**8** mins

1 tbsp coconut or rapeseed oil
juice of 1 lime (around 2 tbsp)
½ tsp crushed dried
    chilli flakes
2 tsp dark soy sauce
3 boneless, skinless chicken
    breasts (each around 175g),
    cut into 16 long, thin strips
lime wedges, to serve
1 green chilli, sliced, to serve
    (optional)

For the satay sauce
60g no-added-sugar
    crunchy peanut butter
    (around 4 tbsp)
1 tbsp dark soy sauce
15g fresh root ginger,
    peeled and finely grated

NON-FAST DAYS
Increase your portion size
and serve with 2–3 heaped
tablespoons of brown rice.

COOK'S TIP
Use metal skewers if
cooking on the barbecue
or under the grill.

Now that nuts are back on the menu, even on a fast day, you can enjoy this tasty and filling satay sauce as a dip or drizzled. We like cooking these on a ridged griddle, but you can also cook them on the barbecue or under the grill. They are delicious served cold and make a great portable meal. Michael used to woolf these down – rich in flavour and protein, and low in carbs.

1. You will need 16 × 20cm bamboo (soaked in water for 15 minutes) or metal skewers.

2. Melt the oil, if using coconut, in a small saucepan very gently, then pour into a bowl. Add the lime juice, chilli flakes, soy sauce and a good grinding of black pepper. Mix well. Add the chicken strips and toss everything together well to coat.

3. Thread the chicken strips on to the skewers. Work quickly as the lime juice will start 'cooking' the chicken. The coconut oil will also begin to solidify.

4. Place a large lightly greased griddle or frying pan over a medium–high heat and cook the chicken for 3–4 minutes on each side, depending on thickness, or until lightly browned and cooked through.

5. Meanwhile, to make the satay sauce, place the peanut butter in a small saucepan with around 4 tablespoons of water, the soy sauce and grated ginger. Heat gently, stirring constantly until the peanut butter softens and the mixture becomes glossy and thickened. Add a little more soy sauce or water to taste, if needed.

6. Serve the chicken with lime wedges, chilli, if using, and the warm sauce in individual dipping bowls or simply drizzled over.

DAIRY FREE

CHICKEN, TURKEY AND DUCK   133

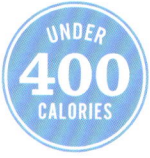

Pesto Chicken Traybake

SERVES **2** | **PREP** **15** mins | **COOK** **40** mins

1 red onion, cut into 10 wedges
2 peppers, any colour,
    deseeded and cut into
    roughly 3cm chunks
1 courgette, trimmed, halved
    lengthways and cut into
    roughly 2cm chunks
3 tsp extra-virgin olive oil
2 skinless chicken breast fillets
    (each around 150g)
2 tbsp sun-dried tomato pesto
½ tsp paprika, any kind
    (optional)

Delicious served hot or cold as a salad, this is a doddle to double up if you are feeding more. We use sun-dried tomato pesto but you could use green basil pesto instead, if you like.

1. Preheat the oven to 200°C/Fan 180°C/Gas 6.

2. Place the onion, peppers and courgette in a large roasting tin. Drizzle with 2 teaspoons of the oil, season with salt and freshly ground black pepper and toss together lightly to coat. Roast for 10 minutes.

3. Meanwhile, place the chicken breasts on a board and cut each one horizontally through the middle so they can be opened out like a book. Spread with the pesto, then close.

4. Remove the tray from the oven and turn all the veg. Nestle the chicken breasts among the vegetables, drizzle over the remaining oil and season with the paprika, if using, and a little salt and lots of pepper. Roast for 20–25 minutes, or until the chicken is cooked through and all the vegetables are tender and lightly browned.

5. Remove from the oven and serve with a crisp green salad or steamed leafy veg.

AIR-FRYER TIP

Preheat the air fryer to 180°C, if needed. Prepare the vegetables and chicken as above. Place the vegetables in the air fryer and cook for 8 minutes (you may need to cook them in two batches). Turn the vegetables (returning the first batch to the air fryer, if necessary) and add the chicken as instructed in Step 4. Air fry for another 16–18 minutes, turning the chicken halfway, until cooked through.

GLUTEN FREE   DAIRY FREE

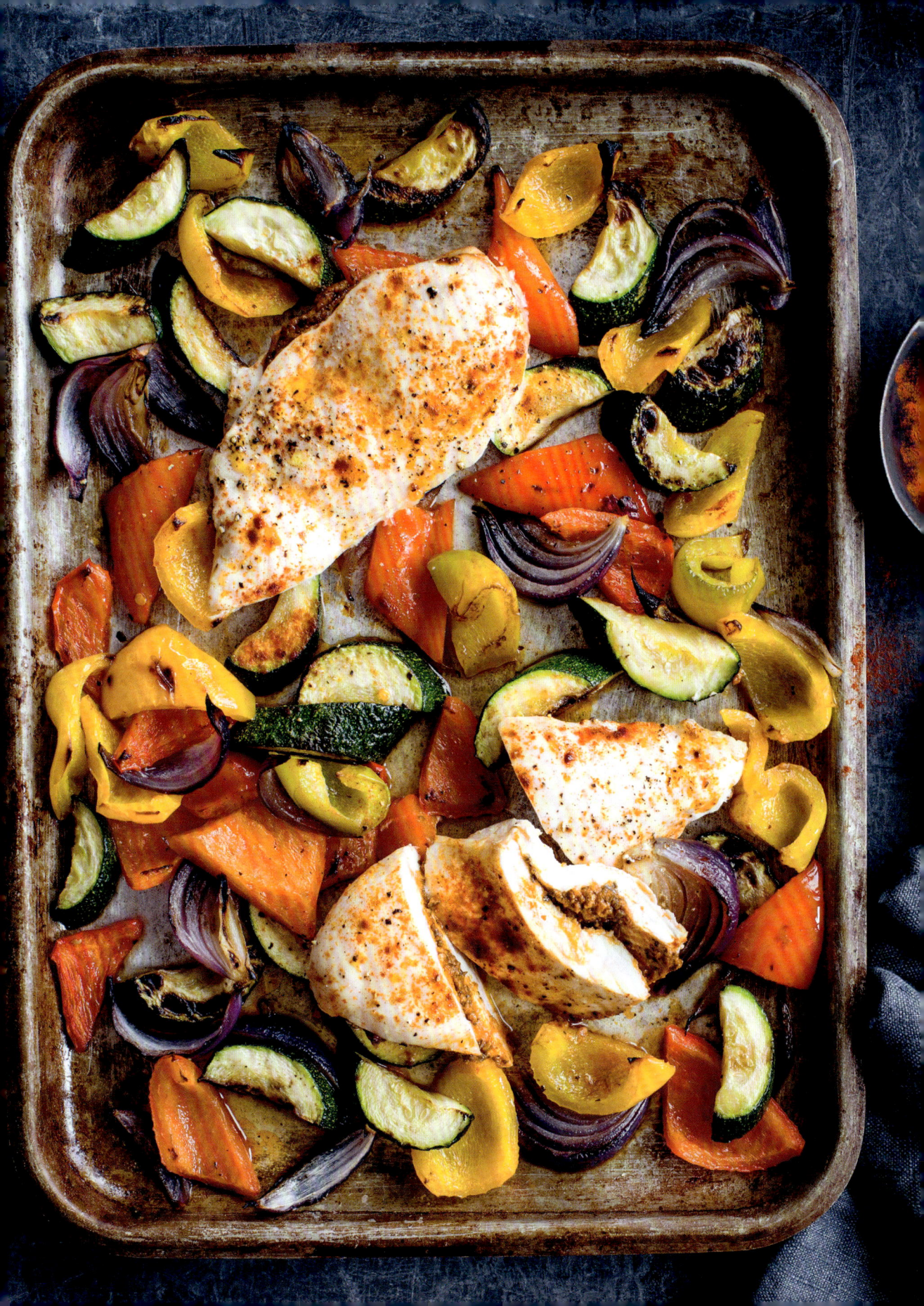

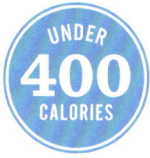

Garden Chicken Casserole

SERVES	PREP	COOK
4	**20** mins	**60** mins

2 tbsp olive oil
6 boneless, skinless chicken
    thighs (around 600g total
    weight), trimmed of fat
    and quartered
1 large onion, finely sliced
3 carrots (around 250g
    total weight), trimmed
    and cut into 1.5cm slices
275g swede, cut into
    2.5cm chunks
500ml chicken stock
    (made with 1 stock cube)
1 tsp mixed dried herbs
2 leeks, trimmed and cut
    into 1.5cm slices
100g frozen peas

A traditional, comforting casserole with delicate flavours. Chicken thighs are simmered in the oven with lots of lovely prebiotic vegetables, so it's not just your waistline that will approve, but your gut bacteria, too.

1. Preheat the oven to 200°C/Fan 180°C/Gas 6.

2. Heat the oil in a flameproof casserole over a moderate heat. Add the chicken and onion, season with a little salt and lots of freshly ground black pepper and fry for 6–8 minutes, stirring regularly, until the chicken is coloured on all sides and the onion is beginning to brown.

3. Add the carrots, swede, stock and herbs. Bring to a simmer then cover with a lid and transfer to the oven for 30 minutes.

4. Remove from the oven and use a ladle to take out around 100ml liquid, including some carrots and swede, and either mash these in a small bowl or put them in a jug and blitz to a purée with a stick blender. Return this to the stew and stir in to thicken the sauce.

5. Add the leeks and peas, cover again and return to the oven for a further 20–30 minutes, or until the chicken is cooked through.

6. Remove from the oven and serve with lightly cooked shredded cabbage or kale.

GLUTEN FREE · NUT FREE · DAIRY FREE

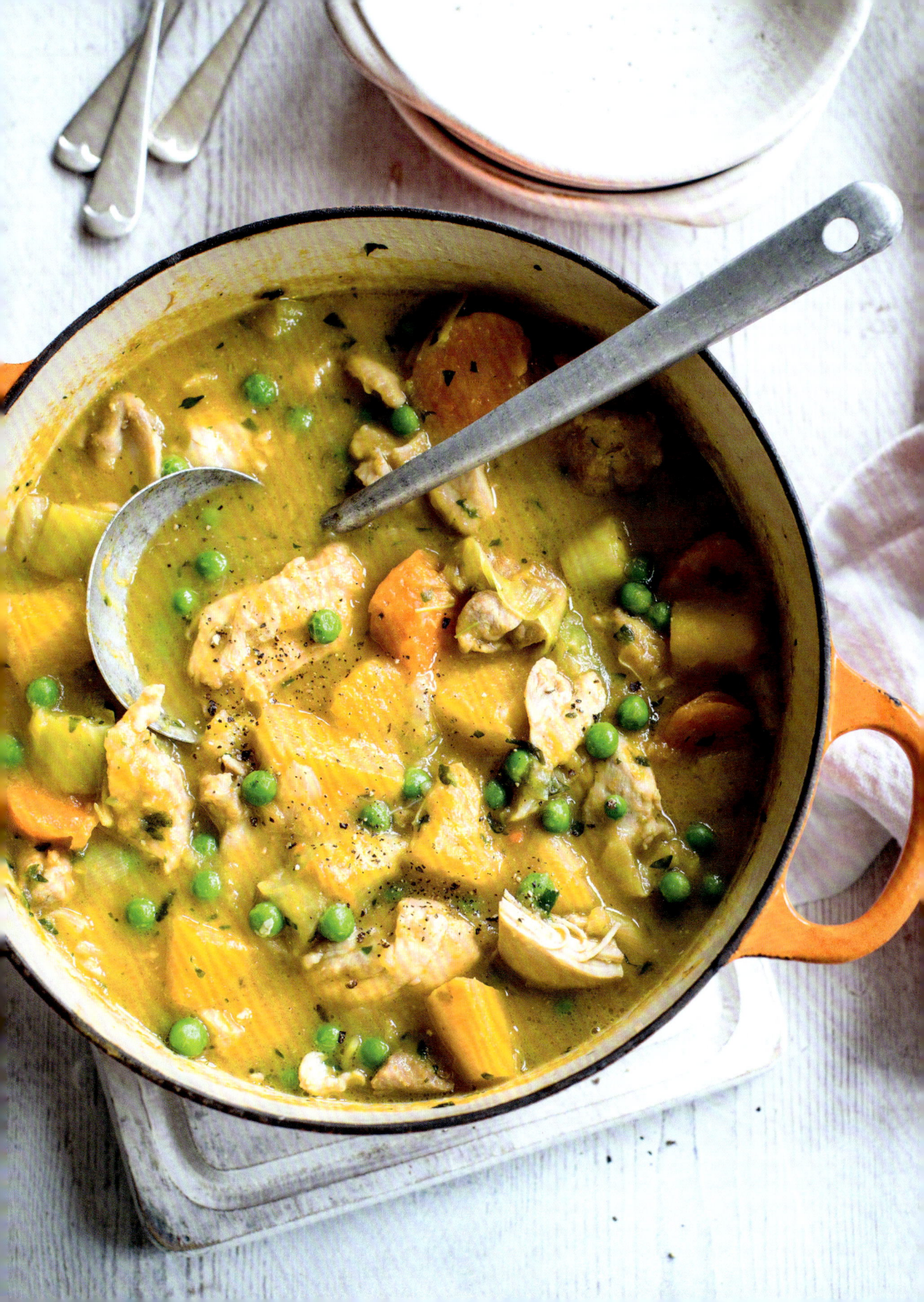

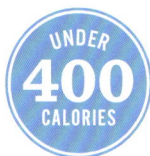

Chicken Katsu Curry

SERVES	PREP	COOK
4	**15** mins	**25** mins

4 skinless chicken breast fillets
(each around 150g)
1 tbsp coconut oil, melted,
or olive or rapeseed oil
50g flaked almonds

For the sauce
1 tbsp olive, coconut
or rapeseed oil
1 onion, roughly chopped
1 garlic clove, finely chopped
15g fresh root ginger,
peeled and finely chopped
1 tsp medium curry powder
¼ tsp Chinese five
spice powder
4 soft dried apricots,
roughly chopped
300ml chicken stock
(made with ½ stock cube)

This nutty, katsu-style curry is nicely low-carb. We top it with flaked almonds instead of breadcrumbs and serve it with a simple sauce flavoured with five spice and sweetened with apricots.

1. Preheat the oven to 200°C/Fan 180°C/Gas 6 and line a large baking tray with non-stick baking paper.

2. Place the chicken breasts on the tray and brush with a little oil. Season with salt and freshly ground black pepper. Sprinkle the almonds on to the chicken, covering as best as you can, but don't worry if a few nuts fall off. Bake for 20–25 minutes, or until the chicken is cooked through and the almonds are lightly toasted.

3. Meanwhile, to make the sauce, place the oil in a small saucepan over a low heat, add the onion, garlic and ginger, and fry for 6–8 minutes, or until softened, stirring regularly. Add the curry powder and five spice, and cook for a few seconds more, stirring. Stir in the apricots and stock and bring to a simmer. Cook for 5 minutes, or until the apricots are softened, stirring regularly.

4. Remove the pan from the heat and blitz the sauce with a stick blender, or let it cool slightly and blitz in a food processor, until very smooth. Season to taste.

5. Serve the chicken with the sauce and a large green salad.

AIR-FRYER TIP
To cook the chicken in an air fryer: preheat the air fryer to 180°C, if needed. Drizzle the chicken with a little oil, season, and air fry for 14 minutes, turning halfway and drizzling with more oil, or until cooked through. Scatter over the almonds in the final 5 minutes.

GLUTEN FREE   DAIRY FREE

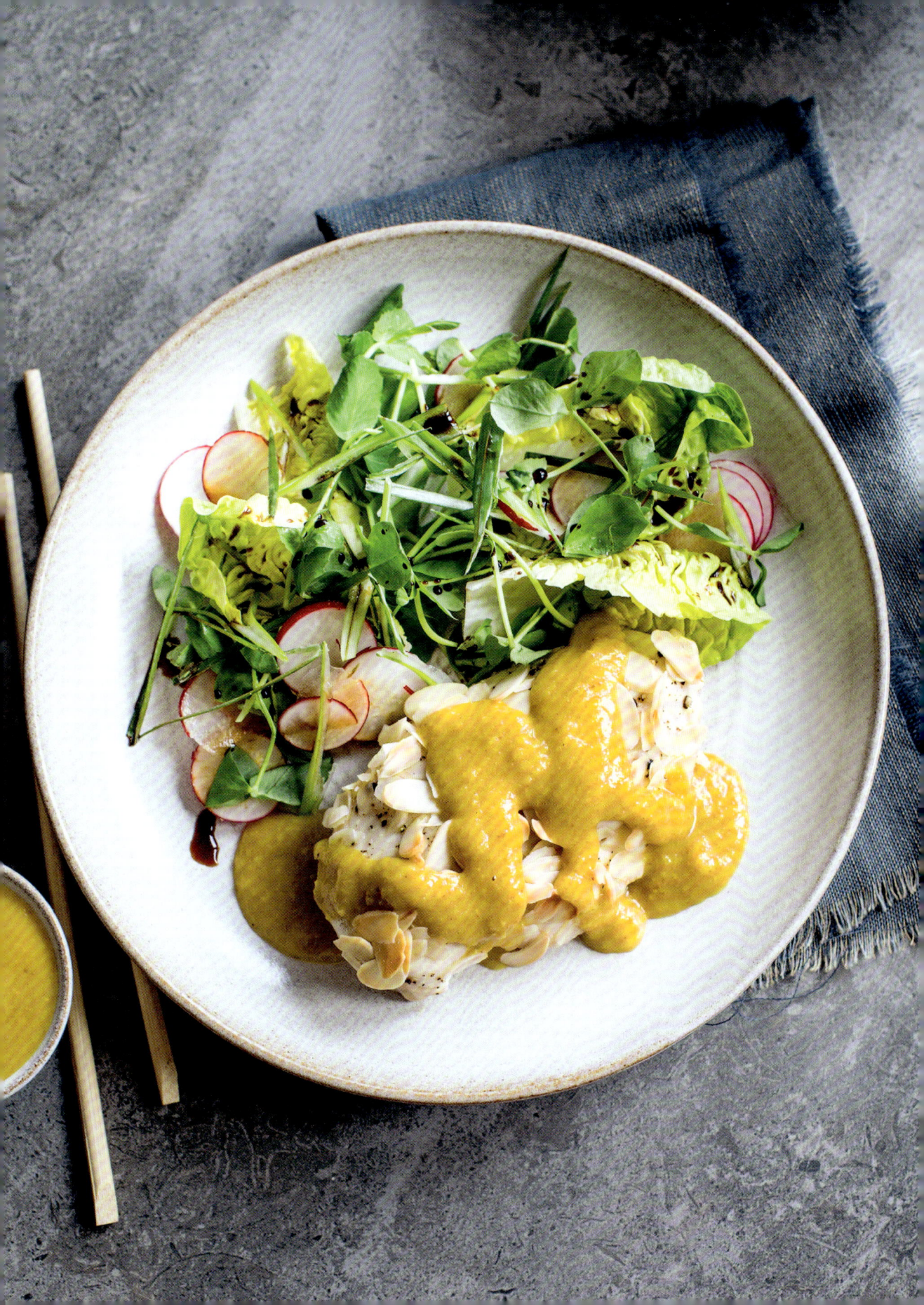

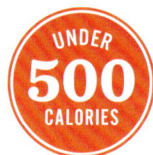

PER SERVING | **426cals** | PROTEIN **57g** | CARBS **23g**

Fastest Spaghetti Bolognese

SERVES	PREP	COOK
4	**15** mins	**23** mins

2 tbsp olive oil
1 onion, finely chopped
200g small mushrooms,
    quartered
500g turkey breast mince
1 × 400g can chopped tomatoes
2 tbsp tomato purée
1 chicken stock cube
1 tsp dried oregano
80g wholewheat spaghetti
2 large courgettes, trimmed
    and spiralized or peeled
    into ribbons, or use a pack
    of courgetti
20g Parmesan, finely grated

NON-FAST DAYS
Mix the Bolognese with
cooked lentils and top
with grated mozzarella.

COOK'S TIP
The Bolognese makes a
great stuffing for peppers.

A brilliantly versatile and quick-to-prepare Bolognese. Made with turkey rather than beef mince, it can be adapted for all sorts of dishes and freezes well. Michael adored a good, protein-rich Bolognese, and was more than happy to switch to courgetti instead of pasta.

1. Heat the oil in a large non-stick frying or sauté pan, add the onion and mushrooms and fry over a medium–high heat for 5 minutes, stirring regularly.

2. Add the turkey and fry for a further 5–8 minutes, or until lightly browned. Tip the tomatoes into the pan with the mince, stir in 400ml water, the tomato purée, crumbled stock cube and oregano. Bring to a simmer and cook for 5–10 minutes, stirring regularly, until thick. Season with salt and freshly ground black pepper.

3. Meanwhile, cook the spaghetti in a large pan of boiling water for 10–12 minutes, or according to the pack instructions. Add the courgette to the pan with the pasta and cook for 30 seconds more.

4. Drain the pasta and courgette, and divide between four warmed bowls or deep plates. Top with the Bolognese, sprinkle with the Parmesan and serve with a green salad or finely sliced steamed greens.

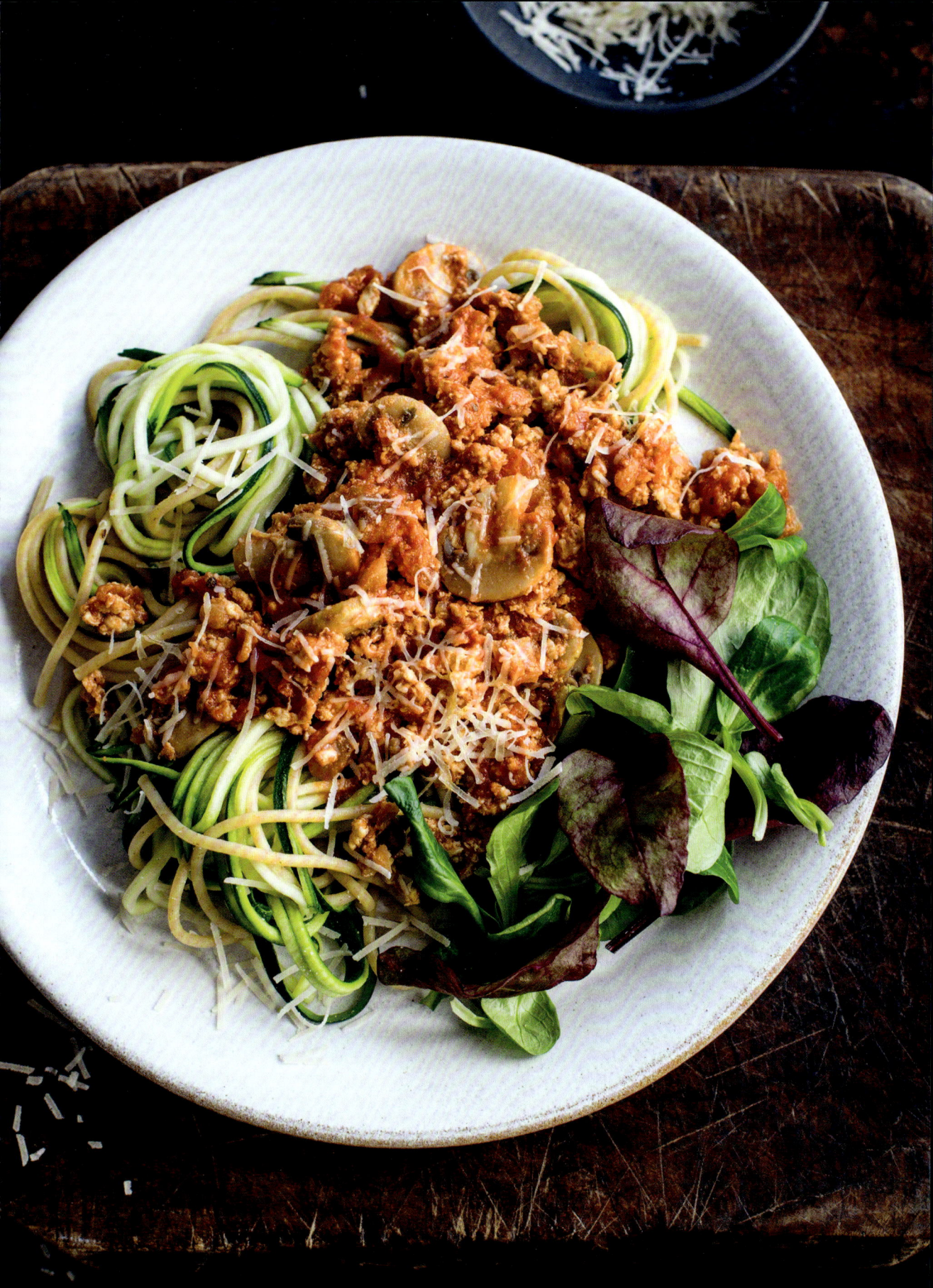

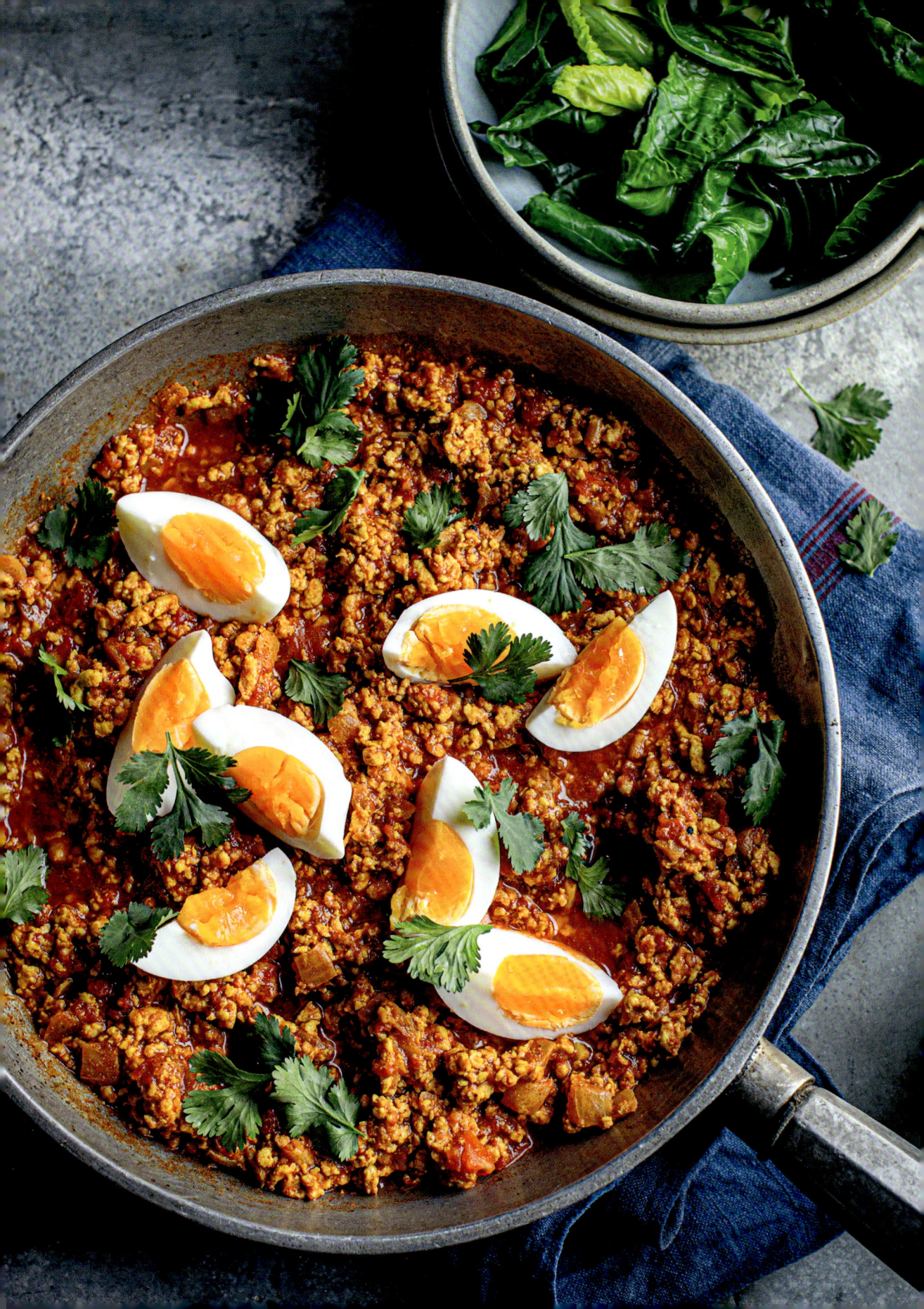

Turkey Keema

SERVES **4**

PREP **10** mins

COOK **20** mins

2 tbsp olive, coconut
    or rapeseed oil
1 onion, finely chopped
500g turkey breast mince
3 tbsp medium Indian curry
    paste, such as rogan josh
    or tikka masala
1 × 400g can chopped tomatoes
1 chicken stock cube
2 large free-range eggs
small handful coriander
    leaves, to serve (optional)

NON-FAST DAYS
Serve with a wholemeal
mini flatbread.

Keema is a traditional Indian mince and pea curry, and is super served with a dollop of full-fat live Greek yoghurt, mixed with grated cucumber and a pinch of cumin seeds.

1. Place the oil in a large, deep frying pan over a medium–high heat, add the onion and turkey, and fry for 8–10 minutes, or until lightly browned, stirring regularly and breaking up the mince.

2. Add the curry paste and cook for 1 minute, stirring constantly. Add the tomatoes, crumbled stock cube and 300ml water, and bring to a simmer. Cook for about 10 minutes, stirring regularly, until thick. Season with salt and freshly ground black pepper.

3. Meanwhile, half fill a saucepan with water and bring to the boil. Gently add the eggs, return to the boil and cook for 8 minutes.

4. Rinse the eggs under cold running water until cool enough to handle, thcn peel and cut them into quarters. Place on top of the turky keema, scatter over the coriander, if using, and serve with a colourful salad or on a bed of finely sliced cooked cabbage.

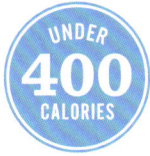

PER SERVING | **377cals** | PROTEIN **56.9g** | CARBS **4.4g**

Piri Piri Roast Chicken with Jalapeño Yoghurt

SERVES	PREP	COOK
4	**12** mins	**90** mins

1 roasted red pepper
  from a jar (around 70g)
1 tbsp piri piri seasoning
2 tbsp olive oil
1 tbsp light soy sauce
1 × 1.5kg whole chicken,
  at room temperature
1 lemon, pierced a few times
  with a fork (optional)

For the jalapeño yoghurt
30g jalapeños from a jar,
  drained
125g full-fat live Greek yoghurt
10g fresh coriander

NON-FAST DAY
Increase the portion
size and/or serve with
2–3 tablespoons cooked
quinoa, wholegrain rice,
bulgur wheat or roasted
butternut squash.

Michael was the master of cooking a whole chicken, ideally with a blast of flavour... If making for fewer than four, simply strip the leftover meat from the bone, store it in the fridge and keep as a base for another quick and easy meal.

1. Preheat the oven to 200°C/Fan 180°C/Gas 6.

2. Place the roasted red pepper, piri piri seasoning, olive oil and soy sauce in a small jug and blitz with a stick blender until smooth. Season with freshly ground black pepper.

3. Pull the skin away from the crown of the chicken, creating a pocket between the flesh and the skin. Add half the piri piri mixture and spread under the skin. Pour the rest over the chicken and rub in. Place the lemon in the cavity of the chicken, if using, then arrange the chicken in a roasting tin. Cover with foil and roast in the oven for 1 hour 10 minutes. Remove the foil and roast for a further 20 minutes.

4. Meanwhile, prepare the jalapeño yoghurt. Place all the ingredients in a small jug and blitz with a stick blender until smooth. Season.

5. Divide the chicken between four plates and serve with the jalapeño yoghurt and a generous portion of greens.

AIR-FRYER TIP
Preheat the air fryer to 170°C, if needed. Prepare the piri piri sauce and chicken as above. Place the chicken in the air fryer, breast-side down (no foil), and cook for 25 minutes. Increase the heat to 180°C. Turn the chicken over, baste with the juices, and air fry for another 25 minutes, or until cooked through.

GLUTEN FREE | NUT FREE

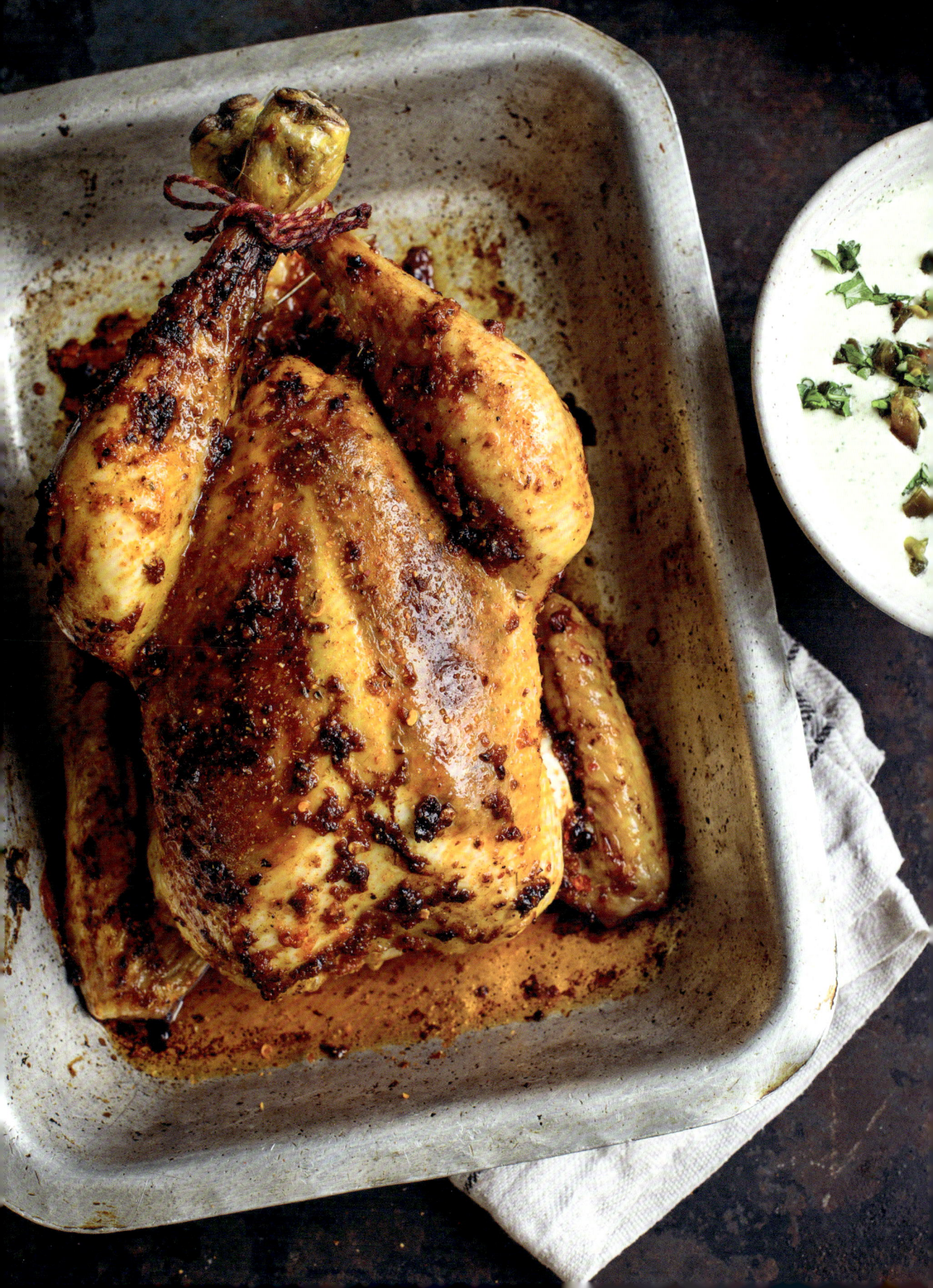

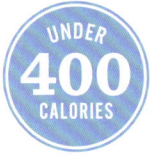

Greek Turkey Burgers with Harissa Yoghurt

SERVES **4** | **PREP** **15** mins | **COOK** **25** mins

½ red onion, finely chopped
40g pitted black olives,
    finely chopped
50g feta cheese, crumbled
40g mature Cheddar, grated
1½ tsp dried oregano
500g turkey thigh mince
1 tbsp olive oil
1 level tbsp harissa paste
4 tbsp full-fat live Greek
    yoghurt
1 head romaine lettuce,
    leaves separated
2 tomatoes, sliced

NON-FAST DAYS
Increase the portion size
and/or serve with cooked
quinoa or bulgur wheat.

You'll love these burgers that are bursting with delicious Mediterranean flavours. If you don't have harissa, sun-dried tomato pesto works well, too. Serve with a generous green salad. You could munch these burgers between two robust lettuce leaves.

1. Preheat the oven to 200°C/Fan 180°C/Gas 6 and line a baking tray with non-stick baking paper.

2. Place the onion, olives, cheeses, oregano, turkey mince, ½ tablespoon of the olive oil and a generous pinch of salt and freshly ground black pepper in a bowl. Use your hands to thoroughly mix everything together.

3. Shape the mixture into 4 burgers and place on the baking tray. Drizzle the remaining olive oil all over and roast in the oven for 25 minutes until cooked through.

4. Meanwhile, mix the harissa and yoghurt together in a small bowl.

5. When the burgers are ready, allow to cool slightly then serve with a couple of lettuce leaves per person and a few slices of tomato.

AIR-FRYER TIP
Preheat the air fryer to 180°C, if needed. Prepare the turkey burgers as above. Put the burgers in an air fryer, drizzle with the remaining oil, and air fry for 20 minutes until cooked through. Serve with the harissa yoghurt as above.

GLUTEN FREE | NUT FREE

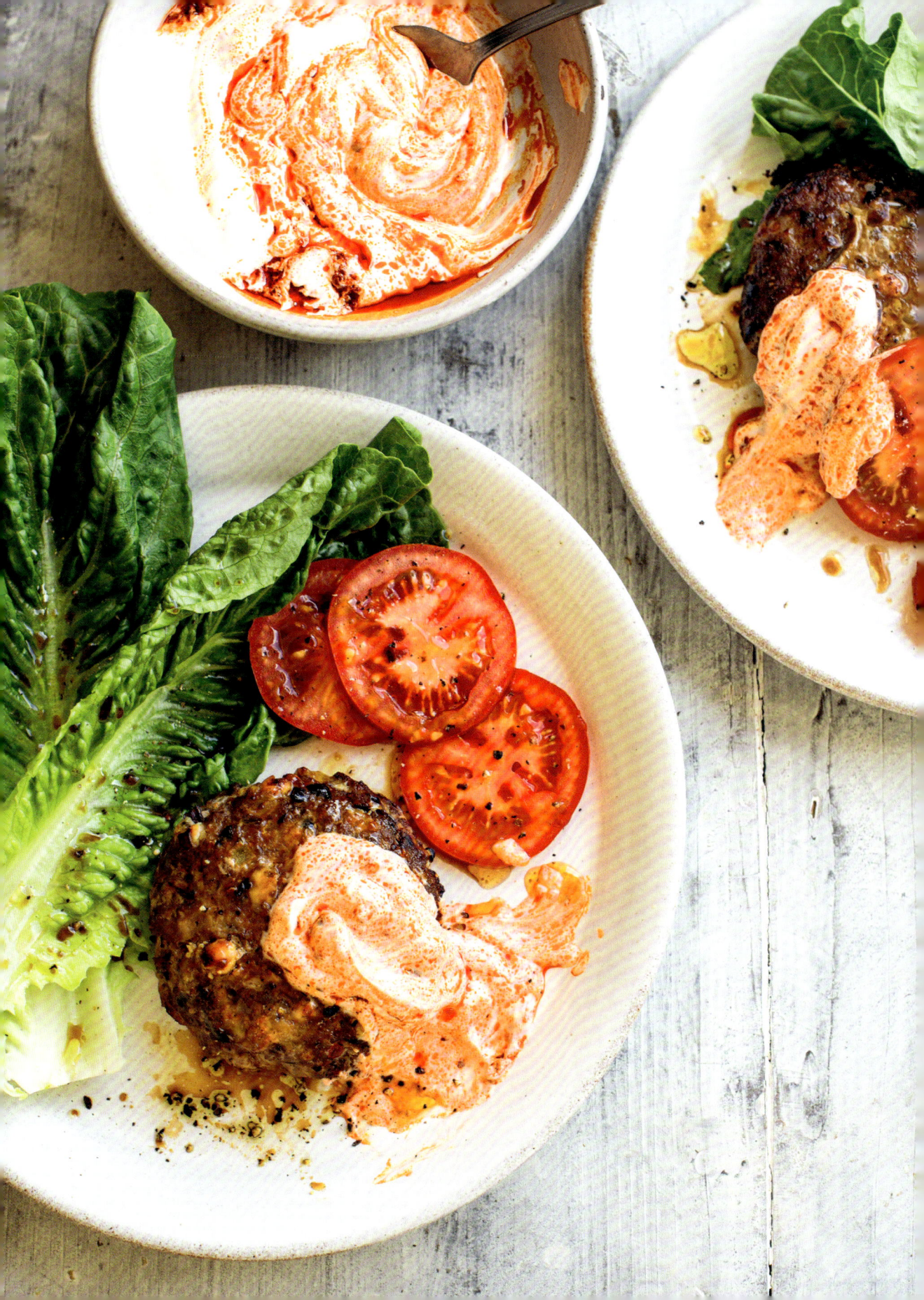

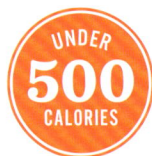

PER SERVING | **460cals** | PROTEIN **48.8g** | CARBS **20.3g**

Duck with Bean Sprout Noodles

SERVES | **PREP** | **COOK**
2 | **15** mins | **20** mins

2 duck breasts
   (around 170g each)
1 onion, finely chopped
1 tsp garam masala
½–1 tsp chilli powder
50g dried apricots,
   roughly chopped
200ml chicken stock
   (made with ½ stock cube)
150g bean sprouts, rinsed
   and drained
100g young spinach leaves

NON-FAST DAYS
Enjoy a larger portion
and/or serve with
2–3 tablespoons cooked
wholegrain rice, quinoa
or wholegrain noodles.

The fruity, tangy and mildly curried sauce contrasts
superbly with the richness of the duck in this recipe.

1. Preheat the oven to 200°C/Fan 180°C/Gas 6.

2. Pat the duck breasts dry, then score the skin with a sharp
knife and season with salt and freshly ground black pepper.

3. Place a frying pan over a high heat and, when hot, place
the duck, skin-side down, in the pan. Fry for 5 minutes, until
the skin is crisp and golden (it will smoke a little). Turn the
breasts and seal on the other side for 1 minute.

4. Transfer them to a baking tray, reserving the fat in the
pan, and roast in the oven for 8–10 minutes for medium
rare (still pink in the middle). Set aside to rest for 5 minutes.

5. Meanwhile, place the frying pan back over a medium
heat and fry the onion for 3–4 minutes, until softened.
Add the garam masala, chilli powder, apricots and stock
and simmer for 2 minutes. Pour the sauce into a jug and
blitz with a stick blender until smooth.

6. Place the bean sprouts and spinach on a baking tray
and cook in the oven for 2–3 minutes, until the spinach
is wilted. Carefully slice the duck and serve on top of
the veg with the sauce spooned over or alongside.

AIR-FRYER TIP
To finish cooking the duck in an air fryer, preheat the
air fryer to 180°C, if needed. Prepare and cook the duck
breasts in the frying pan as instructed in Steps 2–3.
Transfer the browned duck to the air fryer and cook
for 6–8 minutes for medium rare–medium.

GLUTEN FREE   NUT FREE

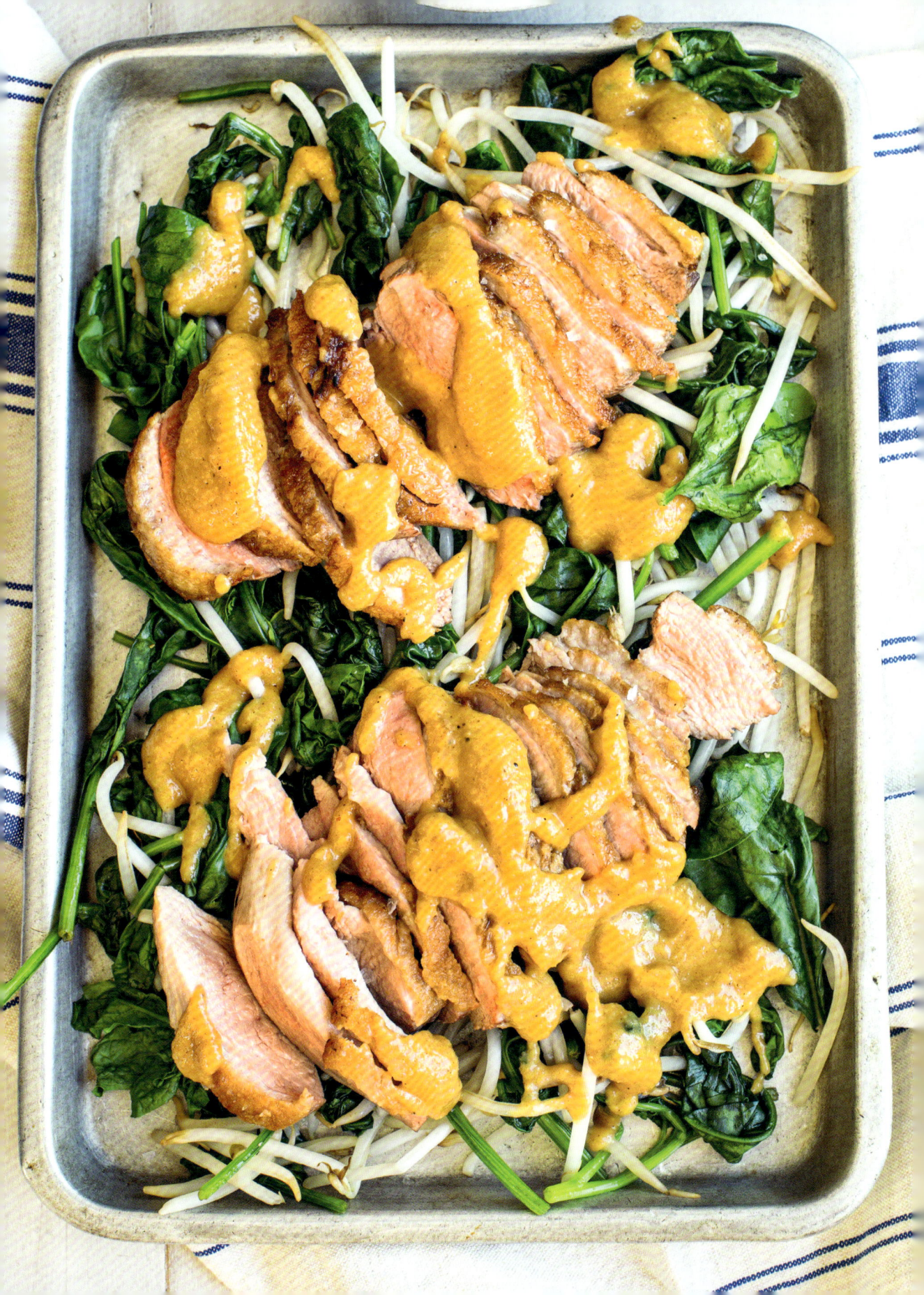

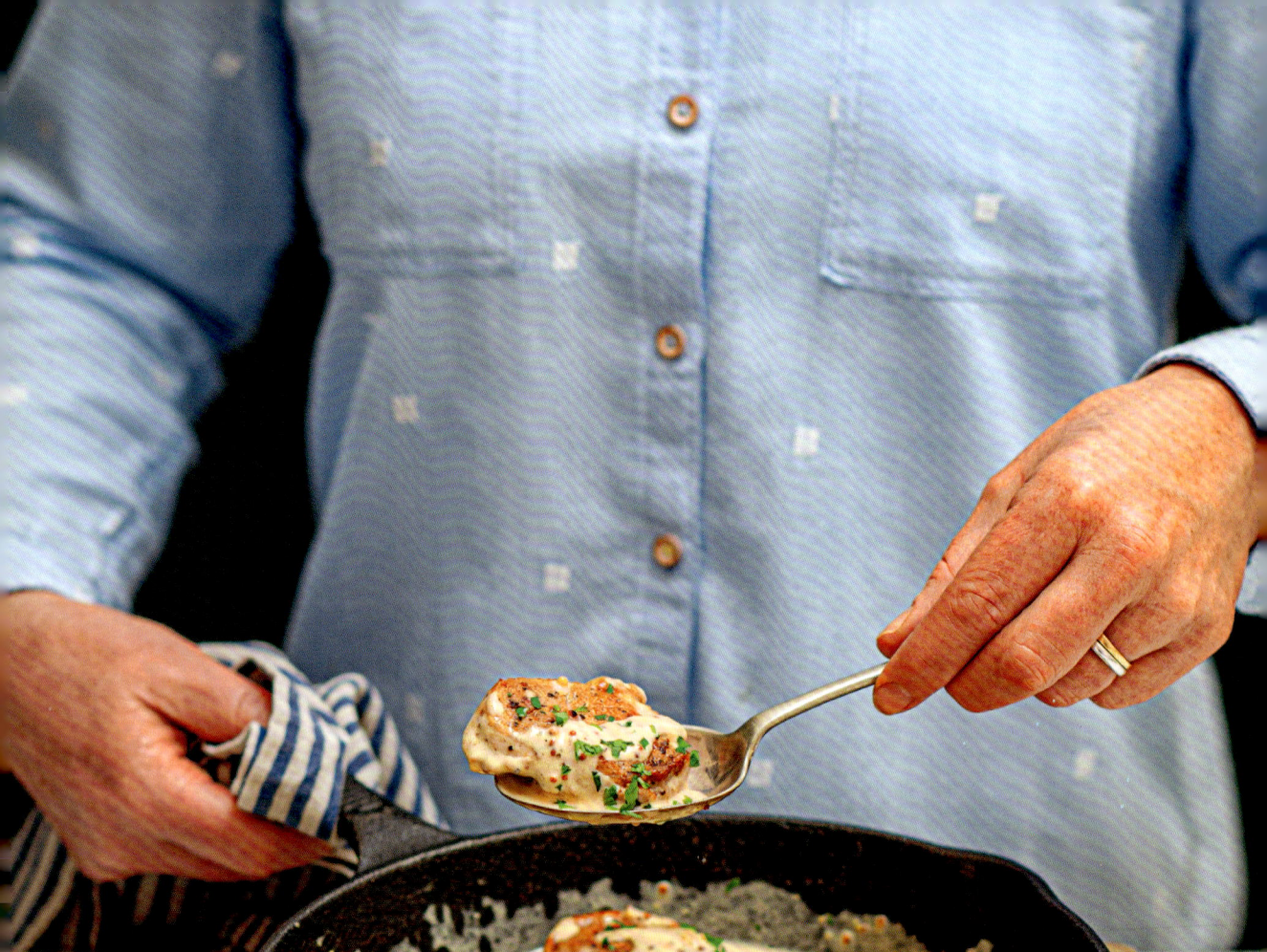

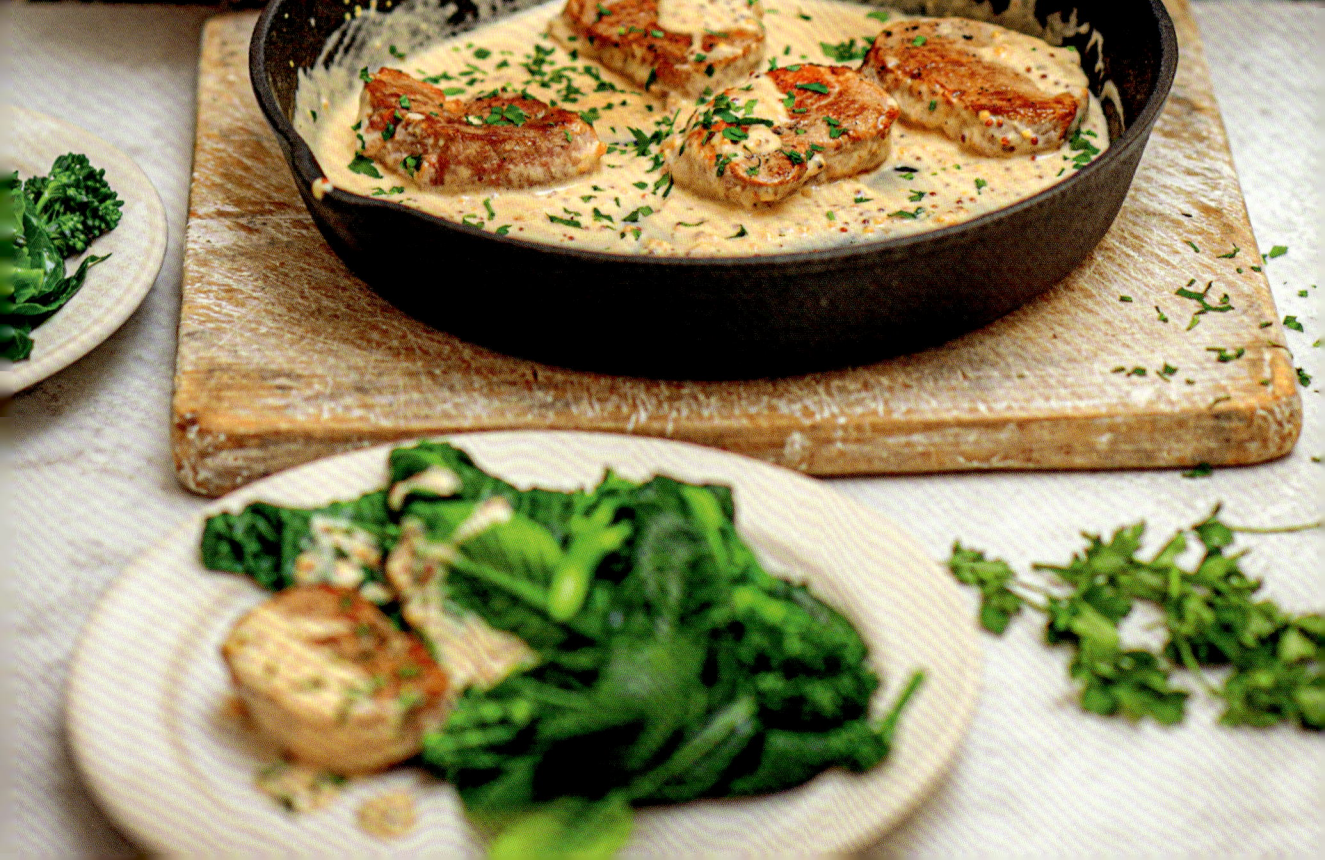

Pork, Lamb and Beef

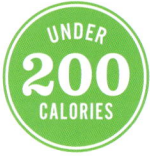

Perfect Pulled Pork

SERVES | **PREP** | **COOK**
6 | **8** hours | **3** hours

1kg pork shoulder joint, rind on

For the marinade
45g tomato purée
    (around 3 tbsp)
30g chipotle paste
    (around 2 tbsp)
juice of 2 large oranges
juice of 2 limes
1 tsp flaked sea salt
1 tsp ground cumin
1 tsp ground allspice
1 tsp coarsely ground
    black pepper

NON-FAST DAYS
Serve in ready-made corn tacos with lots of salad.

COOK'S TIP
You'll find chipotle chilli paste in the World Food section of the supermarket, with other Mexican foods. Or use 2 teaspoons hot smoked paprika instead. If serving fewer people, halve the quantity of pork and marinade and reduce the cooking time slightly.

This succulent, zingy pork reheats beautifully, so can be enjoyed the next day, too. Serve in wraps made from Little Gem or romaine lettuce leaves, and top with some diced cornichons. This goes well with coleslaw (see page 221), but don't forget to add the extra calories.

1. To make the marinade, place the tomato purée, chipotle paste, orange and lime juices, sea salt and spices in a large non-metallic bowl and whisk until combined.

2. Remove any string from the pork and add the meat to the bowl with the marinade. Turn the pork several times until it is well coated, then cover and leave to marinate in the fridge for at least 8 hours or overnight.

3. Preheat the oven to 170°C/Fan 150°C/Gas 3.

4. Place the pork and its marinade in a casserole or roasting tin, cover and bake for about 3 hours, or until the pork falls apart when prodded with a fork. Check after a couple of hours and add some water, if needed, to keep the pork moist.

5. Transfer the pork to a board or warmed platter and shred with two forks, discarding the rind and fat. Serve with a little of the spicy cooking juices spooned over.

GLUTEN FREE · NUT FREE · DAIRY FREE

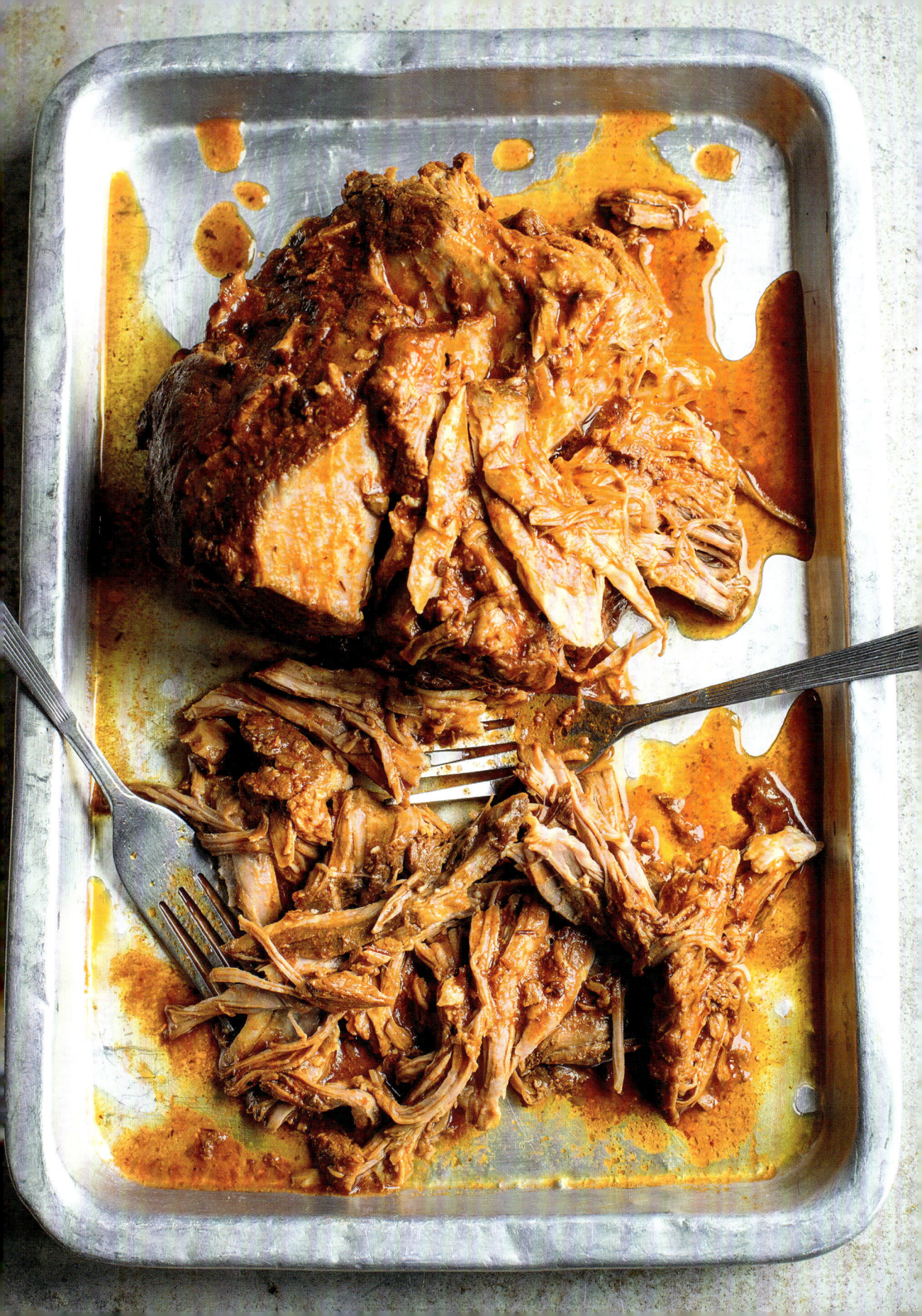

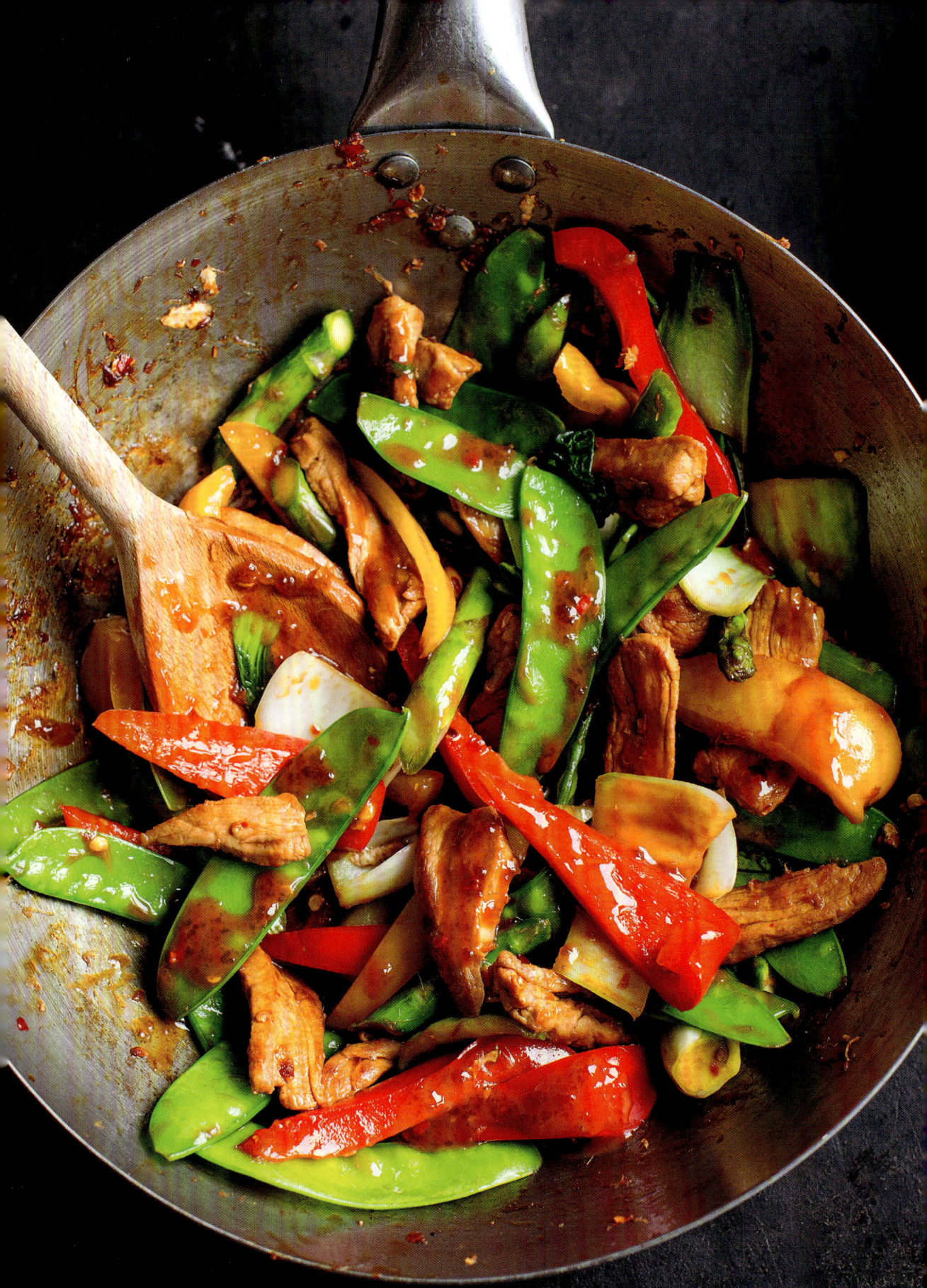

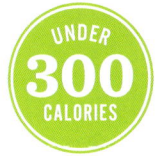

Peppered Pork Stir Fry

SERVES **2**

PREP **5** mins

COOK **9** mins

250g pork tenderloin, trimmed, cut in half lengthways and into 1cm slices
1 tbsp coconut or rapeseed oil
1 × 320–350g pack mixed stir-fry vegetables
15g fresh root ginger, peeled and finely grated

For the spicy sauce
1 tsp cornflour
1 tbsp dark soy sauce
1 tsp runny honey
¼–½ tsp crushed dried chilli flakes, to taste

NON-FAST DAYS
Add cooked wholewheat or soba buckwheat noodles and a little of the noodle water at the same time as the sauce, or serve with a few tablespoons of brown rice.

COOK'S TIP
Freeze any leftover pork from the whole tenderloin – wrap tightly in foil and place in the freezer for up to 3 months. This could also be made with strips of beef, chicken or tofu. The pork in this recipe contributes 154cals per serving – adjust the calories accordingly.

A super-quick, super-tasty stir fry.

1. Season the pork all over with a little salt and a generous amount of freshly ground black pepper.

2. Heat the oil in a large frying pan or wok over a medium–high heat. Add the pork and stir fry, tossing frequently, for 3–4 minutes, or until lightly browned and cooked through.

3. Add the vegetables and stir fry with the pork for 2–3 minutes. Stir in the ginger and cook for a few seconds more.

4. Meanwhile, mix the cornflour with the soy sauce, honey and chilli in a small bowl. Stir into the pan and toss everything together for 1–2 minutes, or until the vegetables are tender and glossy. Serve with a little extra soy sauce, if you like.

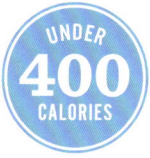

PER SERVING | **308cals** | PROTEIN **35g** | CARBS **23.5g**

Parma Pork with Squash Mash

SERVES	PREP	COOK
3	**5** mins	**90** mins

1kg butternut squash
400g pork tenderloin,
    trimmed
3 slices Parma ham
    or prosciutto

NON-FAST DAYS
Use the quantities to serve
two rather than three, so each
person gets a larger portion.

COOK'S TIP
Roasted squash makes a great
accompaniment to other meals
too. The length of cooking time
will vary according to the size
of the squash. The mashed
squash contains 55cals per
150g serving.

A gorgeous roast using just three ingredients, with a total preparation time of less than 10 minutes. It also reheats really well, so can be warmed up for lunch or supper the following day. Serve with lots of freshly cooked shredded kale, cabbage or other greens.

1. Preheat the oven to 200°C/Fan 180°C/Gas 6 and line a baking tray with foil.

2. Place the whole, unpeeled squash on the baking tray and prick 8–10 times with the tip of a knife. Bake for 1 hour.

3. Meanwhile, season the pork with salt and freshly ground black pepper and wrap it in the Parma ham or prosciutto. Place the pork on the tray alongside the squash and return to the oven for a further 25–30 minutes, or until the pork is cooked and the squash is tender. (You should be able to push a knife into the squash easily.)

4. Transfer the pork to a warm plate, cover with foil and leave to rest. Meanwhile, cut the squash in half vertically and scoop out and discard the seeds. Scoop the flesh out of the skin and place in a bowl. Season and mash well.

5. Place the pork on a board, reserving the resting juices, and slice thickly. Spoon the mash on to warmed plates and top with the pork. Drizzle with the juices to serve.

AIR-FRYER TIP
Preheat the air fryer to 180°C, if needed. Prepare the squash as step 2. Air fry for 55 minutes, turning halfway. Prepare the pork as Step 3 and place in the air fryer alongside the squash. Air fry for 18–20 minutes, turning halfway, until the pork is cooked and golden, and the squash is tender.

GLUTEN FREE · NUT FREE · DAIRY FREE

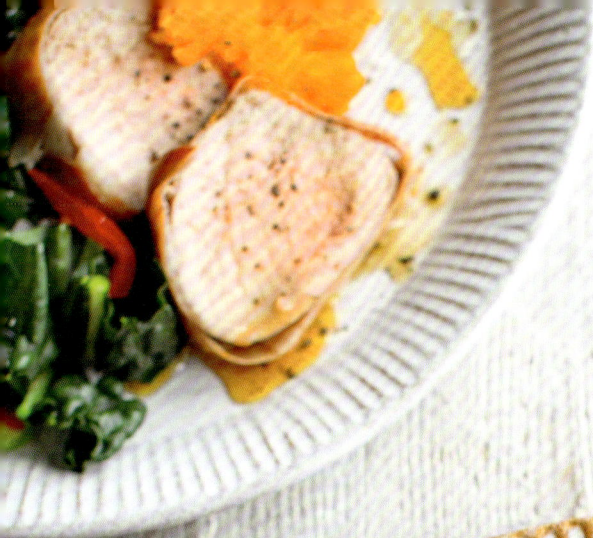

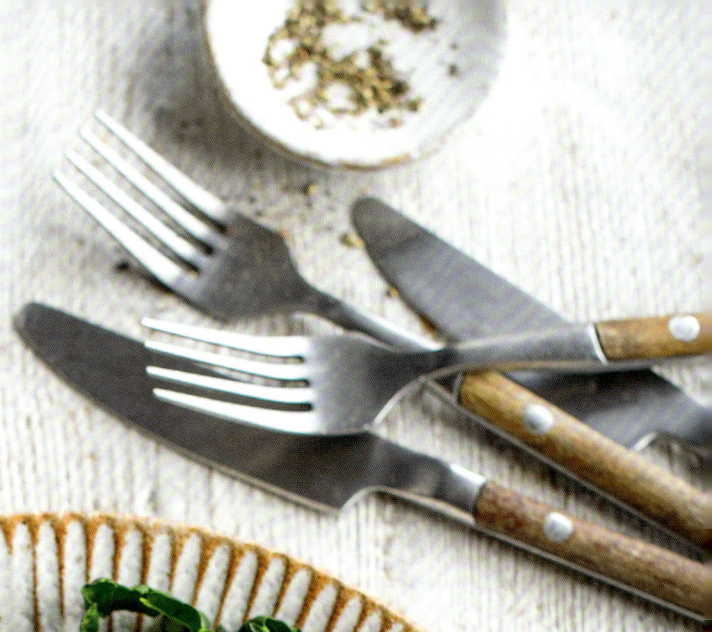

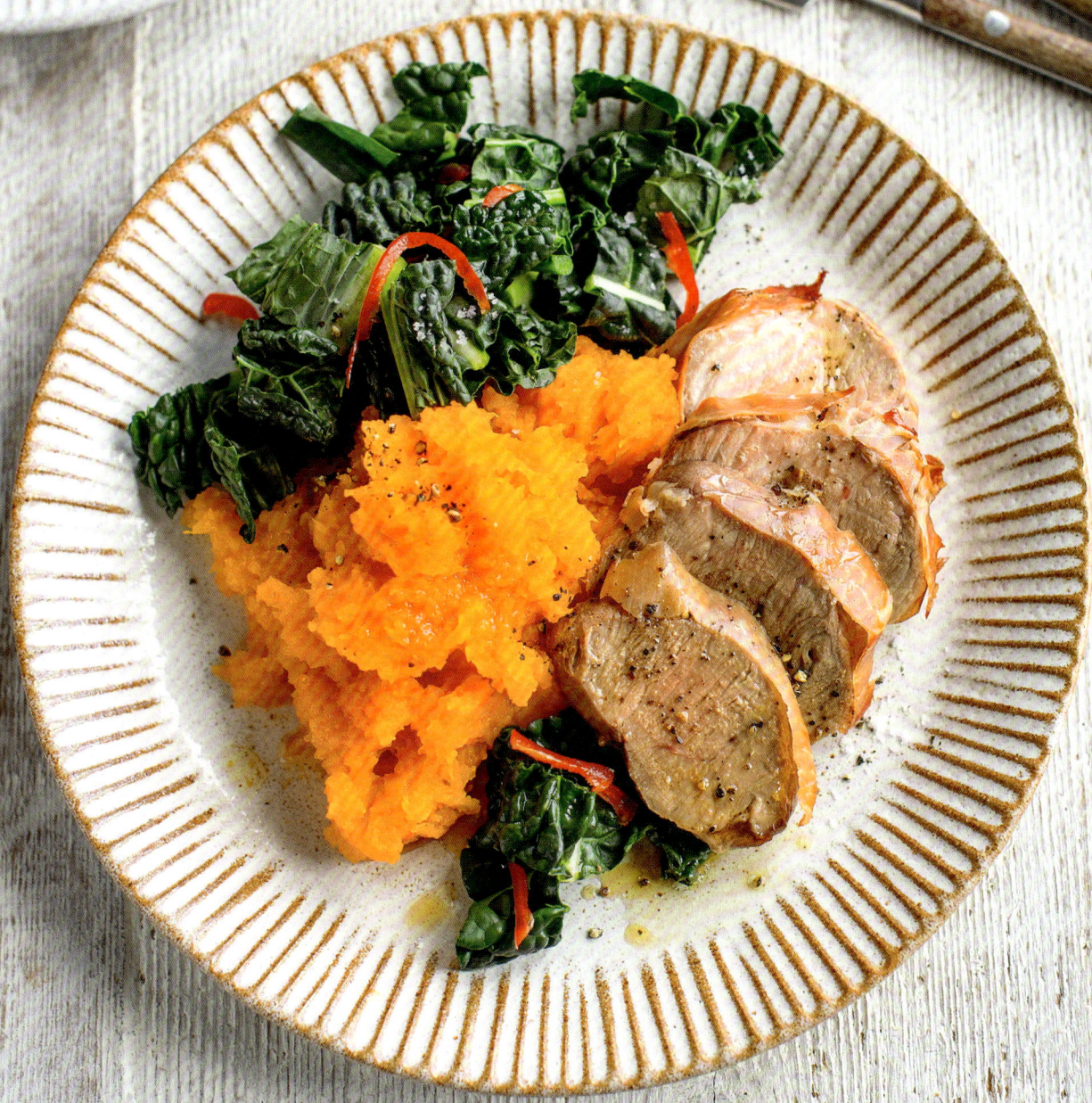

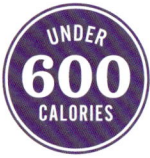

Lamb Chops with Crushed Minted Peas and Feta

SERVES **2** | **PREP** **5** mins | **COOK** **10** mins

2 thick lamb loin chops
   (each around 175g)
   or 4 lamb cutlets
1 tsp olive oil

*For the crushed minted
   peas and feta*
200g frozen peas
1 tbsp olive oil
15g pine nuts, toasted
   (see page 99)
1 red chilli, deseeded
   and finely diced
10g fresh mint, leaves
   finely chopped
50g feta cheese

NON-FAST DAYS
Drizzle with more olive oil or
dress the salad with a no-count
dressing (see page 88–9) and
serve with 2–3 tablespoons
cooked quinoa or pearl barley.

A quick, easy and wonderfully satisfying supper.
Serve with a leafy salad or a generous portion
of wilted spinach (which tastes even better with
a teaspoon of olive oil or butter – add 40cals).

1. Rub the lamb with the oil and season on both sides
with salt and freshly ground black pepper. Place a griddle,
barbecue or frying pan over a medium–high heat. When
hot, add the chops and cook for 3–5 minutes on each side,
depending on thickness, or until done to taste. Turn on
to the fat side for 30 seconds at the end.

2. Meanwhile, to make the minted peas, third fill a
pan with water and bring to the boil. Add the peas and
cook for 3 minutes. Drain the peas then return to the
pan and mash lightly. Add the olive oil, pine nuts and
chilli, sprinkle with the mint and crumble in the feta.
Season with lots of ground black pepper and toss lightly.

3. Divide the lamb and crushed peas between two
plates to serve.

GLUTEN FREE

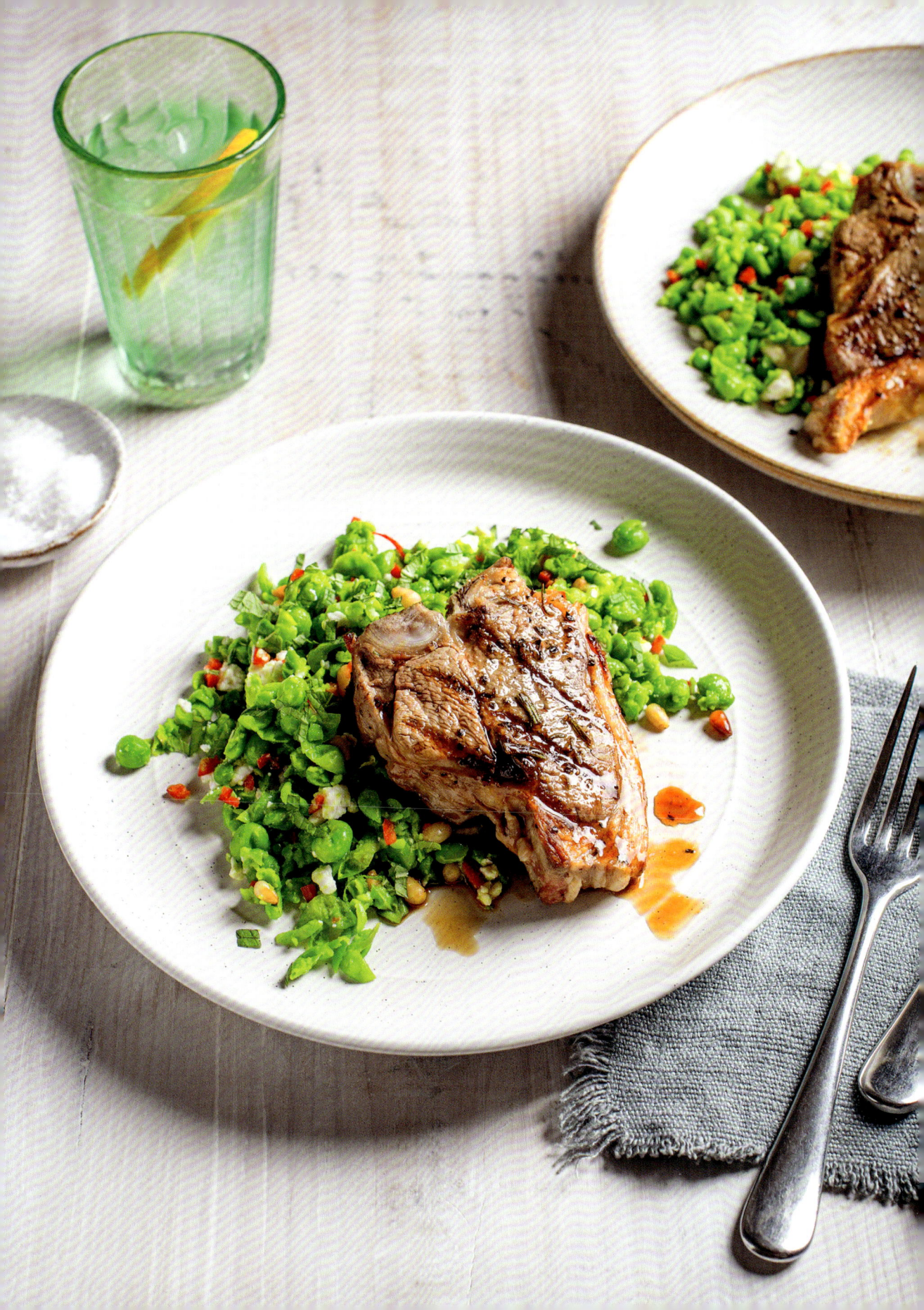

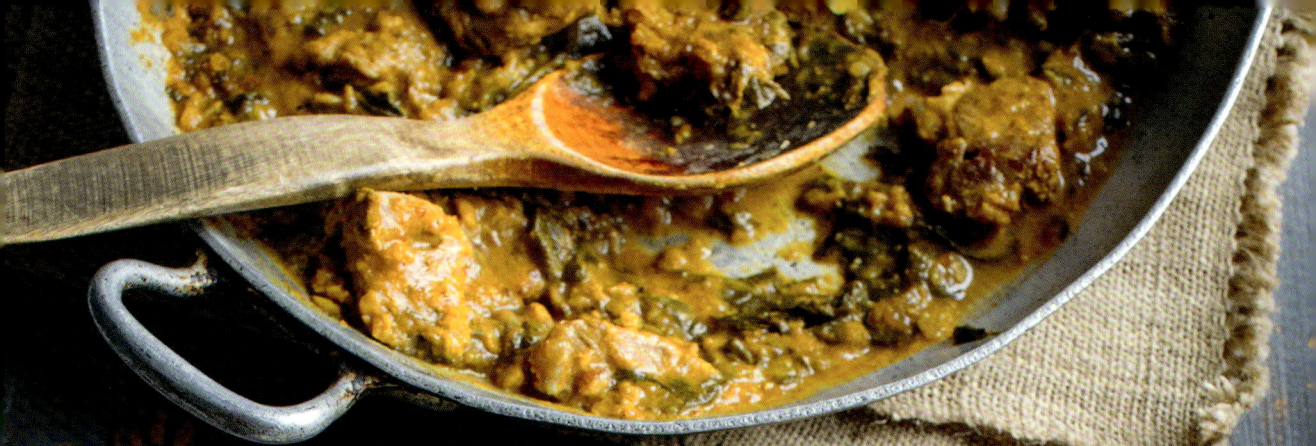

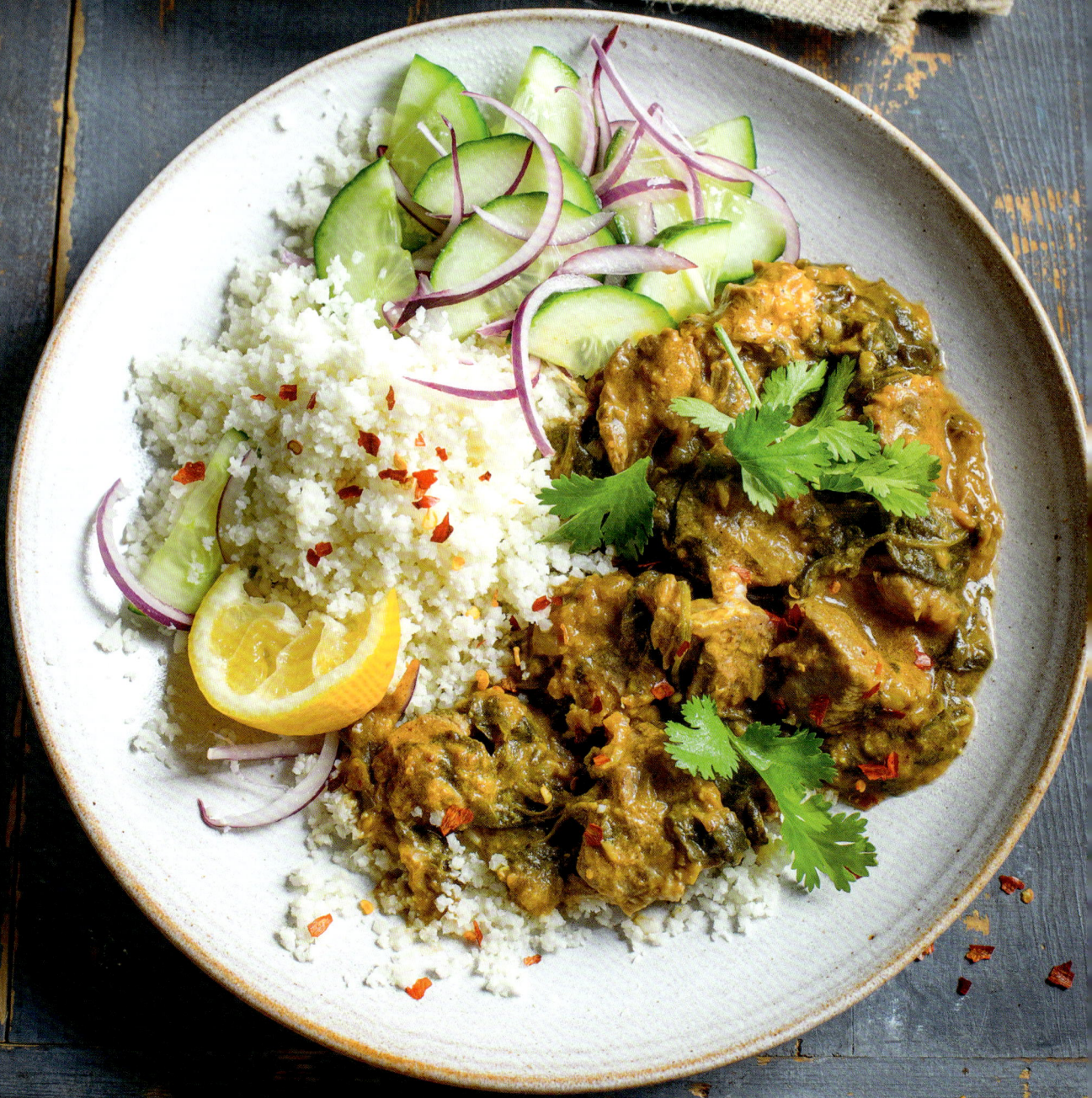

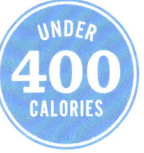

Lamb Saag

SERVES **4** | **PREP** **5** mins | **COOK** **80** mins

1 tbsp coconut or rapeseed oil
1 onion, finely sliced
500g lamb neck fillet, trimmed and cut into 3–4cm chunks
60g (around 4 tbsp) medium Indian curry paste, such as rogan josh or tikka masala
50g dried split red lentils
200g frozen spinach

NON-FAST DAYS
Enjoy a larger portion. Serve with a few tablespoonfuls of brown rice and pickles.

A handy throw-it-all-together curry that you can bung in the oven and forget about. Use a good-quality curry paste for the best results. Serve with cauli-rice (see page 232) and a cucumber and red onion salad.

1. Preheat the oven to 180°C/Fan 160°C/Gas 4.

2. Heat the oil in a flameproof casserole and gently fry the onion for 5 minutes, or until softened and lightly browned.

3. Add the lamb pieces, season with salt and freshly ground black pepper, and cook for 3 minutes, or until coloured on all sides, turning regularly. Stir in the curry paste and cook with the lamb and onion for 1 minute.

4. Add the lentils and spinach and stir in 500ml water. Bring to the boil, cover with a lid and transfer to the oven for 1–1¼ hours, or until the lamb is tender and the sauce is thick.

GLUTEN FREE | NUT FREE | DAIRY FREE | ❄

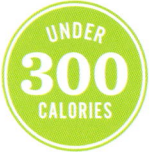

Meatballs in Tomato Sauce

SERVES	PREP	COOK
4	**3** mins	**15** mins

300g small good-quality beef
   meatballs (around 20)
1 tbsp olive oil
1 onion, finely chopped
2 garlic cloves, finely grated
1 × 400g can chopped tomatoes
1 tsp dried oregano
¼–½ tsp crushed dried
   chilli flakes (optional)

NON-FAST DAYS
Serve the meatballs with small
portions of wholegrain pasta,
or bean, lentil or pea pasta,
and sprinkle with a little grated
Parmesan. Serve the Moroccan-
style version (see cook's tip)
with a few tablespoons of
quinoa or brown rice.

COOK'S TIP
For a Moroccan-style version
of the recipe, with 300cals
per serving, fry the onion with
1 diced pepper for 5 minutes
then add 1 teaspoon ground
cumin and fry for a few seconds
before adding 1 tablespoon
harissa paste and 6 quartered
dried apricots, as well as the
tomatoes, water, oregano
and chilli. Finish with a
generous scattering of
freshly chopped coriander.

You can make this dish with the classic Mediterranean
flavours suggested here, or give it a more exotic
Moroccan taste (see cook's tip). Serve with a large
helping of lightly cooked courgetti (see page 106)
and a leafy salad.

1. Preheat the oven to 200°C/Fan 180°C/Gas 6.

2. Place the meatballs on a baking tray and cook in the oven
for 10 minutes.

3. Meanwhile, place the oil in a large frying pan over a
medium heat. Add the onion and fry gently for 5 minutes,
or until softened and lightly browned, stirring regularly.
Add the garlic and cook for a few seconds more, stirring.

4. Tip the tomatoes into the pan, add 200ml water, the
oregano and chilli, if using, and bring to a gentle simmer.
Cook for 5 minutes, stirring.

5. Remove the meatballs from the oven and transfer to
the tomato sauce. Season with salt and freshly ground
black pepper, and cook for a further 5 minutes, or until
the meatballs are thoroughly cooked. Stir regularly and
add a splash of water, if the sauce thickens too much.

AIR-FRYER TIP
To cook the meatballs in an air fryer: preheat the
air fryer to 180°C, if needed. Air fry the meatballs for
8 minutes, turning halfway, until browned. Continue
with the recipe as above.

GLUTEN FREE   NUT FREE   DAIRY FREE

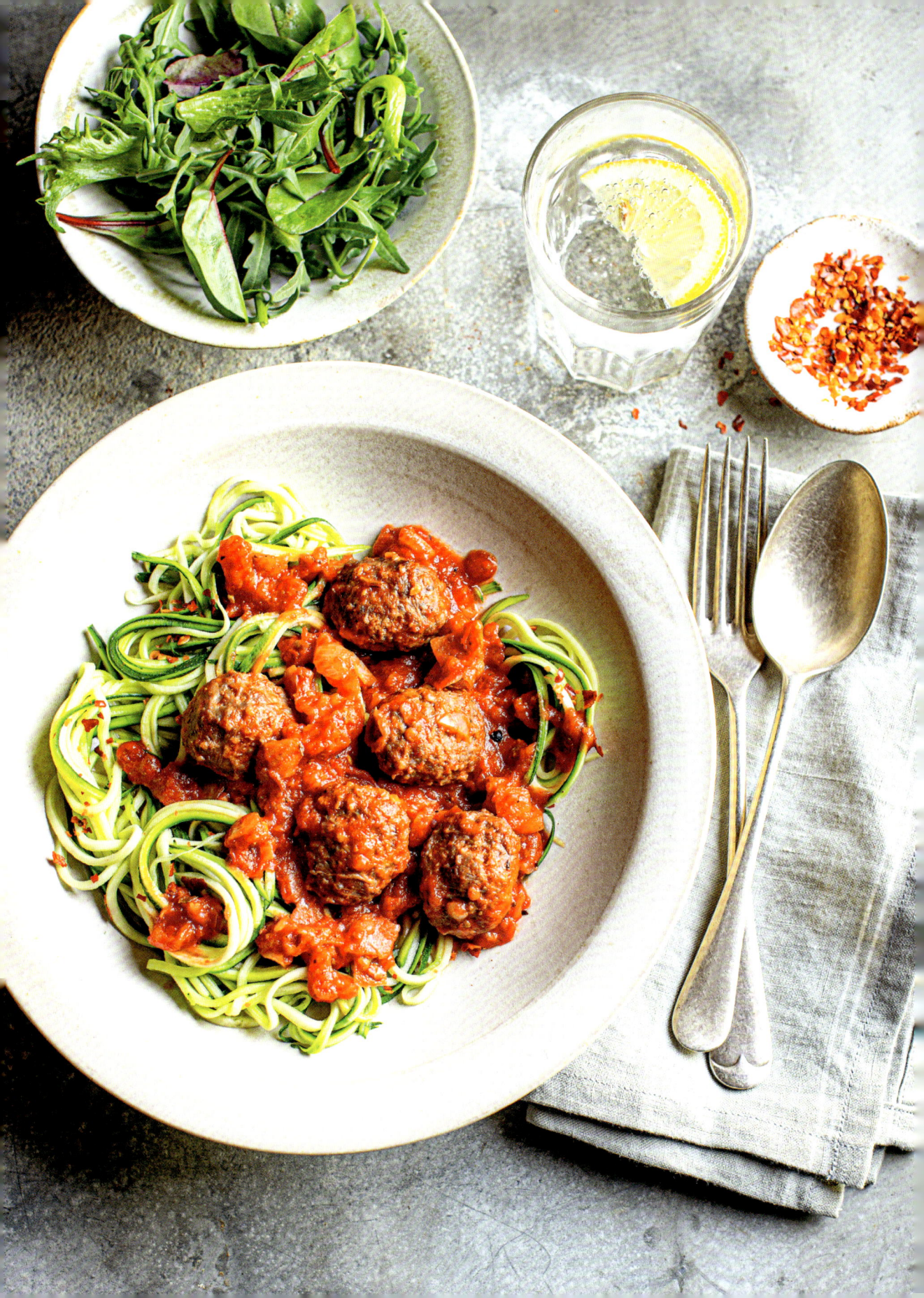

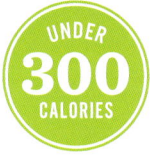

PER SERVING | **288cals** | PROTEIN **34g** | CARBS **1g**

Pork with Mustard and Cider Vinegar

SERVES | **PREP** | **COOK**
2 | **5** mins | **10** mins

1 tbsp olive oil
300g pork medallions, or
   trimmed tenderloin fillet,
   and cut into 6 slices
2 tsp wholegrain mustard
2 tbsp full-fat crème fraîche
1 tbsp apple cider vinegar
10g fresh parsley,
   leaves finely chopped

COOK'S TIP
If you don't like pork,
you could use sliced,
skinless chicken breast
fillets (around 150g)
instead. Made with
chicken, this dish will
have 267cals and 37g
protein per serving.

This family favourite proved a hit on our Channel 4 series *Lose a Stone in 21 Days* and on Instagram, too, where we cooked it with pork steaks, rather than tenderloin. It's simple and luxurious, and Michael thoroughly enjoyed it.

1. Heat the oil in a small frying pan over a moderate heat. Season the pork with salt and freshly ground black pepper, and cook for 3–4 minutes, or until starting to brown. Turn and fry on the other side for a further 3–4 minutes, or until just cooked through.

2. Meanwhile, mix together the mustard, crème fraîche and vinegar in a small bowl. Add half the parsley, a pinch of salt and a generous amount of freshly ground black pepper.

3. Reduce the heat under the pan and pour the mustard sauce over the pork. Stir to incorporate any cooking juices. Add a splash of water and simmer for 1–2 minutes, or until the sauce is hot, stirring occasionally.

4. Remove from the heat, scatter the remaining parsley over the top and serve with mounds of freshly cooked green veg.

GLUTEN FREE | NUT FREE

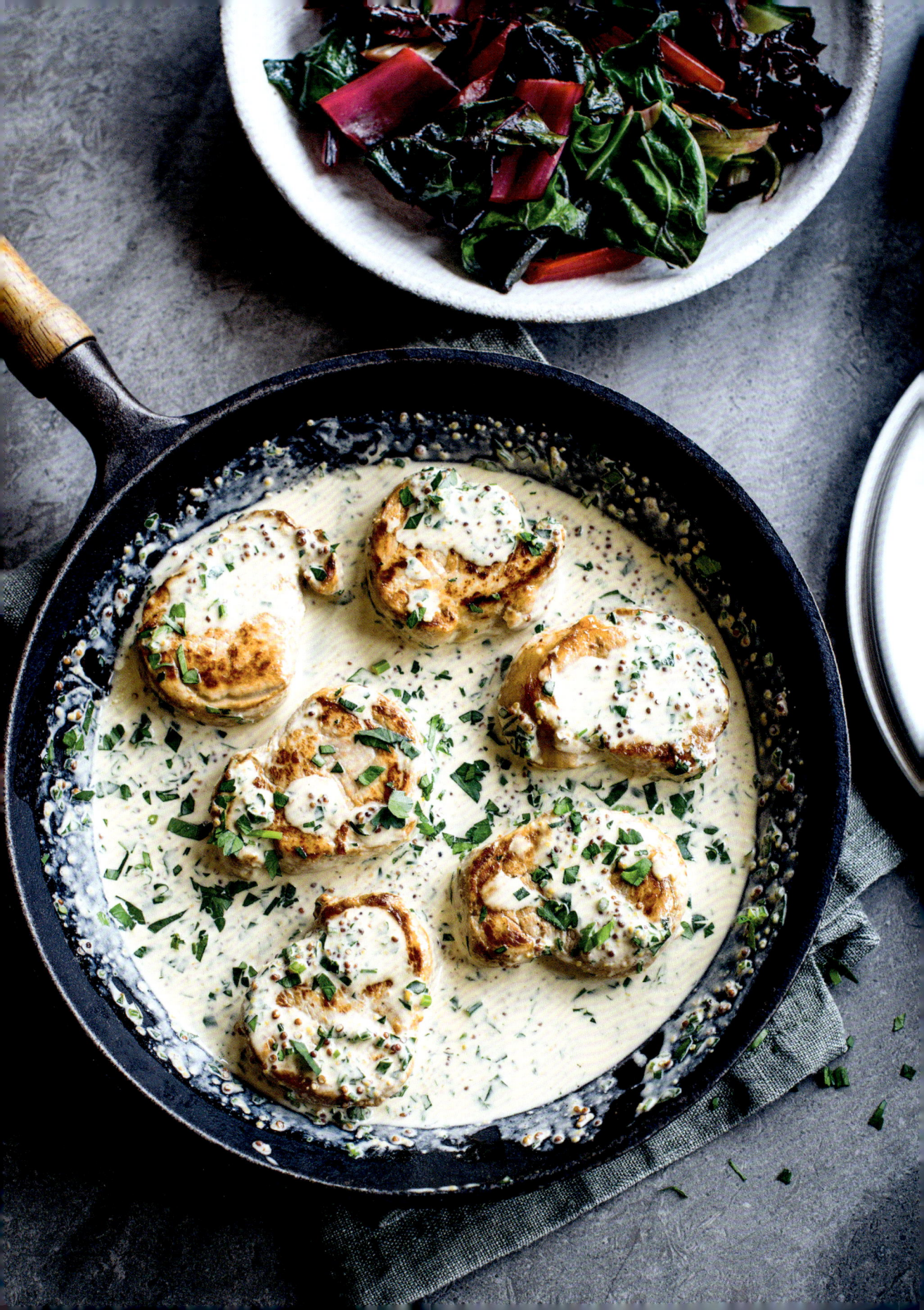

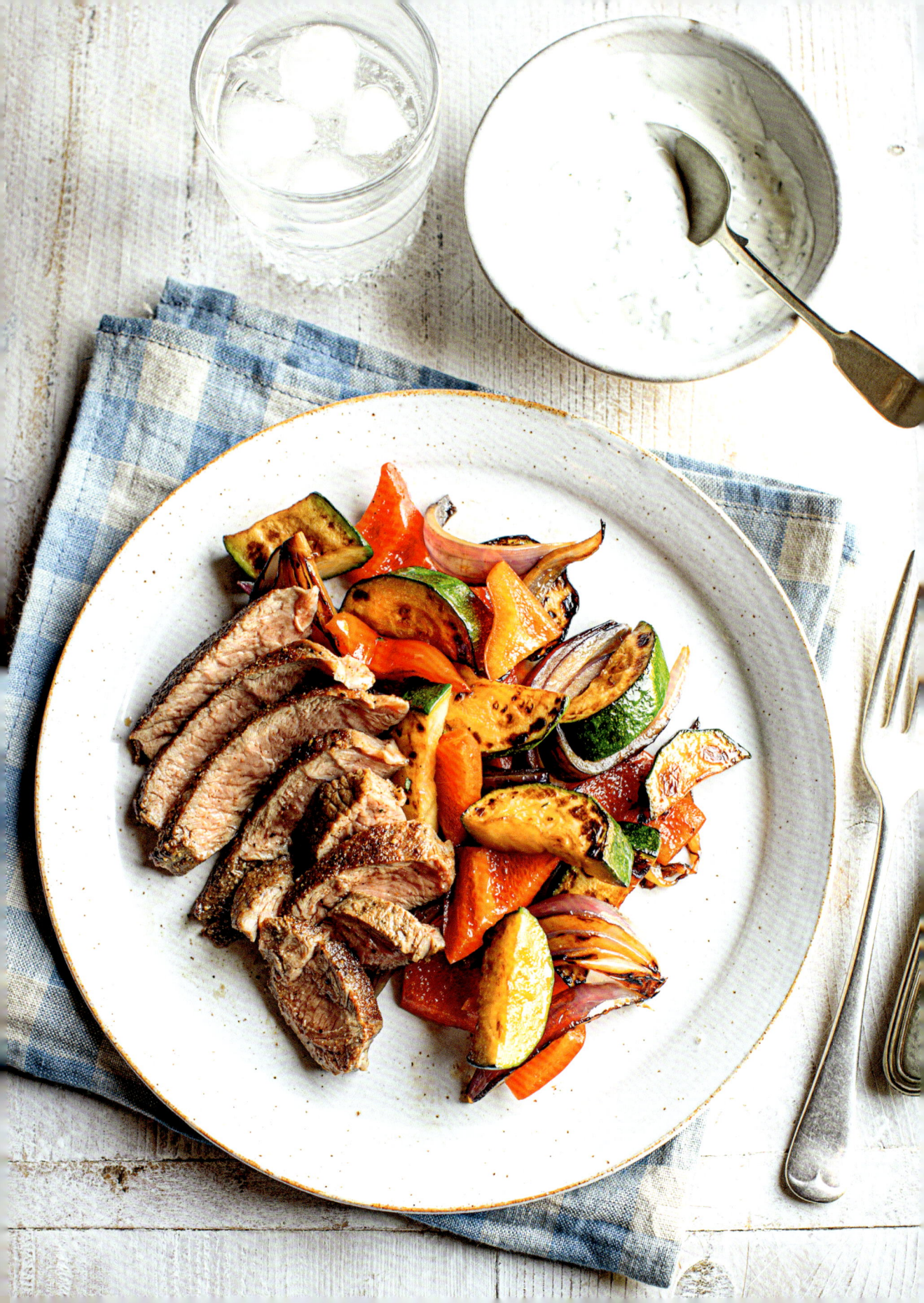

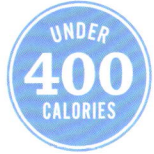

Spiced Lamb and Minted Yoghurt

SERVES **2** | PREP **15** mins | COOK **12** mins

½ tsp ground cumin
½ tsp ground coriander
2 lean boneless lamb leg steaks
    (each around 100g)
2 tbsp olive oil
1 red onion, cut into 12 wedges
1 pepper, any colour,
    deseeded and cut into
    roughly 3cm chunks
1 courgette, trimmed, halved
    lengthways and cut into
    roughly 1.5cm slices

For the minted yoghurt
100g full-fat live
    Greek yoghurt
½ small garlic clove,
    finely grated
2 tbsp finely chopped
    mint leaves

NON-FAST DAYS
Take the lamb steaks out of
the pan once cooked and add
200g canned chickpeas to
the vegetables. Stir fry for
a couple of minutes until hot.

A classic combination of spice-crusted lamb
with colourful Mediterranean vegetables.

1. Mix the cumin, coriander, a pinch of salt and lots
of freshly ground black pepper on a plate. Coat the lamb
steaks on both sides with the spice mix, then set aside.

2. To make the minted yoghurt, combine the yoghurt,
garlic and mint in a small bowl and add just enough
cold water to make a drizzly consistency.

3. Heat 1 tablespoon of the oil in a large frying pan over
a low heat. Add the onion, pepper and courgette, and fry
gently for 4–5 minutes, stirring regularly.

4. Push all the vegetables to one side of the pan, add the
remaining oil and fry the steaks over a medium heat for
3–4 minutes on each side, or until done to taste. (Turn the
vegetables occasionally while the lamb is cooking so they
don't burn.)

5. Leave to stand for 5 minutes, then divide between
two plates and drizzle with the minted yoghurt to serve.

AIR-FRYER TIP

Preheat the air fryer to 180°C, if needed. Toss the
prepared vegetables in 1½ tablespoons of the olive
oil and season. Air fry for 18 minutes, turning halfway
(you may need to cook them in batches). Meanwhile,
prepare the lamb as Step 1 and the minted yoghurt as
Step 2. Remove the vegetables and keep warm. Turn the
air fryer to 190°C. Drizzle the lamb with the remaining
oil and air fry for 4–5 minutes on each side, or until done
to taste. Leave to rest for 5 minutes before serving as
above. (Note: If you have a large air fryer, you may be
able to cook the vegetables and lamb together on 190°C.
Cook the for 16–18 minutes.)

GLUTEN FREE   NUT FREE

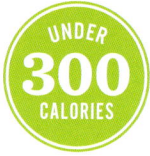

Classic Burger with Celeriac Chips

SERVES | PREP | COOK
4 | **15** mins | **30** mins

½ onion, coarsely grated
    or very finely chopped
1 garlic clove, finely grated
1 carrot (around 100g),
    trimmed and finely grated
400g lean minced beef
    (around 10% fat)
½ tsp flaked sea salt
½ tsp dried mixed herbs

For the celeriac chips
750g celeriac, peeled
    (around 600g peeled weight)
1 tbsp olive or rapeseed oil

NON-FAST DAYS
Top the burgers with
slices of blue cheese
and pop under the grill.

COOK'S TIP
We use a few cherry
tomatoes in the salad for
colour, but any more than
that and you would need
to include the calories
if you are on a fast day.

Adding grated carrot to burgers makes them extra juicy and boosts the fibre. Michael still indulged in the occasional protein-packed burger, and swapped starchy potato for celeriac chips.

1. Preheat the oven to 220°C/Fan 200°C/Gas 7.

2. To make the celeriac chips, carefully cut the celeriac into roughly 1.5cm slices, then into chips. Place in a bowl with the oil, some salt and lots of freshly ground black pepper. Toss well. Scatter over a baking tray and bake for 20 minutes. Turn the chips and return to the oven for a further 5–10 minutes, or until tender and lightly browned.

3. Meanwhile, put the onion, garlic, carrot, beef, salt and dried mixed herbs in a bowl, season with lots of ground black pepper and combine thoroughly with your hands.

4. Divide the mixture into 4 balls and flatten into burger shapes. Make them a little flatter than you think they should be, as they will shrink as they cook.

5. Place a large frying pan over a medium heat. Add the burgers and cook for 10 minutes, or until lightly browned and cooked through, turning occasionally.

6. Divide the chips between four warmed plates and serve a burger alongside.

AIR-FRYER TIP

To cook the chips in an air fryer: preheat the air fryer to 200°C. Prepare the celeriac as Step 2, and air fry for 13–15 minutes, turning halfway, until tender and lightly browned.

GLUTEN FREE | NUT FREE | DAIRY FREE

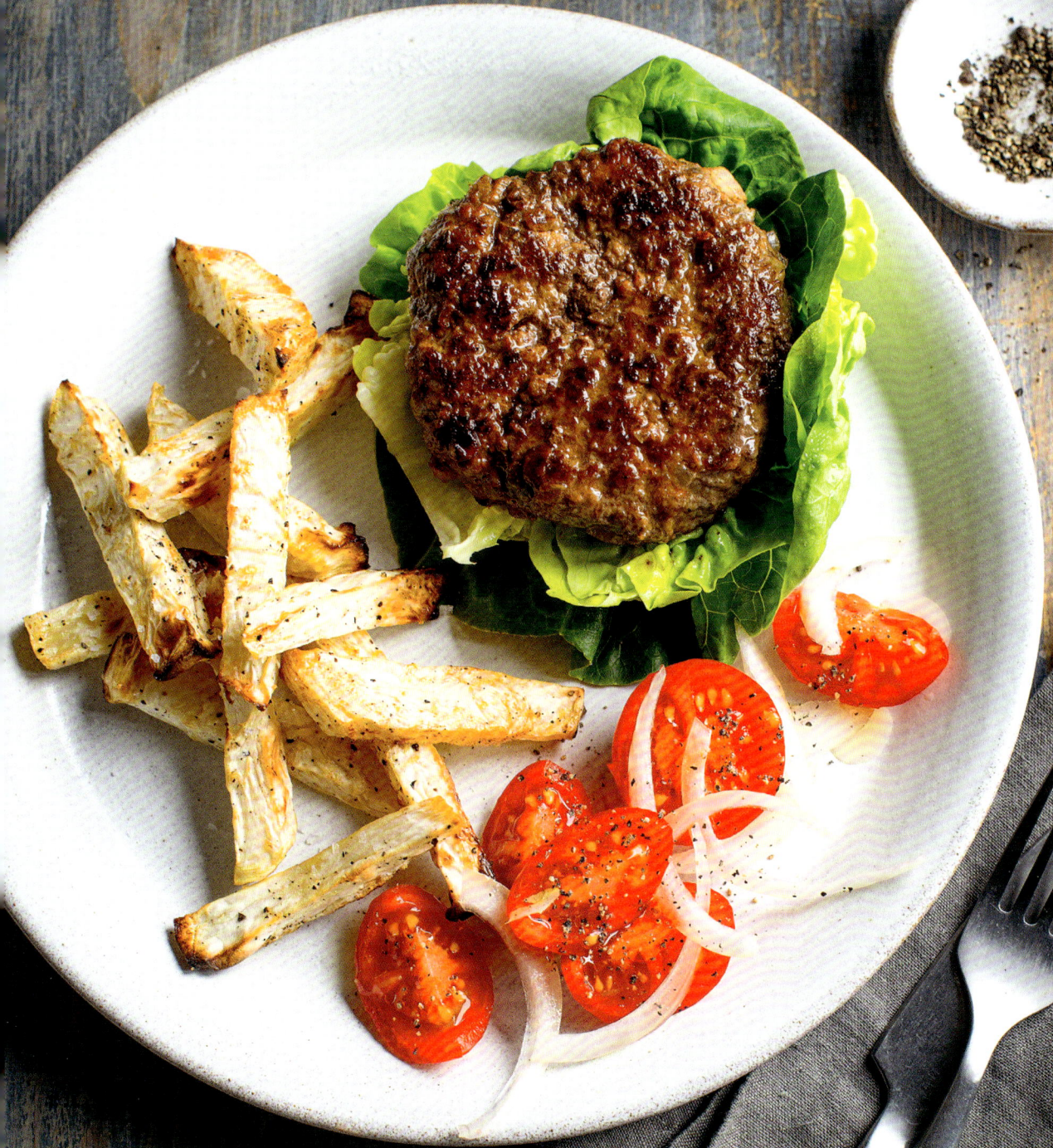

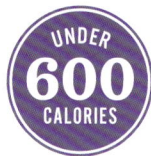

PER SERVING | **525cals** | PROTEIN **22.7g** | CARBS **15.2g**

One-pan Sausage Casserole

SERVES | PREP | COOK
2 | **10** mins | **10** mins

4 good-quality sausages
   (around 270g total weight)
2 tbsp olive oil
½ onion, thinly sliced
200g butternut squash,
   peeled and cut into
   1cm pieces
½ tsp dried thyme
150g cavolo nero, central stalks
   removed and leaves sliced
1 tbsp apple cider vinegar
½ tsp crushed dried chilli
   flakes (optional)

NON-FAST DAY
Increase the portion size and/
or serve with 2–3 tablespoons
cooked pearl barley or quinoa.

Oh, the joy of easy one-pan cooking!

1. Use a knife to split the skin on each sausage and discard.
Cut the sausage meat into 2cm pieces.

2. Heat the oil in a large frying pan over a high heat and
add the sausage pieces, onion and squash. Cook for a few
minutes until slightly browned.

3. Reduce the heat to medium, stir in the thyme and cook
for 3 minutes. Add the greens, cider vinegar and chilli, if
using, and cook for a final 4 minutes to soften the greens.
Season with salt and freshly ground black pepper to taste.

GLUTEN FREE | NUT FREE | DAIRY FREE

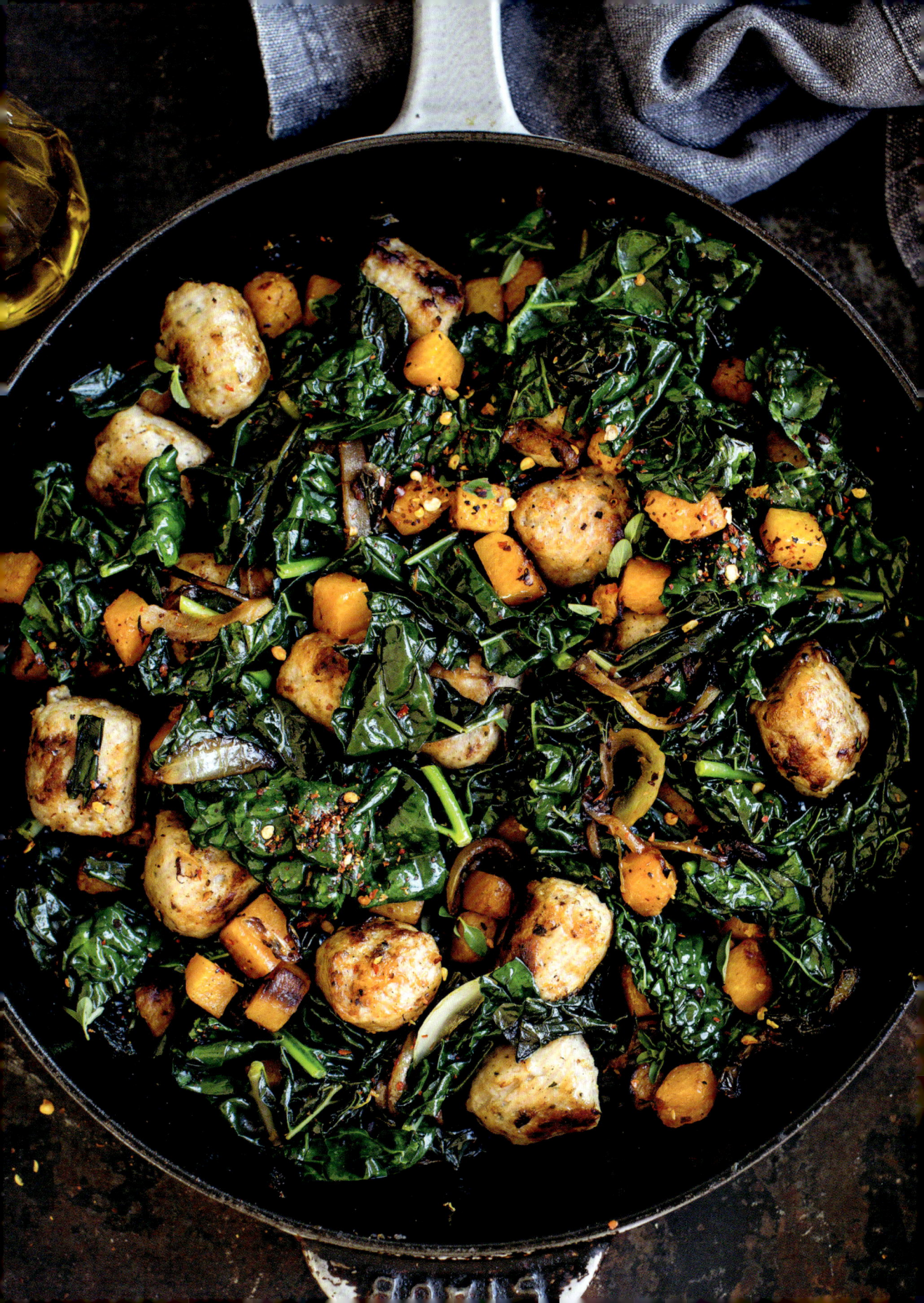

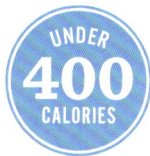

| PER SERVING | **346cals** | PROTEIN **30g** | CARBS **5g**

Simple Steak and Salad

SERVES | PREP | COOK
2 | **10** mins | **10** mins

1 × 225g lean sirloin beef
  steak, cut in half
1 tbsp olive oil
150g button chestnut
  mushrooms, halved
  or sliced if large

For the salad
100g mixed leaves
½ yellow pepper,
  deseeded and sliced
10 cherry tomatoes, halved
⅓ cucumber (around 135g),
  sliced
2 spring onions, trimmed
  and finely sliced

For the balsamic dressing
2 tbsp extra-virgin olive oil
2 tsp balsamic vinegar

NON-FAST DAYS
Serve with roasted butternut
squash wedges, add a generous
spoonful of full-fat crème
fraîche to the mushrooms
just before the end of their
cooking time and double up
on the dressing ingredients.

A juicy steak with a colourful dressed salad is
a fantastic, easy, low-carb combination, which
provides a good protein boost on a fast day.

1. To make the salad, toss all the ingredients in a bowl.

2. Season the beef all over with salt and lots of freshly
ground black pepper.

3. Heat the oil in a large frying pan over a medium–high
heat. Add the steaks and fry for 3–4 minutes on each side,
or until done to taste. Place the steaks on two warmed
plates and leave to rest.

4. Add the mushrooms to the pan and cook for
2–3 minutes, or until browned, stirring regularly.
Spoon on top of the steaks.

5. Drizzle the oil and vinegar over the salad and toss
lightly. Serve alongside the steak and mushrooms.

GLUTEN FREE · NUT FREE · DAIRY FREE

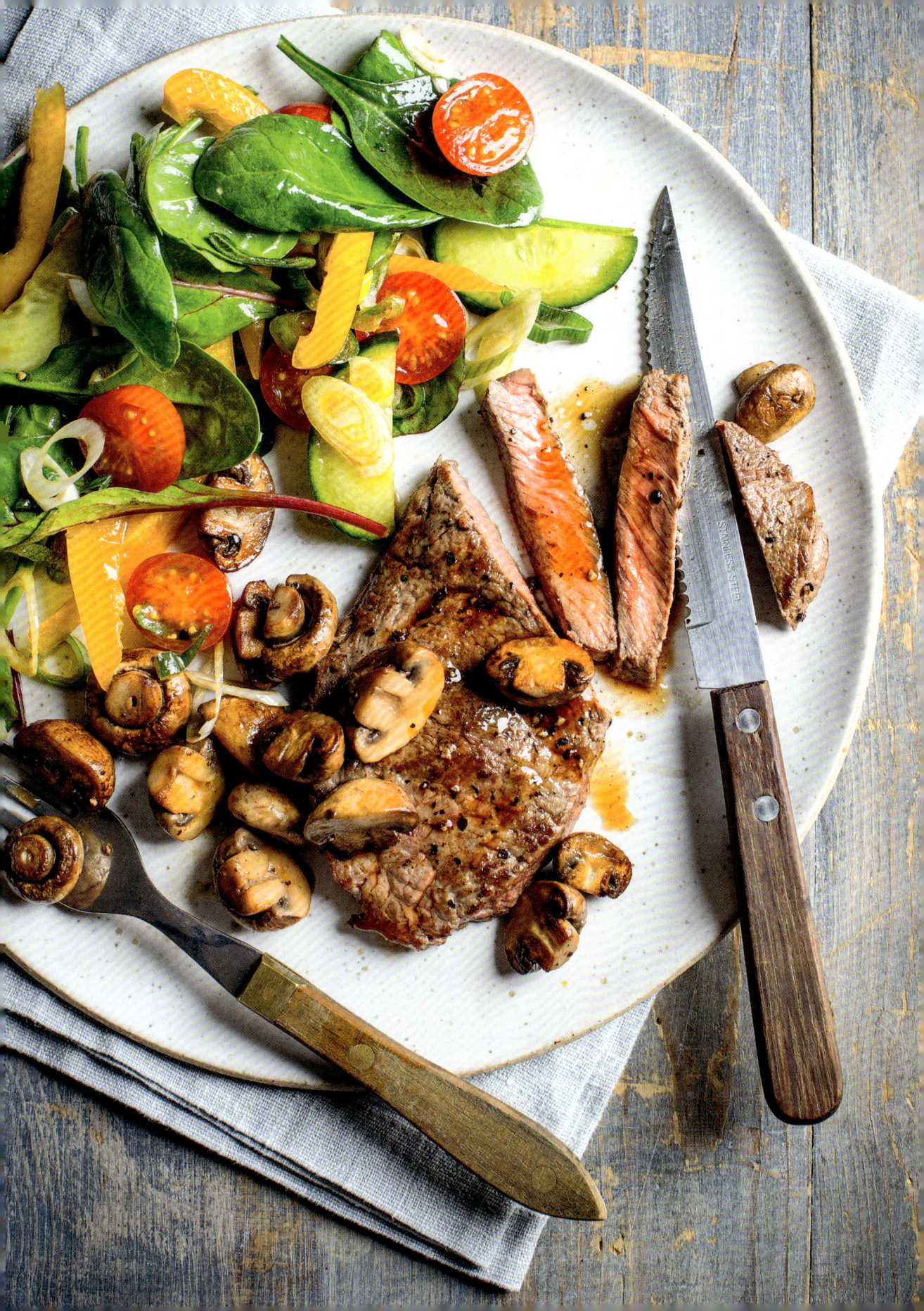

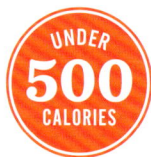

PER SERVING | **482cals** | PROTEIN **39.6g** | CARBS **19.3g**

Navarin of Lamb with Mangetout

SERVES	PREP	COOK
2	**10** mins	**105** mins

2 tbsp olive oil
350g diced lamb shoulder
1 red onion, sliced
2 garlic cloves, finely chopped
6 thyme sprigs, leaves
    picked (or 1 tsp dried)
1 tbsp tomato purée
1 beef stock cube
250g butternut squash,
    peeled and sliced
100g mangetout

NON-FAST DAY
Increase the portion size and
serve with 2–3 tablespoons
wholegrains, such as pearl
barley or bulgur wheat.

Traditionally a navarin of lamb is made using root vegetables. Here, lighter, less starchy spring vegetables are used instead – you could also try green beans, runner beans or sliced Savoy cabbage. A deeply satisfying stew which is easy to put together.

1. Preheat the oven to 180°C/Fan 160°C/Gas 4.

2. Place ½ tablespoon of the oil in a heavy-based medium ovenproof saucepan that has a lid over a high heat. When hot, place a single layer of diced lamb in the pan (it is important not to overcrowd the pan, or the meat will stew). Brown the meat for a couple of minutes, then turn. Remove the meat from the pan and repeat with the remaining lamb and another ½ tablespoon of the oil. Remove the second batch and set aside.

3. Add the remaining oil to the pan and stir in the onion. Reduce the heat, add a splash of water, cover with a lid and sweat for 3 minutes. Add the garlic and thyme and cook uncovered for 30 seconds. Stir in the tomato purée, crumble in the stock cube and pour in 400ml water. Return the lamb to the pan, bring to a simmer, then cover with the lid and transfer to the oven for 1½ hours. Halfway through the cooking time, add the butternut squash and season with salt and freshly ground black pepper.

4. Remove from the oven and add the mangetout – the heat from the stew will be enough to cook them.

GLUTEN FREE · NUT FREE · DAIRY FREE · ❄

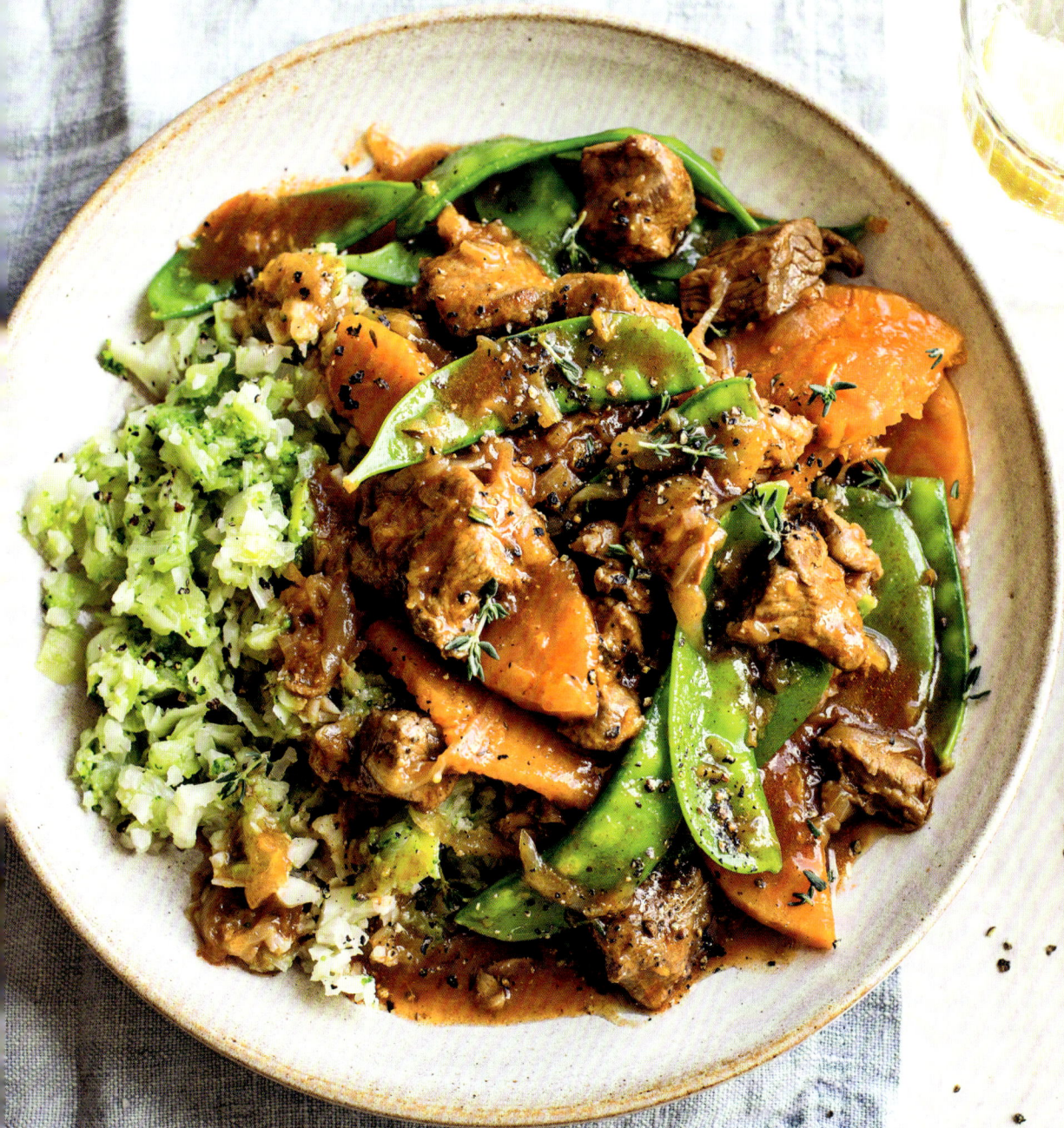

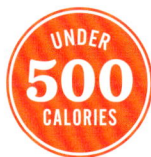

PER SERVING | **415cals** | PROTEIN **38.9g** | CARBS **6.8g**

Tandoori Lamb Cutlets with Garlic and Ginger Spinach

SERVES **2** | PREP **10** mins | COOK **12** mins

2 tbsp full-fat live Greek
  yoghurt
1 tbsp tandoori powder
4 lamb chops
  (around 75g each)
1 tbsp olive oil
1 garlic clove,
  roughly chopped
10g fresh root ginger,
  peeled and grated
350g young spinach leaves
15g cashew nuts,
  roughly chopped

NON-FAST DAY
Increase the portion
size and serve with
2–3 tablespoons cooked
wholegrains, such as
brown rice.

Thanks to tandoori seasoning, lamb chops just got more interesting. This is a simple dish packed with flavour.

1. Preheat the grill to its highest setting and line a baking tray with non-stick baking paper.

2. Mix the yoghurt with the tandoori powder in a large bowl and season with salt and freshly ground black pepper. Add the lamb chops and toss to coat. Place on the prepared baking tray and cook under the grill for 6 minutes on each side. Set aside to rest for a couple of minutes.

3. Meanwhile, place the olive oil in a large frying pan over a medium heat. Add the garlic and ginger, and sauté for 1 minute. Add the spinach and stir to wilt the leaves – this will take 1–2 minutes. Season and keep warm.

4. Divide the spinach between two warm plates, scatter the cashew nuts all over and place the lamb chops on top to serve.

GLUTEN FREE   NUT FREE

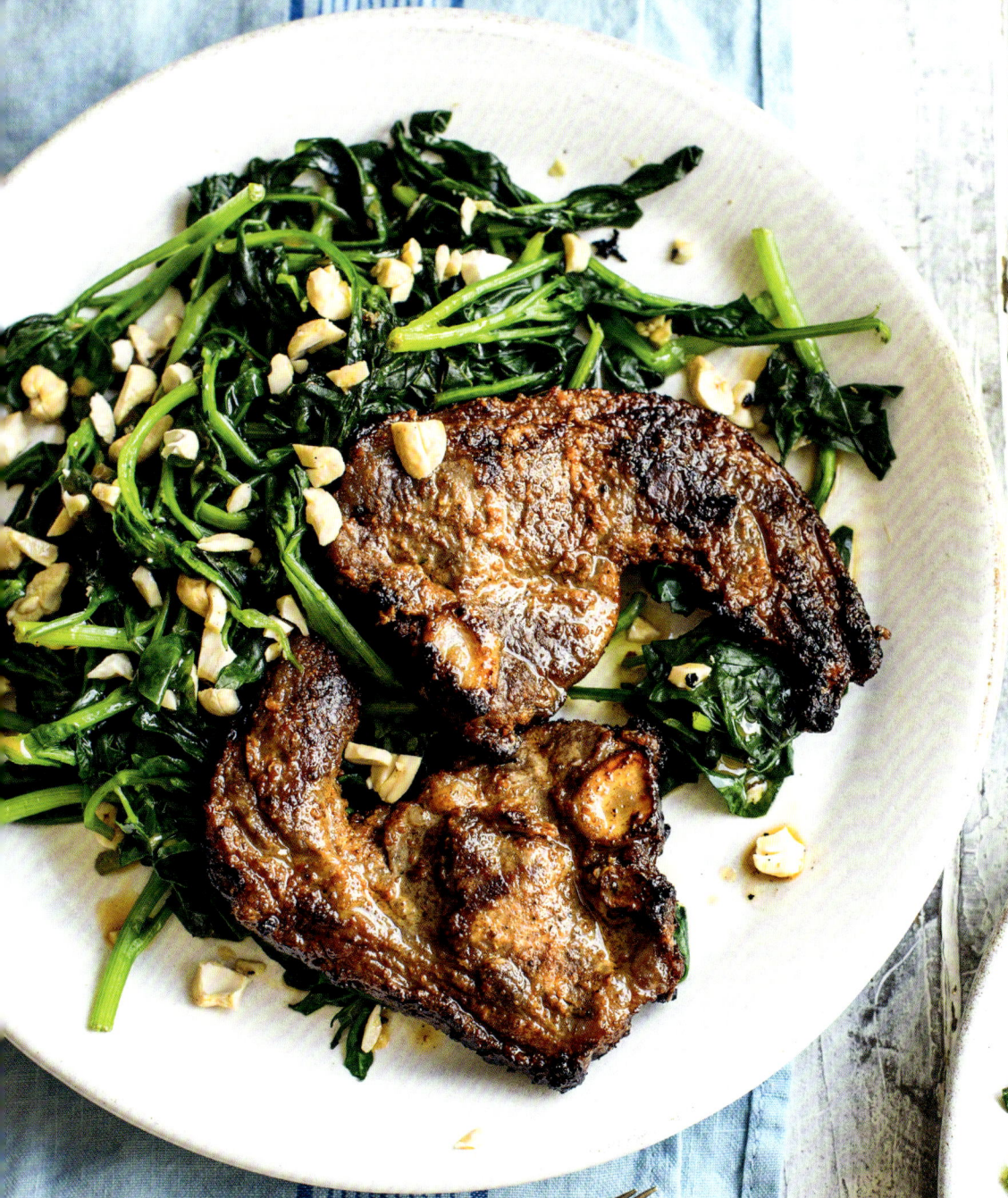

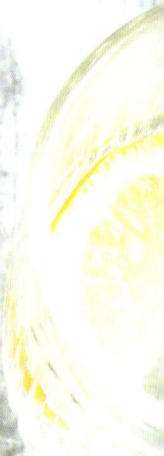

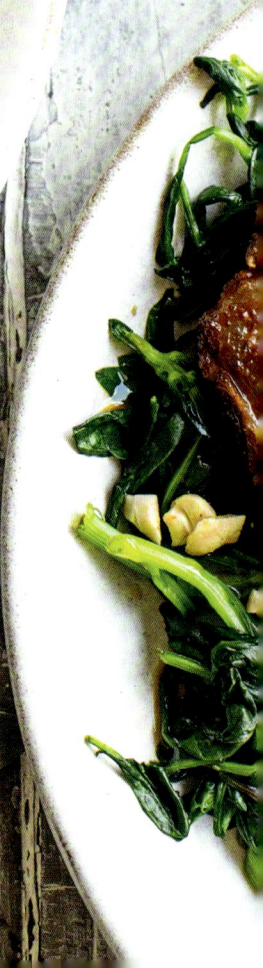

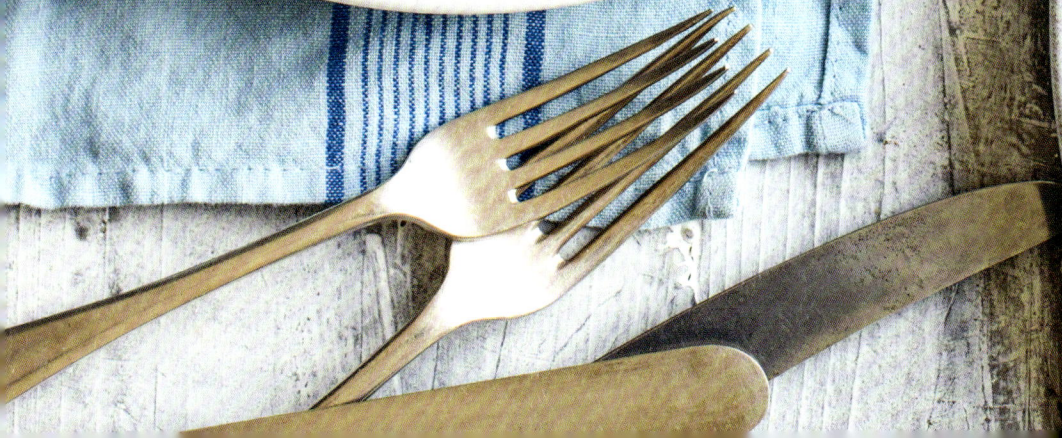

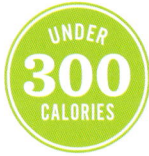

Beef and Black Bean Stir Fry

SERVES **2** | PREP **10** mins | COOK **8** mins

250g beef frying steak,
    trimmed and cut into
    1.5cm thin strips
1 tbsp olive or rapeseed oil
1 onion, cut into thin wedges
2 small peppers, any colour,
    deseeded and cut into
    1.5cm slices
1 garlic clove, finely chopped
10g fresh root ginger,
    peeled and cut into
    thin matchsticks
3 tbsp black bean stir-fry
    sauce, from a jar or sachet
    (around 40g)
1 red chilli, finely sliced, or
    1 tsp crushed dried chilli
    flakes, to serve (optional)

COOK'S TIP
Frying steak from
the supermarket is
less expensive than
a premium cut, but
you could use sirloin
or rump steak instead.

Stir fries were particularly popular with Michael, as they are speedy and full of flavour. As a cheat, you can swap the veg for a packet of supermarket, ready-prepared stir-fry veggies.

1. Season the beef well with a little salt and lots of freshly ground black pepper.

2. Heat 2 teaspoons of the oil in a large frying pan or wok over a high heat. Add the beef and stir fry for 1 minute, or until lightly browned but not cooked through. Transfer the beef to a plate and set aside.

3. Return the pan to the heat and add the remaining oil, onion and peppers, and stir fry for 4 minutes, or until just softened. Add the garlic and ginger, and cook for 1 minute more.

4. Pour over the black bean sauce, then return the beef to the pan. Add 4 tablespoons cold water and cook for 1–2 minutes, or until the beef is hot and glossy, stirring regularly.

5. Scatter the chilli over the top, if using, and serve with steamed sliced cabbage or courgetti (see page 106).

GLUTEN FREE · NUT FREE · DAIRY FREE

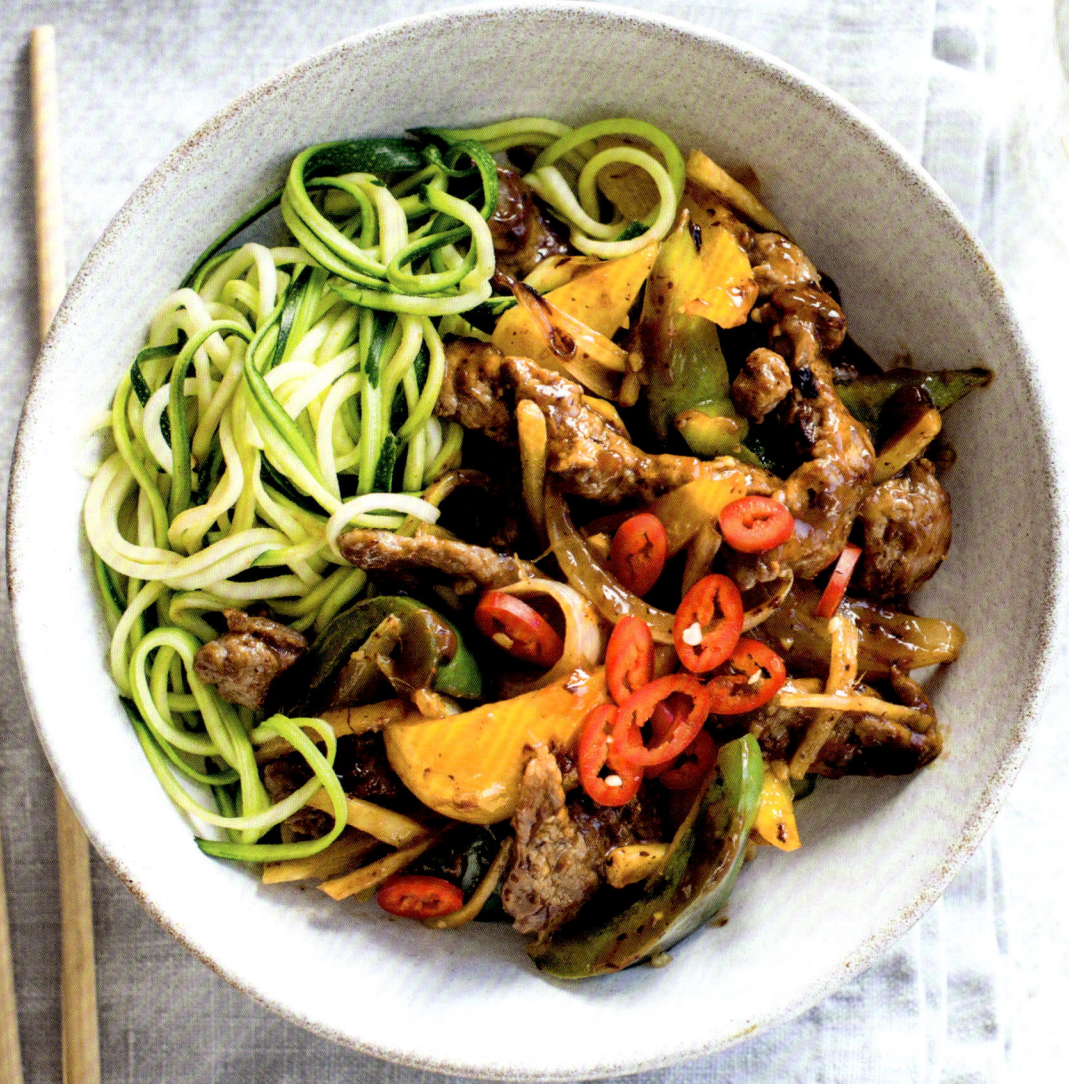

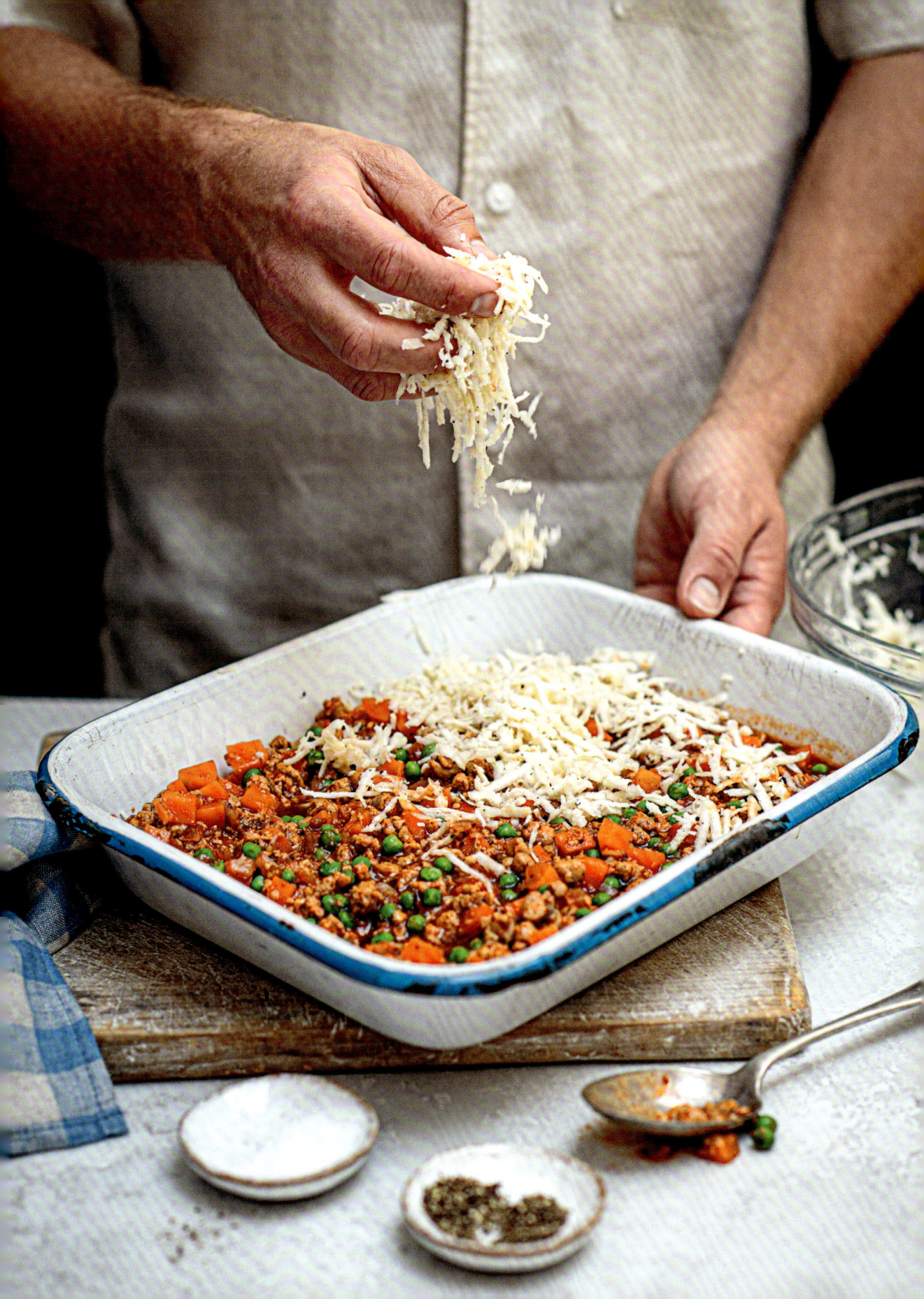

Meat-free

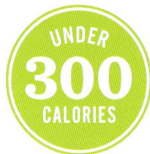

Garlic and Herb Stuffed Mushrooms

SERVES	PREP	COOK
2	**10** mins	**15** mins

1 tbsp olive oil, plus
   extra for greasing
4 large, flat mushrooms,
   such as Portobello
25g wholegrain breadcrumbs
25g ground almonds
10g Parmesan, finely grated
85g medium-fat garlic
   and herb soft cheese
   (such as Philadelphia)
small handful fresh thyme
   leaves (optional)

NON-FAST DAYS
Increase the portion size.
Sprinkle the mushrooms
with a couple of tablespoons
of flaked almonds before
baking. Drizzle with olive
oil to serve.

COOK'S TIP
To make your own crumbs,
simply blitz some wholegrain
bread in a food processor.
Any extra can be frozen
for another time.

A lovely light lunch or supper. Mushrooms are low
in starchy carbs and have been found to reduce the
risk of cognitive decline. Serve with a generous mixed
leaf salad, drizzled with a little balsamic vinegar.

1. Preheat the oven to 200°C/Fan 180°C/Gas 6 and lightly
grease a small baking tray.

2. Twist the stalk out of each mushroom and place the
mushrooms, dark-side up, on the prepared tray.

3. Mix the breadcrumbs with the almonds and Parmesan
in a small bowl and season with salt and lots of freshly
ground black pepper. Using half the breadcrumbs, sprinkle
some into each mushroom, then dot with small pieces
of the soft cheese. Top with the remaining breadcrumbs,
drizzle with the oil and bake for 12–15 minutes, or until
the mushrooms are tender and the crumbs are crisp.

4. Divide the mushrooms between two plates, sprinkle
with fresh thyme, if using, and serve.

AIR-FRYER TIP

Preheat the air fryer to 180°C, if needed. Prepare
the mushrooms and stuffing as Steps 2–3. Air fry the
mushrooms for 10–13 minutes, or until the mushrooms
are tender and the crumbs are crisp.

VEGGIE

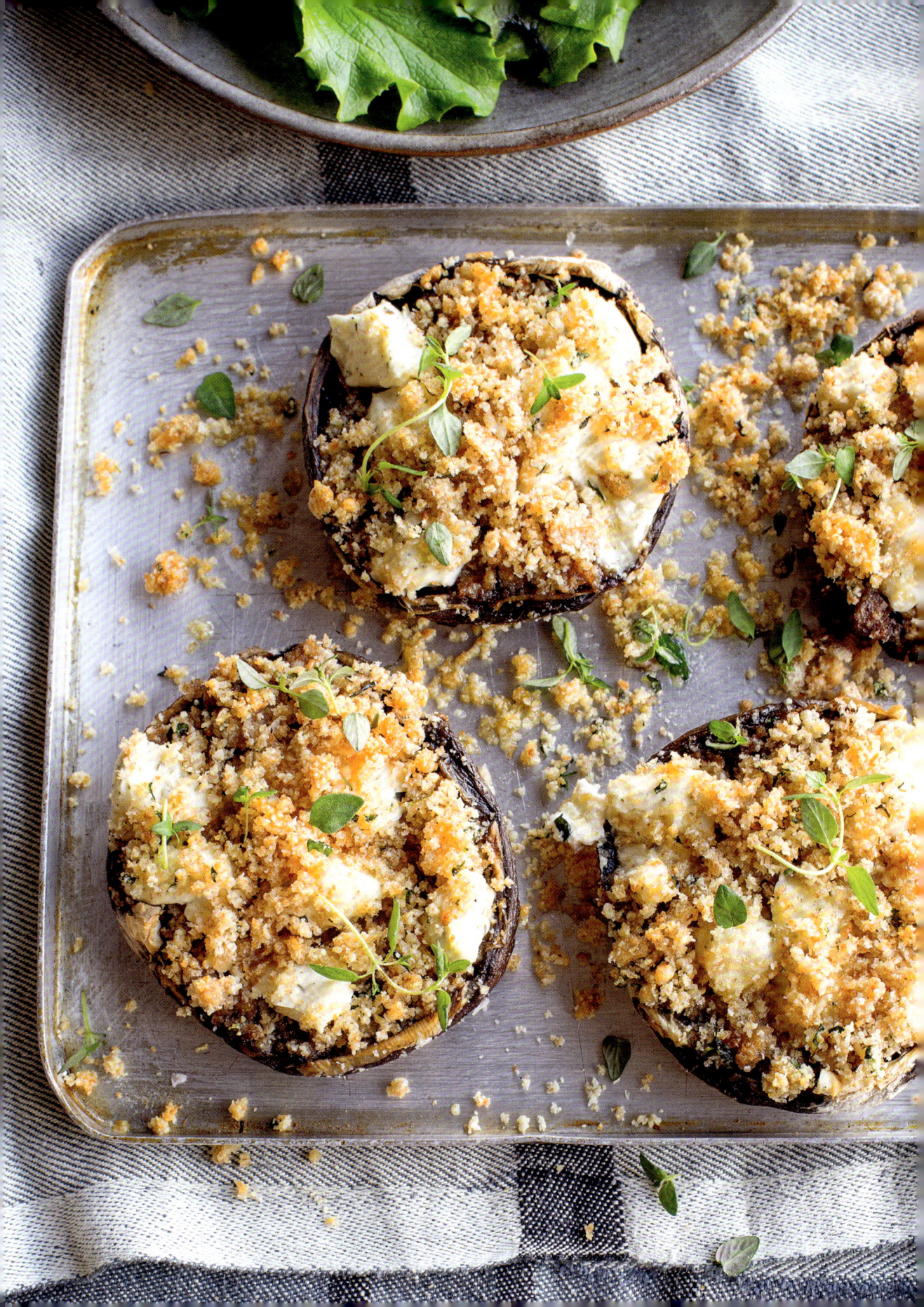

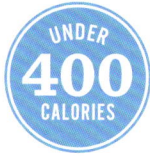

PER SERVING | **346cals** | PROTEIN **18g** | CARBS **26g**

Spicy Bean Chilli

SERVES **4** | PREP **10** mins | COOK **24** mins

2 tbsp olive oil
1 onion, thinly sliced
1–1½ tsp hot smoked paprika
   (to taste)
1 tsp ground cumin
1 tsp ground coriander
1 × 400g can chopped tomatoes
1 × 400g can black beans or
   red kidney beans, drained
1 × 400g can mixed
   beans, drained
300ml vegetable stock
   (made with 1 stock cube)
1 tbsp tomato purée
1 tsp dried oregano
   or mixed dried herbs
75g mature Cheddar, grated
100g full-fat live
   Greek yoghurt

NON-FAST DAYS
Serve with brown rice and top
with sliced avocado. Drizzle the
salad with a No-count dressing
(see pages 88–9), or a splash
of balsamic vinegar and
glug of olive oil.

COOK'S TIP
If you have IBS, you might need
to reduce the bean portions or
skip this recipe. For extra depth
of flavour, add a tablespoon of
cocoa powder (11cals per
serving) with the dried herbs.

A rich, spicy chilli made with a mixture of different beans to give you plenty of fibre and slow-release complex carbs. Your microbiome will love it, too. Serve with a large mixed salad.

1. Heat the oil in a large, deep frying pan, wide-based saucepan or shallow flameproof casserole over a low heat. Add the onion and fry gently for 3–4 minutes, or until softened, stirring frequently. Add the smoked paprika, cumin and coriander, and cook for a few seconds, stirring.

2. Stir in the tomatoes, beans, vegetable stock, tomato purée and dried herbs, season with salt and freshly ground black pepper, and bring to a simmer. Cover loosely with a lid and cook for 15–20 minutes, or until the sauce has reduced and thickened, stirring occasionally.

3. Serve topped with the Cheddar and generous spoonfuls of Greek yoghurt.

VEGGIE · GLUTEN FREE · NUT FREE

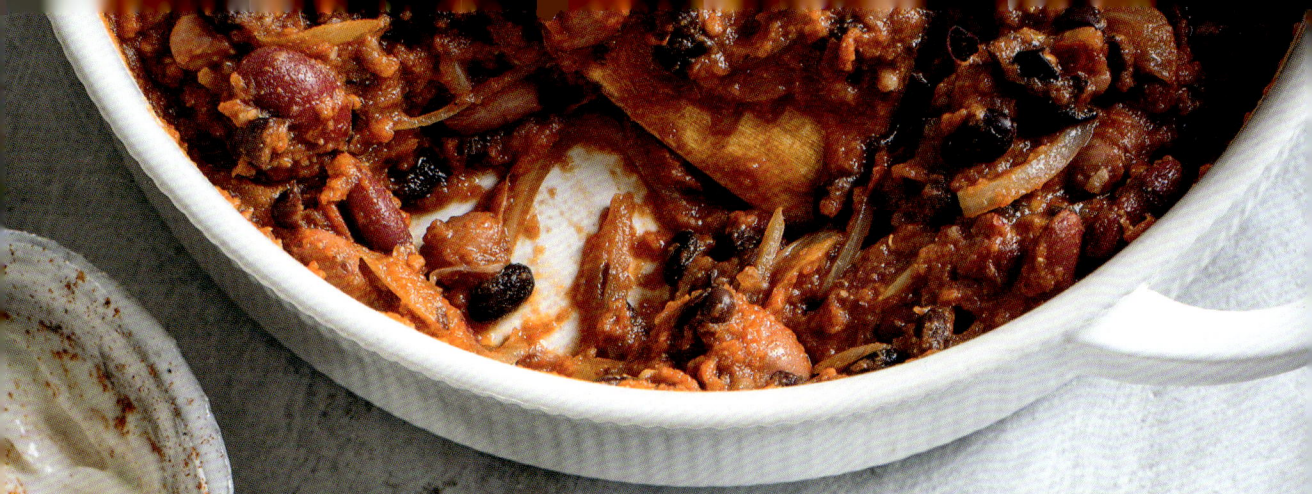

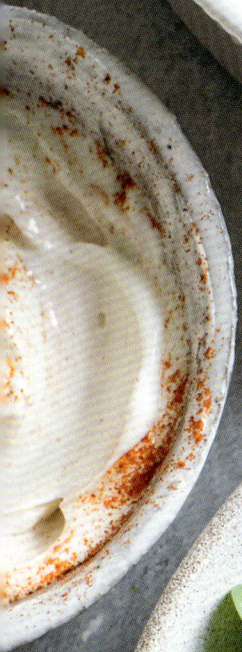

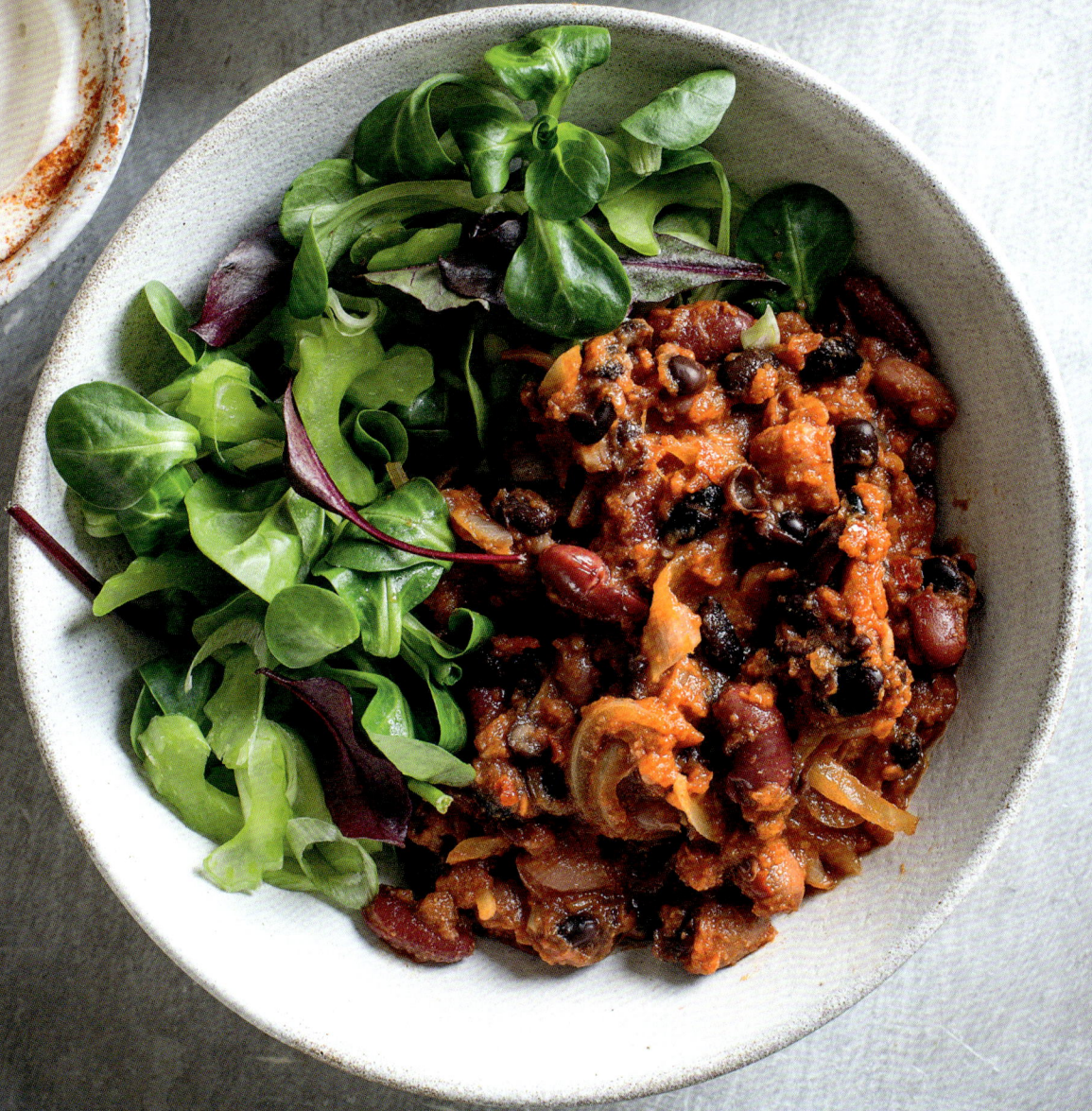

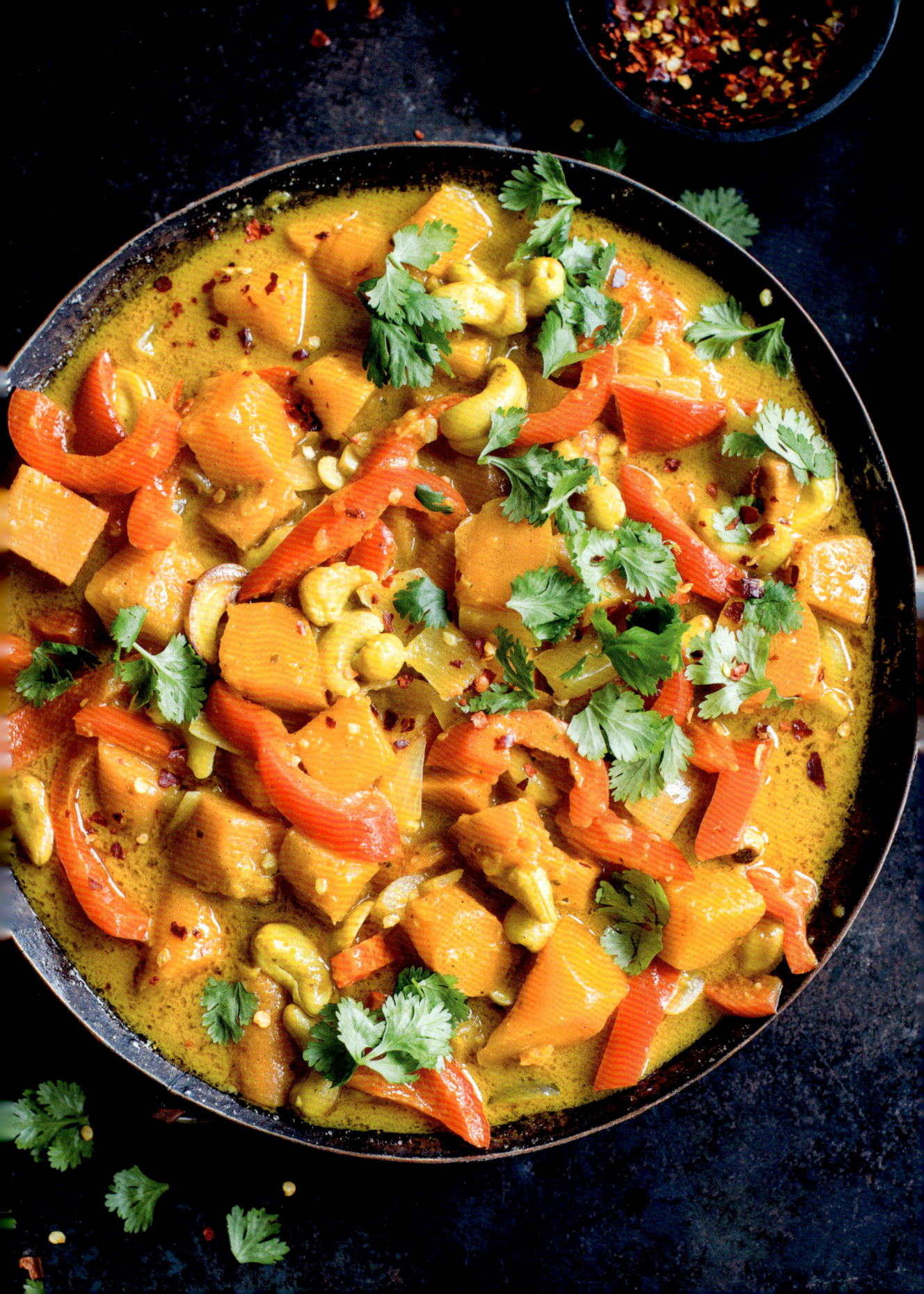

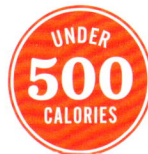

Creamy Cashew and Squash Curry

SERVES **4**

PREP **15** mins

COOK **40** mins

1 tbsp olive, coconut
   or rapeseed oil
1 large onion, roughly chopped
100g cashew nuts
2 large garlic cloves,
   finely chopped
3 tbsp medium Indian
   curry paste
300g butternut squash, peeled
   and cut into 2.5cm chunks
3 medium carrots, trimmed
   and cut into 2.5cm chunks
1 × 400ml can full-fat
   coconut milk
2 peppers, any colour,
   deseeded and sliced
small handful coriander
   leaves, to serve (optional)
small pinch crushed dried
   chilli flakes, to serve
   (optional)

COOK'S TIP
This curry is a great base
for fish or chicken – fry 300g
chicken breast chunks with
the onions in step 1, or add
300g white fish chunks for
the last 5 minutes of the
cooking time.

A vegetable curry packed with golden vegetables
and cashews. Serve with a generous portion of
leafy green veg. If you like a little more heat, stir in
½–1 teaspoon crushed dried chilli flakes for the last
5 minutes of the cooking time. This is an all-round
family favourite and is great for feeding a crowd.

1. Heat the oil in a large, wide-based saucepan over a
medium heat. Add the onion and cashews, and fry for
5 minutes, or until the onion is softened, stirring regularly.

2. Add the garlic and curry paste, and cook for 1 minute,
stirring constantly.

3. Add the squash and carrots, pour over the coconut
milk and refill the can with water. Pour this water into
the pan and stir well. Cover with a lid, bring to a gentle
simmer and cook for about 25 minutes, or until the
vegetables are almost tender, stirring occasionally.

4. Add the peppers, return to a simmer and cook,
uncovered, for a further 5 minutes, stirring once or twice.

5. Season with salt and freshly ground black pepper,
and scatter with fresh coriander and chilli flakes,
if using, to serve.

VEGAN | GLUTEN FREE | DAIRY FREE

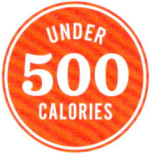

Roasted Vegetable Pasta with Mozzarella

SERVES	PREP	COOK
2	10 mins	35 mins

2 peppers, any colour,
    deseeded and cut into
    roughly 2cm chunks
1 courgette, trimmed,
    quartered lengthways
    and cut into roughly
    2cm chunks
1 large red onion,
    cut into wedges
2 tbsp olive oil
12 cherry tomatoes, halved
½ tsp crushed dried chilli
    flakes (to taste)
50g dried bean, pea, lentil
    or wholewheat penne pasta
50g young spinach leaves
125g mozzarella pearls (mini
    balls), drained and halved

NON-FAST DAYS
Sprinkle 25g lightly toasted
pine nuts or walnuts over
the pasta and serve with
freshly grated Parmesan
and a large mixed salad,
tossed with a No-count
dressing (see pages 88–9).

A comforting, rich dish that's a doddle to prepare. It is best cooked with bean, pea or lentil pasta, which is higher in both protein and fibre, and is available in most supermarkets.

1. Preheat the oven to 200°C/Fan 180°C/Gas 6.

2. Place the peppers, courgette and onion in a large baking tray. Drizzle with the oil, season with salt and lots of freshly ground black pepper and toss together to coat. Roast in the oven for 20 minutes.

3. Remove from the oven and turn all the vegetables. Add the tomatoes and sprinkle with the chilli flakes. Cook for a further 10 minutes, or until lightly browned.

4. Meanwhile, cook the pasta according to the packet instructions, stirring occasionally. Drain the pasta and return to the pan.

5. Add the spinach, roasted vegetables and mozzarella pearls to the pan with the pasta, toss everything together and season with more black pepper. Cook for about 1 minute, stirring, until the mozzarella begins to melt and the spinach wilts.

AIR-FRYER TIP
To cook the vegetables in an air fryer: preheat the air fryer to 180°C, if needed. Place the vegetables in an even layer in the air fryer (you may need to cook them in two batches), drizzle with oil and season. Air fry for 18 minutes. Turn the vegetables, add the tomatoes and chilli flakes. Air fry for another 6–7 minutes, until soft and lightly browned. Continue with the recipe as above.

VEGGIE   NUT FREE

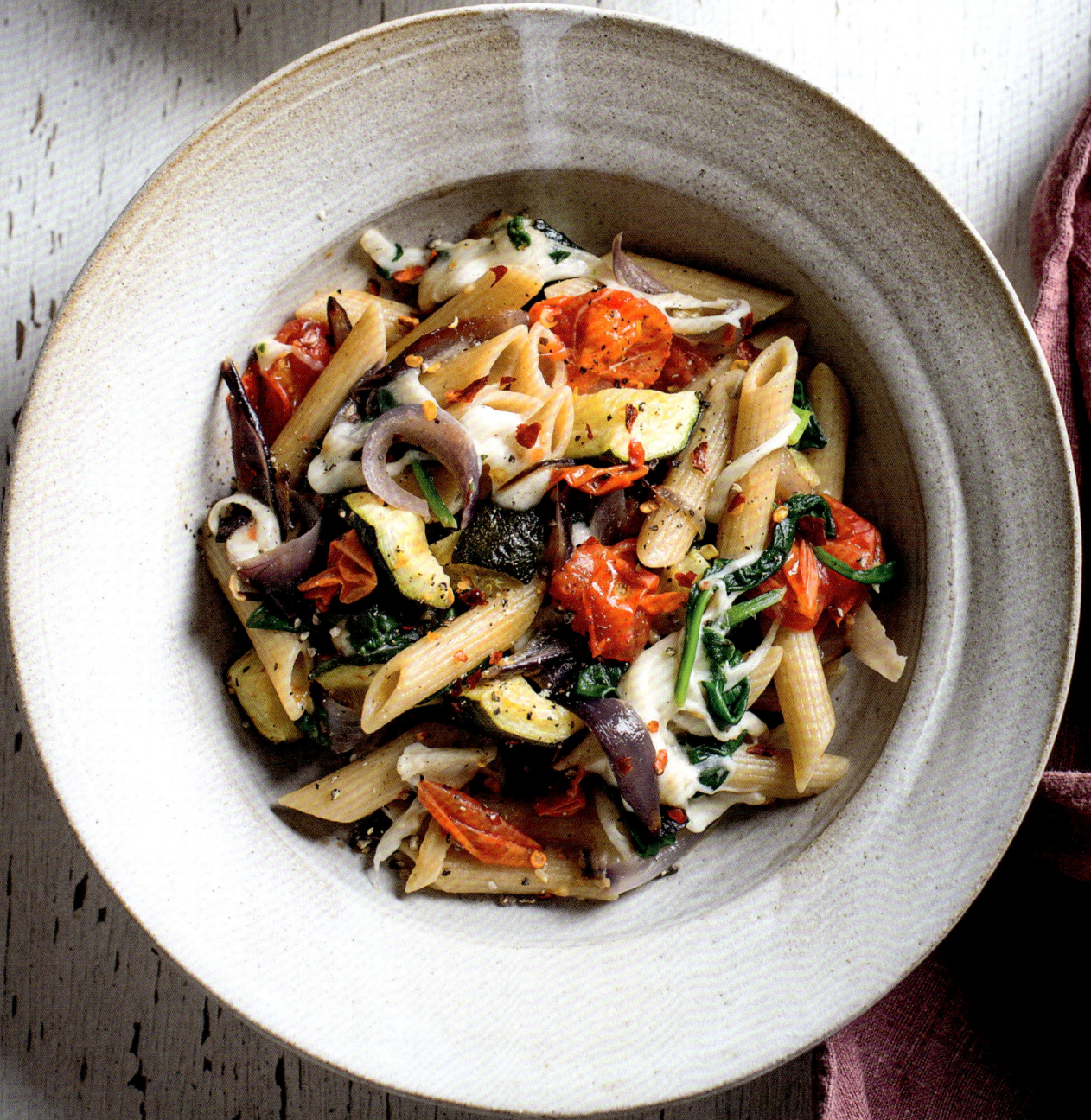

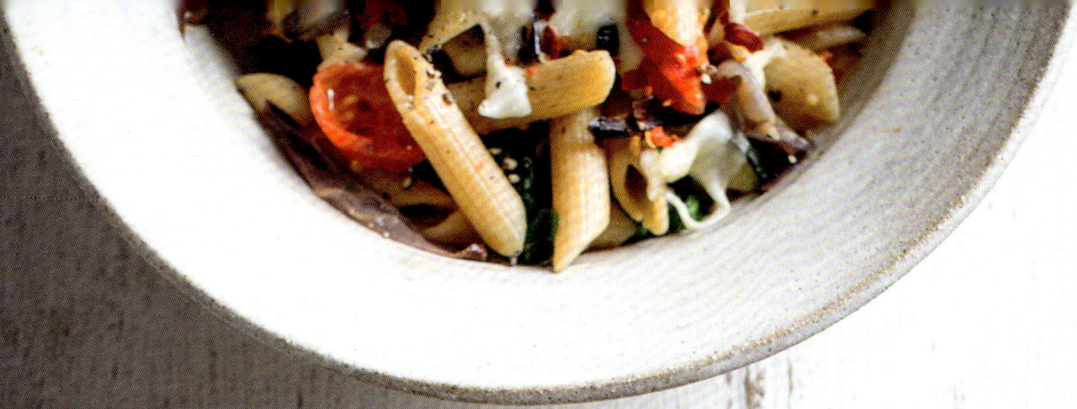

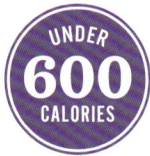

PER SERVING | **570cals** | PROTEIN **22g** | CARBS **28.5g**

Creamy Cashew and Tofu Curry with Cauli-rice

SERVES	PREP	COOK
4	**10** mins	**30** mins

2 tbsp coconut or rapeseed oil
1 aubergine (around 225g),
    cut into roughly 2cm chunks
1 red onion, cut into 12 wedges
350g butternut squash,
    peeled and cut into
    roughly 2cm chunks
4 tbsp Thai red or
    green curry paste
1 × 400ml can full-fat
    coconut milk
100g cashew nuts,
    roughly chopped
1 large pepper, any colour,
    deseeded and cut into
    roughly 2cm chunks
20g fresh coriander, leaves
    roughly chopped
280g firm, or extra-firm
    tofu, drained and cut
    into roughly 2cm cubes
300g cauli-rice
    (see page 232; optional)

NON-FAST DAYS
Serve with a small
portion of brown rice
or wholewheat noodles.

Thai-style curries always seem to go down well and this one is low on carbs and high in flavour. If you don't like tofu, try Quorn pieces instead. Please note, some curry pastes contain fish sauce. If you're serving the curry without the cauli-rice, you only need to count 548cals.

1. Heat 1 tablespoon of the oil in a large frying pan or flameproof casserole over a high heat. Add the aubergine and stir fry for 4–5 minutes, until golden brown. Transfer to a bowl.

2. Reduce the heat, add the remaining oil, onion and squash to the pan and fry gently for 5 minutes, stirring regularly. Add the curry paste and cook for 1 minute, stirring constantly.

3. Stir in the coconut milk, half the nuts, the pepper and 100ml water. Season with salt and freshly ground black pepper. Cover the pan loosely with a lid, bring to a gentle simmer and cook for 10 minutes, stirring occasionally.

4. Return the aubergine to the pan, along with half the coriander, and bring back to a simmer. Add the tofu, cover and cook for a further 5–6 minutes, until the aubergine is softened and the tofu hot. Add a splash more water, if the curry reduces too much.

5. Sprinkle with the reserved coriander and cashew nuts, and serve with freshly cooked cauli-rice, if using.

VEGAN | GLUTEN FREE | DAIRY FREE

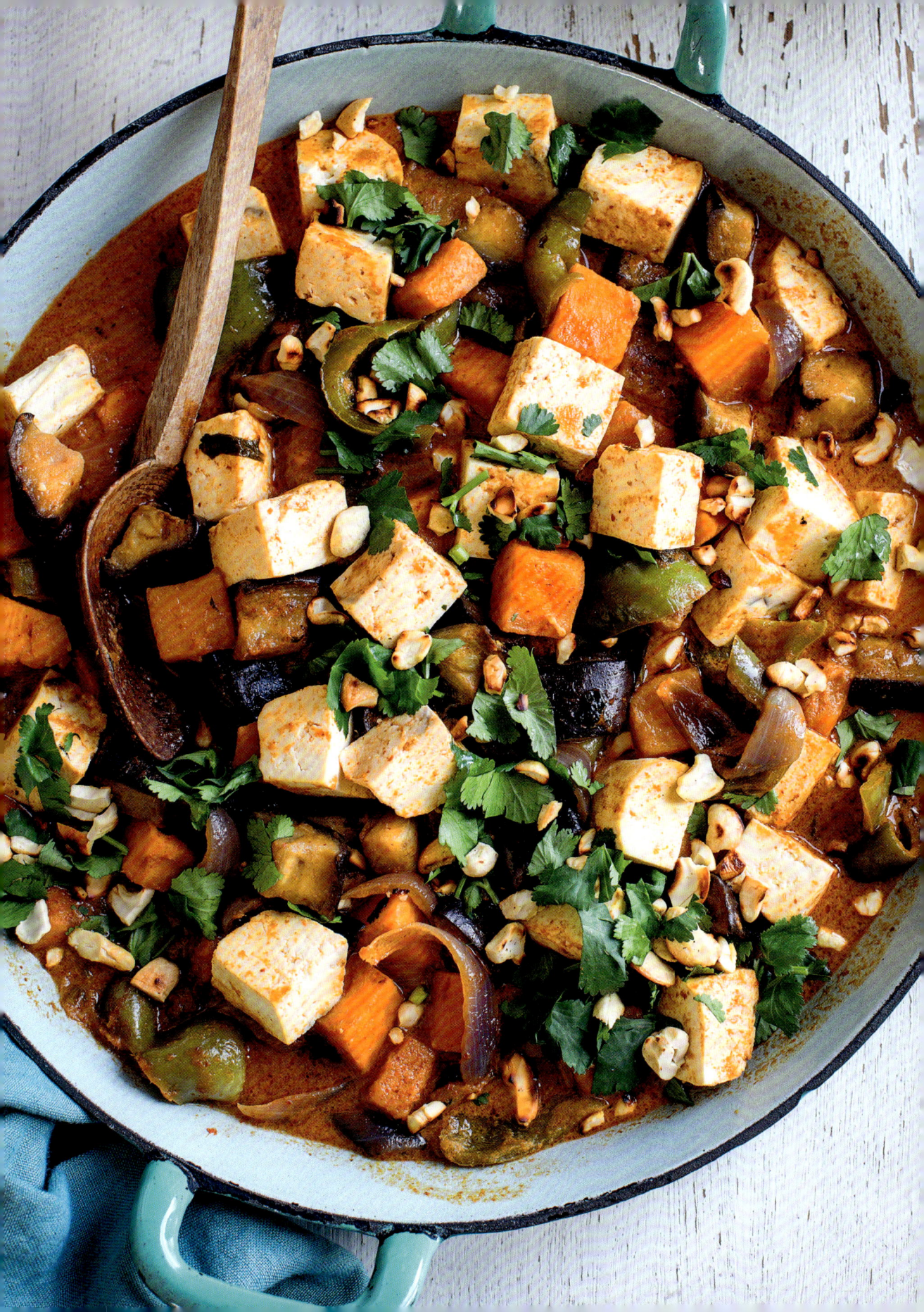

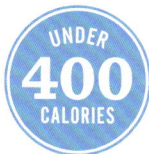

Ratatouille and Halloumi Bake

SERVES	PREP	COOK
4	**8** mins	**50** mins

2 red or yellow peppers,
   deseeded and cut into
   roughly 2cm chunks
1 aubergine (around 250g),
   cut into roughly 2cm chunks
1 onion, cut into 12 wedges
3 tbsp olive oil
2 garlic cloves, crushed
handful fresh basil leaves,
   thinly sliced, plus extra
   to serve
1 × 400g can chopped
   tomatoes with herbs
1 × 225g pack halloumi,
   cut into 8 slices

NON-FAST DAYS
Add a 400g can of drained
and rinsed cannellini beans
to the ratatouille at the same
time as the canned tomatoes.
Drizzle the halloumi and
vegetables generously with
olive oil when you serve.

COOK'S TIP
If you don't have canned
tomatoes with added herbs,
simply stir ½ teaspoon dried
oregano through the tomatoes
before adding to the vegetables.

This ratatouille is wonderfully versatile and delicious served warm or cold. It can be easily reheated in the microwave, so also makes a handy packed lunch. A protein-rich traybake was right up Michael's street.

1. Preheat the oven to 220°C/Fan 200°C/Gas 7.

2. Place the peppers, aubergine and onion in a bowl, add 2 tablespoons of the oil and season with salt and freshly ground black pepper. Toss everything together to coat, then scatter into a shallow baking dish. Bake for 25 minutes.

3. Remove the dish from the oven, turn the vegetables, then cook for a further 5–10 minutes, or until well softened and lightly browned.

4. Remove the dish from the oven again, stir in the garlic, basil and tomatoes, arrange the halloumi on top and drizzle with the remaining oil. Season with more ground black pepper and return to the oven for a final 15 minutes, or until the halloumi is hot and lightly browned.

5. Scatter with fresh basil and serve with a large leafy salad.

AIR-FRYER TIP
Preheat the air fryer to 190°C, if needed. Prepare the vegetables as Step 2. Place the vegetables in an even layer in the air fryer (you may need to cook them in batches). Air fry for 18 minutes, turning halfway, or until softened and lightly browned. Add the garlic, basil and tomatoes, stir until combined and return to the air fryer for 10 minutes, or until the sauce is heated through. Stir again, place the halloumi on top, drizzle with the remaining oil and season. Air fry for another 3–5 minutes until the halloumi is hot and lightly browned.

VEGGIE • GLUTEN FREE • NUT FREE

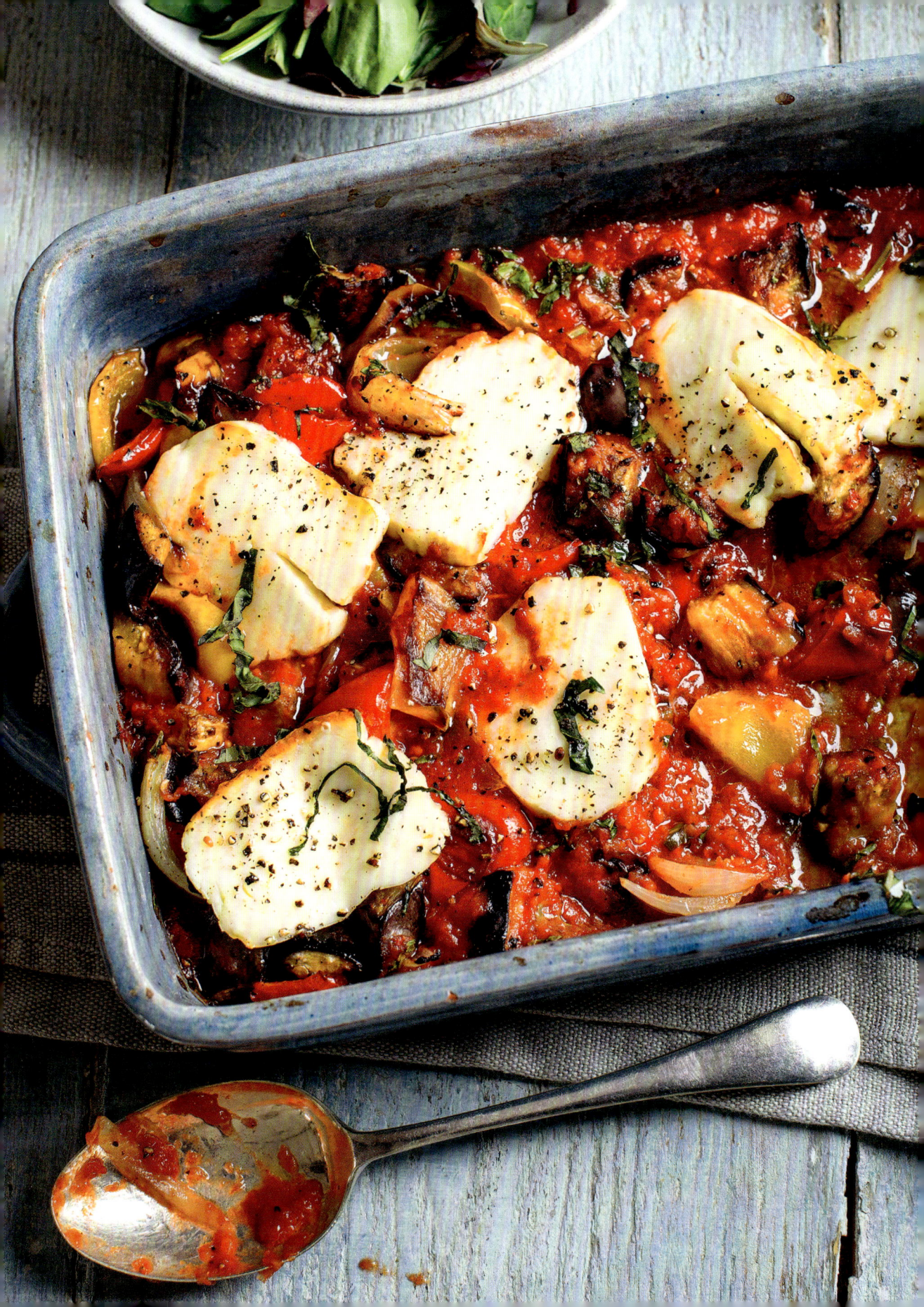

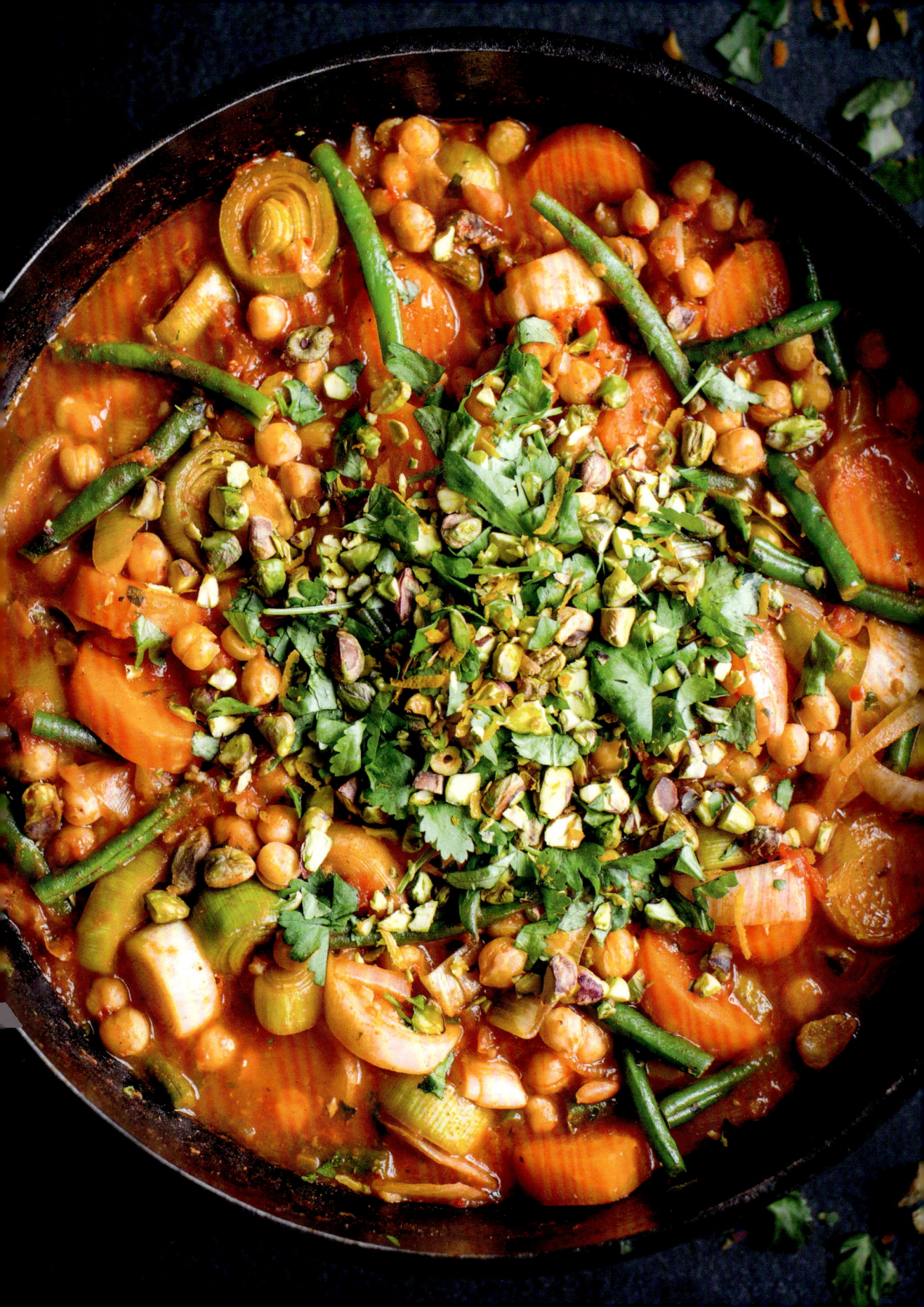

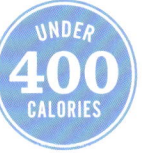

Chickpea and Pistachio Pot

SERVES | PREP | COOK
4 | **15** mins | **30** mins

1 tbsp olive oil
1 large onion, finely sliced
2 garlic cloves, crushed
2 carrots (around 200g),
   trimmed and cut into
   roughly 5mm slices
1 × 400g can chopped tomatoes
2 × 400g cans chickpeas,
   drained
2 tbsp harissa paste
1 vegetable stock cube
100g pistachio nuts
1 tsp dried mixed herbs
2 slender leeks, trimmed and
   cut into around 1cm slices
100g fine green beans,
   trimmed and cut in half
20g bunch coriander,
   leaves chopped
finely grated zest of ½ orange

NON-FAST DAYS
Increase the portion size
and drizzle liberally with
olive oil. Serve with a small
portion of quinoa or mixed
brown and wild rice.

A golden vegetable stew with a tangy orange and
nut topping. Serve with leafy greens.

1. Heat the oil in a large saucepan or flameproof casserole
over a low heat. Add the onion and fry gently for 5 minutes,
or until softened and lightly browned, stirring occasionally.
Add the garlic and cook for a few seconds more.

2. Stir in the carrots, tomatoes, chickpeas and harissa.
Add 450ml water and crumble over the stock cube. Tip in
half the nuts and the dried herbs, season with a little salt
and lots of freshly ground black pepper and stir well.
Bring to a gentle simmer and cook for 10 minutes,
stirring occasionally.

3. Add the sliced leeks, green beans and half the coriander,
and cook for 5–10 minutes, or until all the vegetables are
tender and the sauce has thickened slightly, stirring
regularly.

4. Roughly chop the remaining nuts and mix with the
remaining coriander and the orange zest.

5. Spoon the vegetables into a warm serving dish and
sprinkle the nut mixture over the top to serve.

VEGAN   GLUTEN FREE   DAIRY FREE   ❄

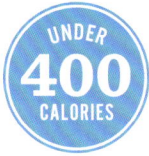

PER SERVING | **306cals** | PROTEIN **14g** | CARBS **29g**

Leek and Goat's Cheese Barley Risotto

SERVES	PREP	COOK
4	**10** mins	**65** mins

1 tbsp olive oil
1 onion, finely chopped
2 garlic cloves, crushed
120g pearl barley
1 bay leaf
1 vegetable stock cube
2 medium leeks (around 375g),
    trimmed and cut into
    roughly 5mm slices
50g Parmesan, finely grated
100g goat's cheese, rind
    removed if you prefer
fresh thyme leaves,
    to serve (optional)

NON-FAST DAYS
Increase the portion size.

COOK'S TIP
Look out for quick-cook barley, or a mixture of quick-cook barley and other grains; this will only take around 20 minutes to cook, but you'll need to reduce the amount of water in the recipe.

The pearl barley adds a wonderful nutty taste and creamy texture to this risotto. Serve with freshly cooked long-stemmed broccoli or kale.

1. Heat the oil in a large saucepan over a low heat. Add the onion and fry gently for 3–5 minutes, or until softened and lightly browned, stirring regularly. Add the garlic and cook for a few seconds more.

2. Add the pearl barley and bay leaf, and crumble over the stock cube. Pour in 900ml cold water, cover loosely and bring to the boil. Reduce the heat to a gentle simmer and cook for 40–50 minutes, or until tender, stirring occasionally. Add extra water, if the barley absorbs more than expected. It should be nice and saucy.

3. Add the sliced leeks and cook for 5 minutes, or until tender, then stir in the Parmesan and season to taste with salt and lots of freshly ground black pepper.

4. Spoon the risotto on to warmed plates or bowls and crumble the goat's cheese on top. Sprinkle with thyme leaves, if using, to serve.

VEGGIE   NUT FREE

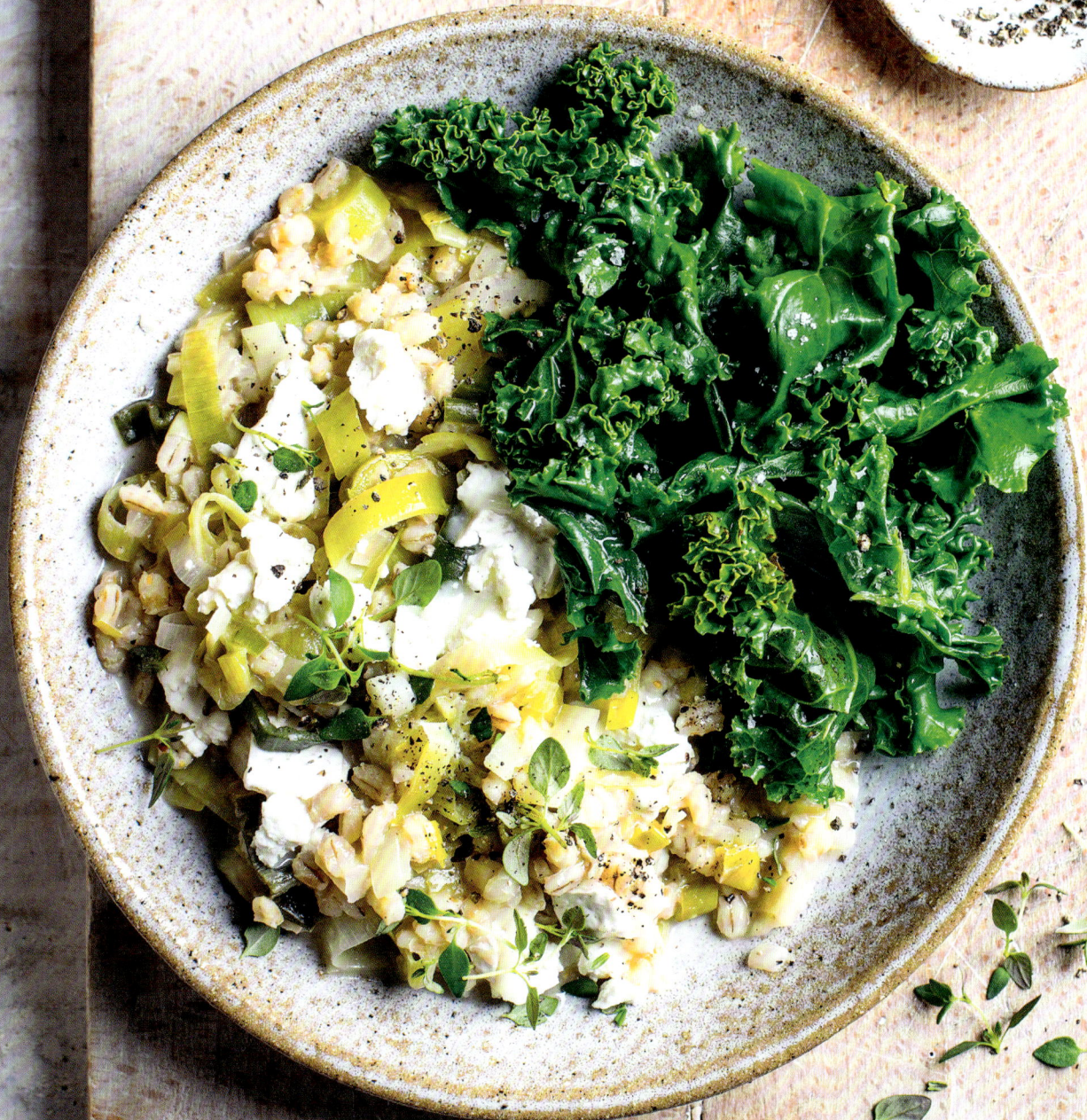

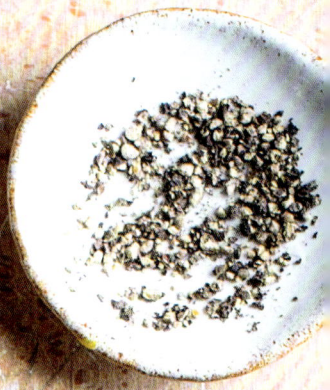

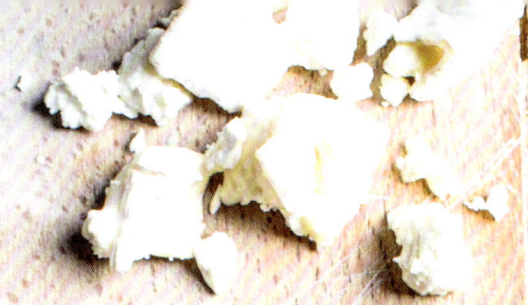

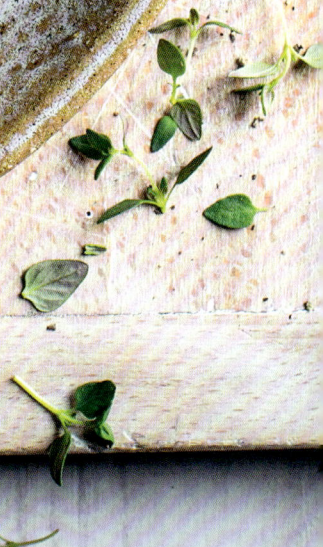

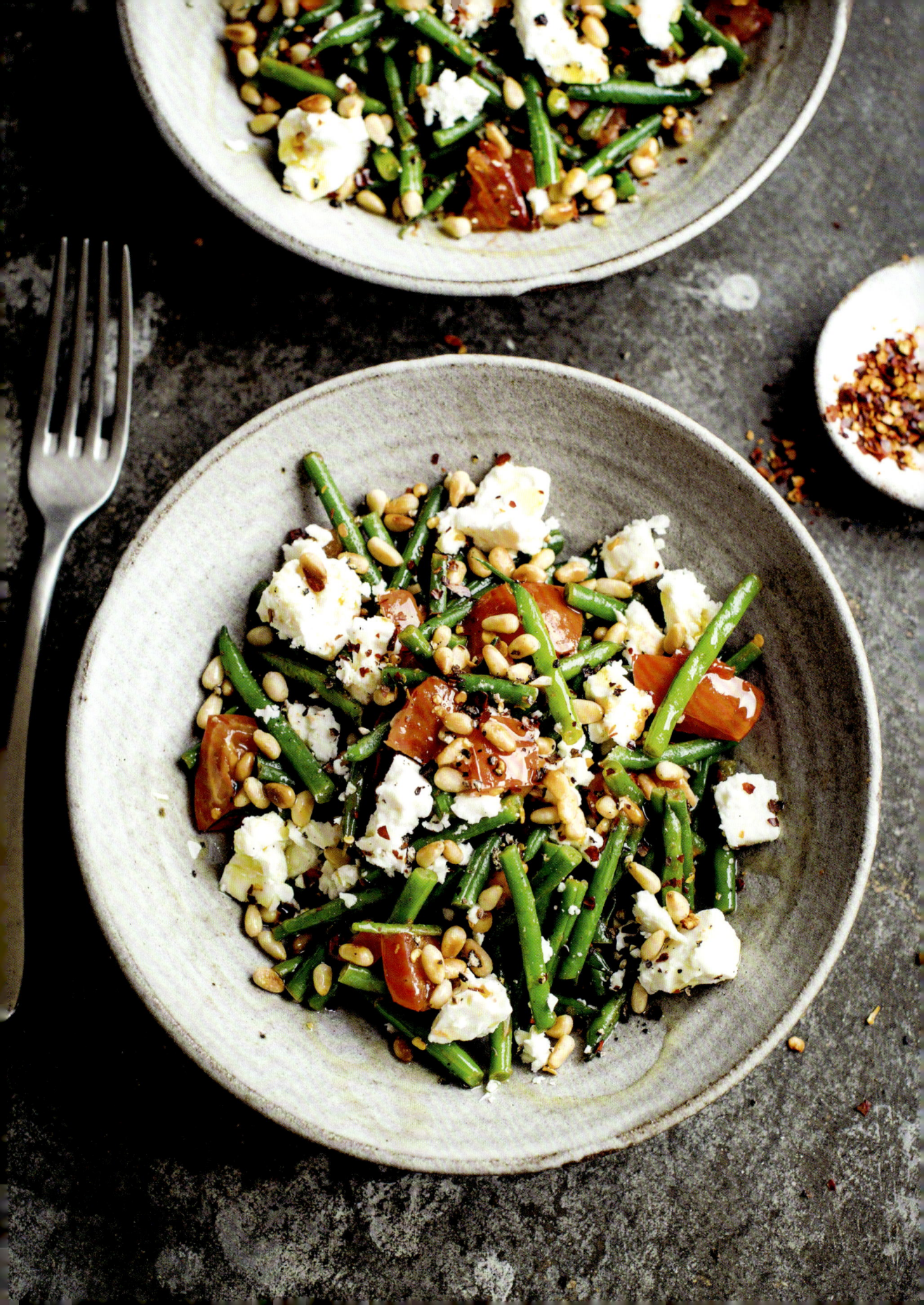

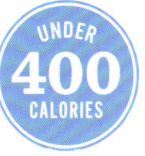

French Bean Bowl with Feta and Pine Nuts

SERVES **2** | **PREP** **10** mins | **COOK** **10** mins

2 tbsp pine nuts
   (or other seeds)
180g French beans,
   topped, tailed and
   cut into 2cm pieces
1 tbsp olive oil
2 tomatoes, cut into
   2cm pieces
1 garlic clove,
   finely chopped
100g feta cheese,
   roughly crumbled
pinch crushed dried chilli
   flakes, to serve (optional)

NON-FAST DAY
Increase the portion size.

Although not a great gardener, I do like growing beans. Beans are a good source of soluble and insoluble fibre, and their juicy crunch contrasts beautifully here with the salty, creamy feta. I try to keep a pack of feta in the fridge – it's great for adding a flavourful protein boost to salads and oven bakes. This dish would work well in a lunchbox.

1. Place the pine nuts in a dry frying pan over a medium heat and toast for 1–2 minutes, or until turning golden. Remove from the pan and set aside.

2. Return the pan to the heat, add the beans and oil, and fry for a couple of minutes, stirring occasionally. Stir in the tomatoes and cook for 4 minutes. Add the garlic and cook for 1 minute more.

3. Remove from the heat and scatter the feta and pine nuts all over the beans and tomatoes.

4. Allow to rest for a minute or so, to let the feta soften, then divide between two bowls and season with plenty of freshly ground black pepper and a pinch of chilli flakes, if using, to serve.

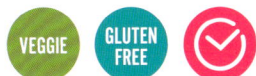

VEGGIE   GLUTEN FREE

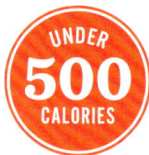

| PER SERVING | **421cals** | PROTEIN **21.3g** | CARBS **28.2g**

One-pan Miso Aubergine with Peanuts

SERVES	PREP	COOK
2	**10** mins	**40** mins

2 medium aubergines
2 tsp extra-virgin olive oil
2 tbsp miso paste
1 tbsp dark soy sauce
20g fresh root ginger,
    peeled and finely grated
½ tsp crushed dried
    chilli flakes
50g peanuts or cashew nuts,
    roughly chopped
2 spring onions, trimmed
    and finely sliced
100g frozen edamame
1 red chilli, deseeded and
    finely sliced, to serve

COOK'S TIP
If you don't have any fresh
ginger, use 1 tablespoon ginger
purée or 1 teaspoon ground
ginger instead.

Michael enjoyed sweet umami flavours, and this fried
aubergine almost tastes like steak, while the nuts and
edamame deliver a protein boost. It makes a filling
supper for two or can be shared between four. It is
delicious with a Chinese leaf salad or steamed broccoli.

1. Preheat the oven to 200°C/Fan 180°C/Gas 6 and line
a baking tray with foil.

2. Cut the aubergines in half lengthways and score the flesh
in a criss-cross pattern, without cutting all the way through
to the skin. Place on the baking tray, cut-side up, and brush
with the oil. Bake for about 30 minutes, or until softened
and lightly browned.

3. Meanwhile, mix the miso paste with the soy sauce,
ginger and chilli flakes in a small bowl. In a separate bowl,
combine the peanuts and spring onions.

4. Remove the tray from the oven and spread the
aubergines with the miso mixture. Sprinkle the peanuts on
top and scatter the frozen edamame on the tray around the
aubergines. Return to the oven for 8–10 minutes, or until
the peanuts are lightly browned and the edamame are hot.

5. Scatter over the spring onion and chilli to serve.

AIR-FRYER TIP
Preheat the air fryer to 180°C, if needed. Prepare the
aubergine as Step 2. Brush with oil and air fry for 20
minutes, or until softened and lightly browned. (You
may need to cook them in batches.) Prepare the miso
mixture and spread over the cut side of the aubergines.
Scatter with the peanuts and edamame and air fry for
another 6–8 minutes. Scatter with the spring onions
and chilli to serve.

VEGAN   DAIRY FREE

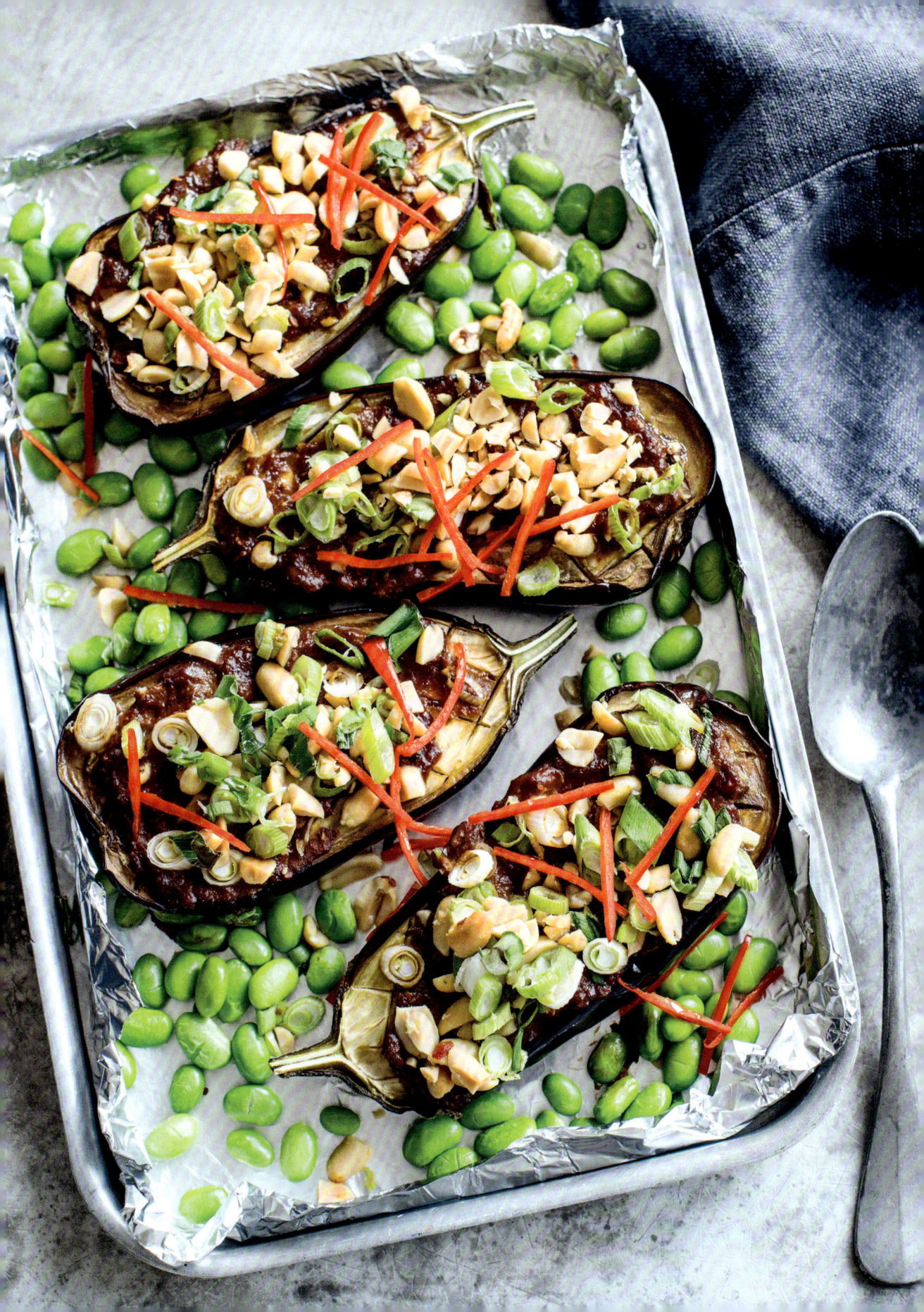

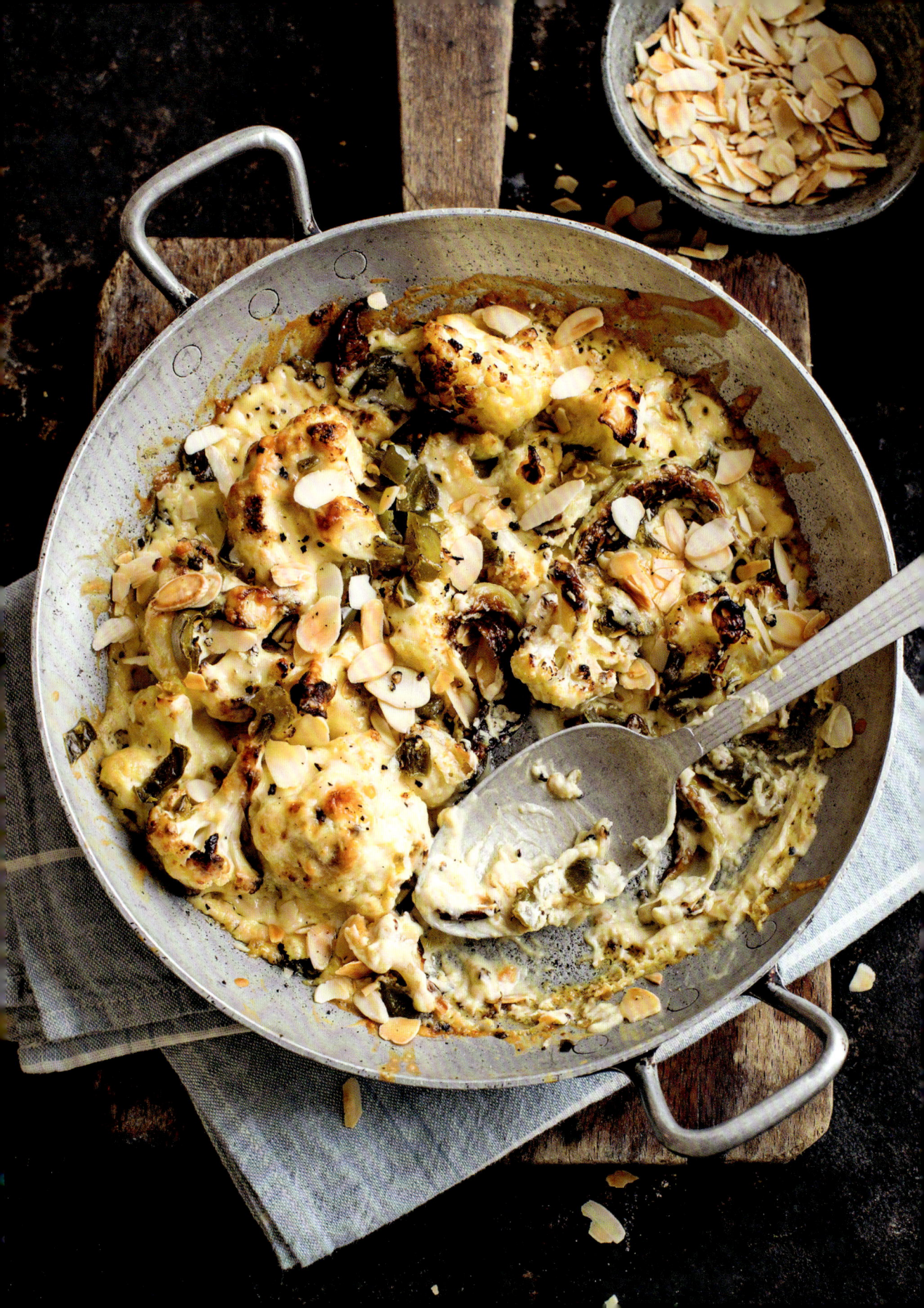

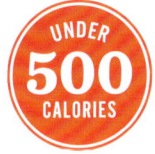

Cauli Cheese with Jalapeño Peppers

SERVES	PREP	COOK
2	**10** mins	**30** mins

½ cauliflower
1 tbsp olive oil
70g full-fat cream cheese
1 tbsp Dijon mustard
1½ tbsp milk
60g mature Cheddar, grated
30g jalapeños from a jar,
    roughly chopped
2 tbsp toasted flaked almonds
    (around 35g)

NON-FAST DAY
Serve a larger portion
and add extra cheese.

COOK'S TIP
For non-vegetarians,
this dish is lovely
served with cured hams,
diced bacon or chorizo
(see protein top-ups
on page 271).

Forget stodgy bechamel sauce, this quick and fuss-free version of cauliflower cheese is juicy and creamy, and nicely balanced by a mild spicy kick from the jalapeño peppers. A fabulous, easy mid-week meal. Serve with steamed greens or a colourful leafy salad if you like.

1. Preheat the oven to 200°C/Fan 180°C/Gas 6.

2. Break the cauliflower into small florets, and chop the stalk into chunks. Place in a baking dish and toss with the olive oil. Season with salt and freshly ground black pepper and roast in the oven for 15 minutes.

3. Meanwhile, in a small bowl, mix together the cream cheese, mustard, milk and half of the Cheddar. Remove the dish from the oven and stir in the cream cheese mixture.

4. Scatter the jalapeños all over, along with the remaining grated cheese. Season with a little more salt and lots of freshly ground black pepper and return to the oven for a further 10–15 minutes, until golden and bubbling.

5. Garnish with the flaked almonds to serve.

AIR-FRYER TIP
Preheat the air fryer to 180°C, if needed. Toss the prepared cauliflower with the oil and season. Place in the air fryer and cook for 13–15 minutes, or until softened and lightly browned. Prepare the cheese sauce as Step 3 and spoon over the cauliflower. Scatter over the jalapeños, remaining cheese and season. Air fry for another 8–10 minutes, until golden and bubbling.

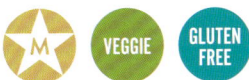

VEGGIE   GLUTEN FREE

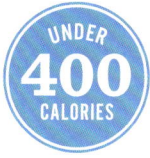

PER SERVING | **304cals** | PROTEIN **13.8g** | CARBS **14g**

Halloumi Skewers with Simple Coleslaw

SERVES	PREP	COOK
4	**15** mins	**10** mins

1 × 225g pack halloumi,
    cut into 12 pieces
1 small courgette, trimmed
    and cut into 12 pieces
1 small red pepper, deseeded
    and cut into 12 wedges
½ red onion, cut into 12 wedges
1½ tbsp olive oil
1 × portion Simple Coleslaw
    (see page 221)

NON-FAST DAY
Double the portion size and
serve with 2–3 tablespoons
cooked wholegrains, such
as quinoa, bulgur wheat
or brown rice.

COOK'S TIP
Use metal skewers if
cooking on the barbecue
or under the grill.

Halloumi, unlike most other cheeses, remains firm when fried or griddled, and browns beautifully, making it ideal to add flavour and protein to kebabs. This gorgeous summery dish will also work really well on a barbecue. If you are serving the halloumi skewers without the coleslaw, you only need to count 226cals.

1. You will need 4 × 20cm bamboo (soaked in water for 15 minutes) or metal skewers.

2. Divide the ingredients between the skewers and drizzle with the olive oil. Season with a small pinch of salt and freshly ground black pepper.

3. Place a griddle pan over a high heat and, when hot, add the skewers and cook on each side until the veggies are slightly charred and the halloumi is soft.

4. Serve with a leafy green salad.

VEGGIE   GLUTEN FREE   NUT FREE

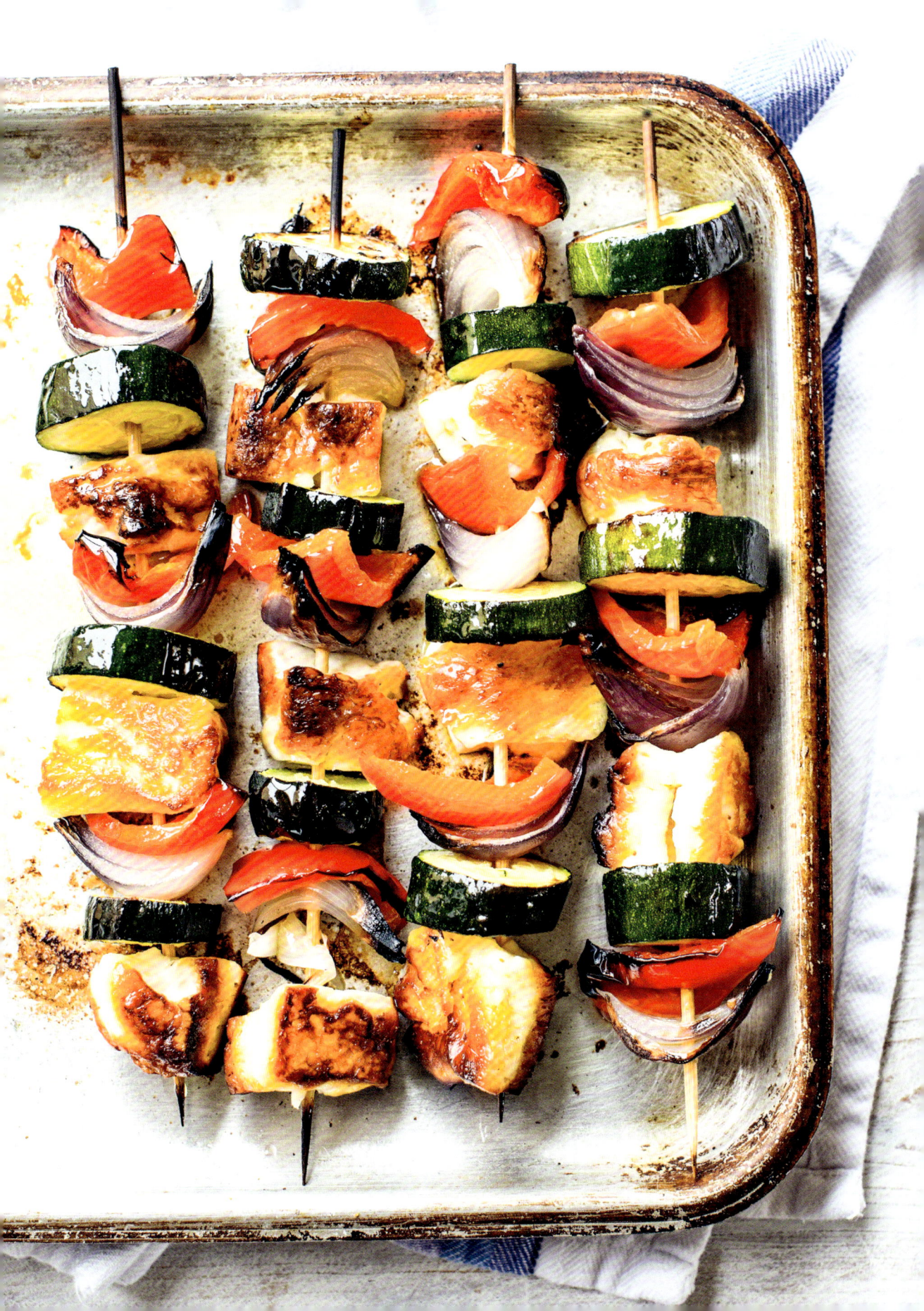

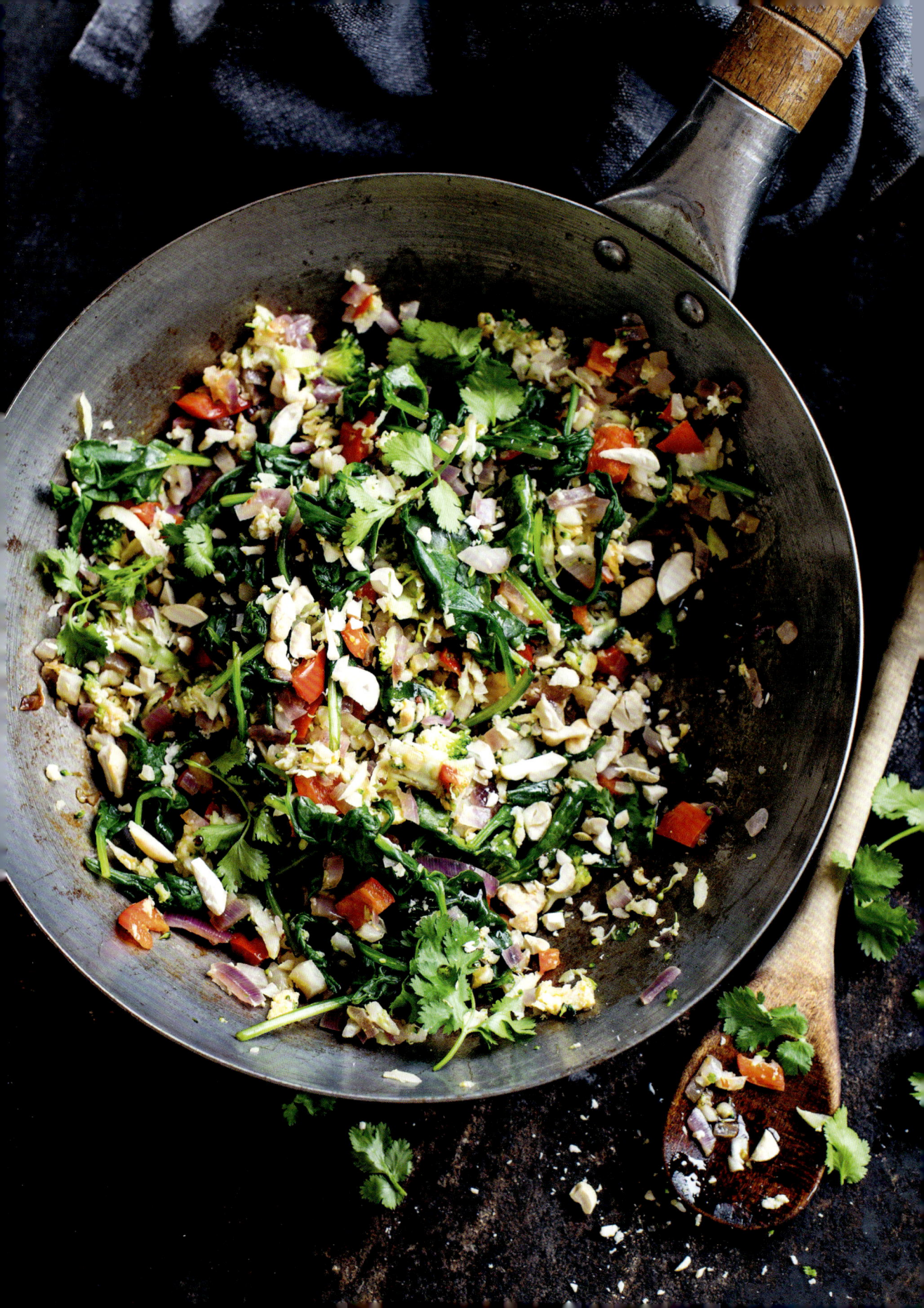

Egg-fried Cauli and Broccoli Rice

SERVES
2

PREP
10
mins

COOK
10
mins

1 tbsp olive oil
1 red onion, finely chopped
1 small red pepper,
   deseeded and diced
1 garlic clove, roughly chopped
1 small red chilli, finely sliced
   (or ½–1 tsp crushed dried
   chilli flakes)
¼ cauliflower, coarsely grated
100g broccoli, coarsely grated
50g young spinach leaves
2 medium free-range eggs
1½ tbsp light soy sauce
10g fresh coriander,
   roughly chopped
10g cashew nuts,
   roughly chopped

NON-FAST DAY
Enjoy a larger portion
and add some protein
top-ups (see page 271).

This colourful plant-based version of egg-fried rice is a great way to introduce a variety of vegetables into a meal and use up odds and ends from the fridge.

1. Place the oil in a wok or large frying pan over a high heat and, when hot, add the onion and pepper. Stir fry for 2 minutes, then add the garlic and chilli and fry for a further 30 seconds.

2. Stir in the cauliflower and broccoli and stir fry for 3–4 minutes, until hot and just starting to soften. Add the spinach and stir to wilt.

3. Push everything to one side of the pan and crack in the eggs. Stir until starting to scramble, then mix everything together, adding the soy sauce. Cook for 1 minute.

4. Add the coriander and garnish with cashews to serve.

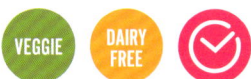

VEGGIE DAIRY FREE

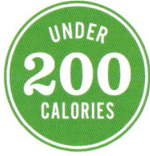

PER SERVING | **200cals** | PROTEIN **8g** | CARBS **15g**

Indian-inspired Chickpea Patties

SERVES | PREP | COOK
4 | **15** mins | **10** mins

2 tbsp coconut or rapeseed oil
1 red onion, finely chopped
15g fresh root ginger,
   peeled and finely grated
2 garlic cloves, finely grated
1½ tsp medium curry
   powder or garam masala
1–2 tsp crushed dried chilli
   flakes (optional)
1 × 400g can chickpeas,
   drained
1 tbsp tahini
20g peanuts, coarsely ground
1 tbsp plain wholemeal flour
15g fresh coriander, leaves
   finely chopped, plus extra
   to serve
1 red chilli, finely sliced,
   to serve (optional)
lime wedges, to serve

COOK'S TIP
To grind the peanuts,
use a food processor, spice
grinder or stick blender.
You can also bash them
in a pestle and mortar,
or very finely chop them
on a board.

Enjoy these mildly spiced patties with a lightly dressed green salad and yoghurt (adding the extra calories – see page 271). They are also delicious served cold or as part of a packed lunch.

1. Heat 1 tablespoon of the oil in a saucepan over a low–medium heat. Add the onion and fry for 4 minutes, or until beginning to soften, stirring regularly.

2. Add the ginger, garlic, curry powder or garam masala, and chilli flakes, if using, and cook for 1 minute, stirring constantly.

3. Remove from the heat, tip the chickpeas into the pan, add the tahini and peanuts, and mash with a potato masher, until the chickpeas turn to a thick paste and clump together (this should take a couple of minutes).

4. Transfer to a bowl, season well with salt and freshly ground black pepper, and add the flour and chopped coriander. Mix well, then form into 8 patties, pressing together firmly so they hold their shape.

5. Heat the remaining oil in a large frying pan over a medium heat. Add the patties and fry for about 2½ minutes on each side, or until golden brown and crisp.

6. Serve 2 patties per person with some chilli, if using, a lime wedge, coriander leaves and a large green salad.

VEGAN   DAIRY FREE   ❄

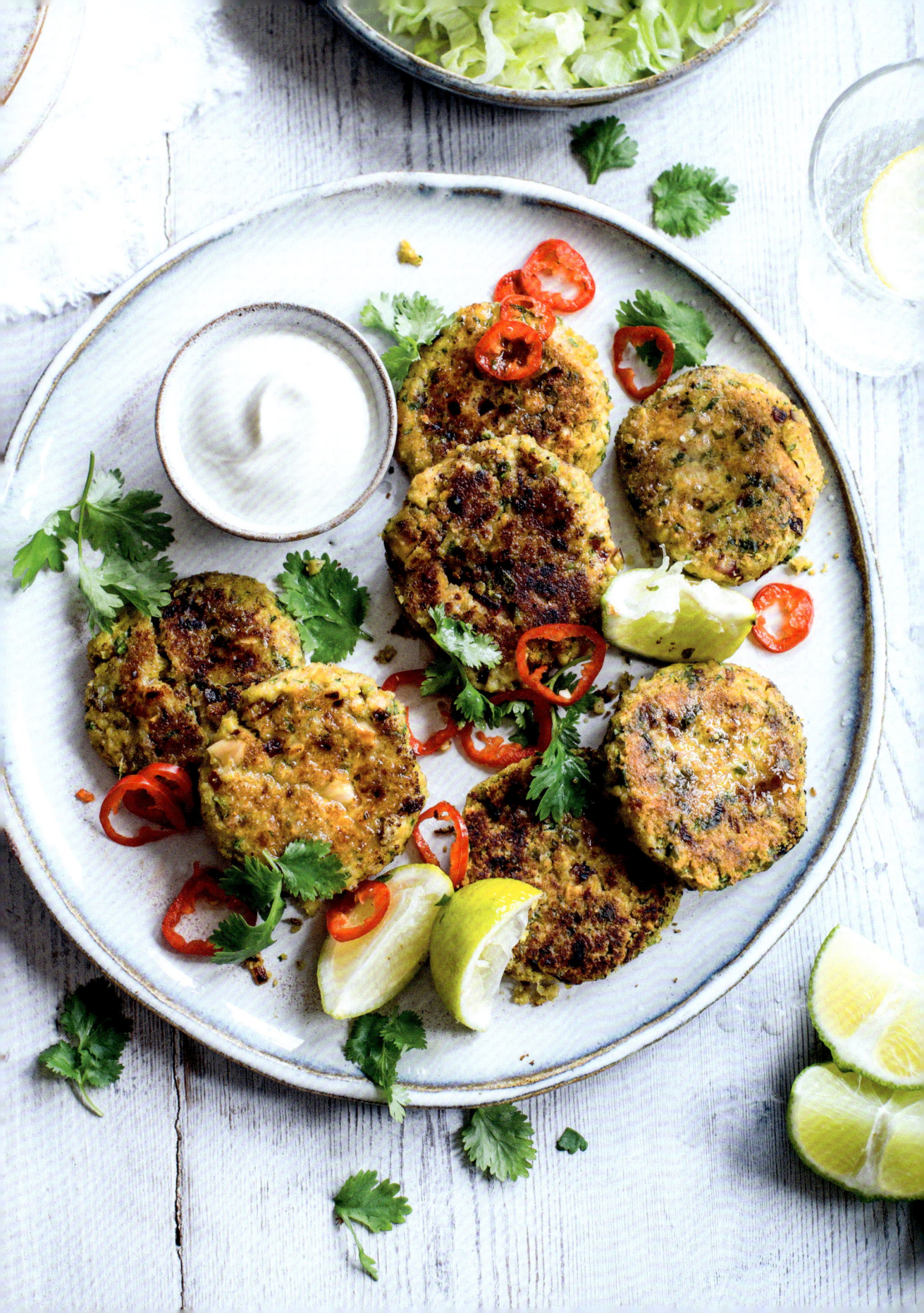

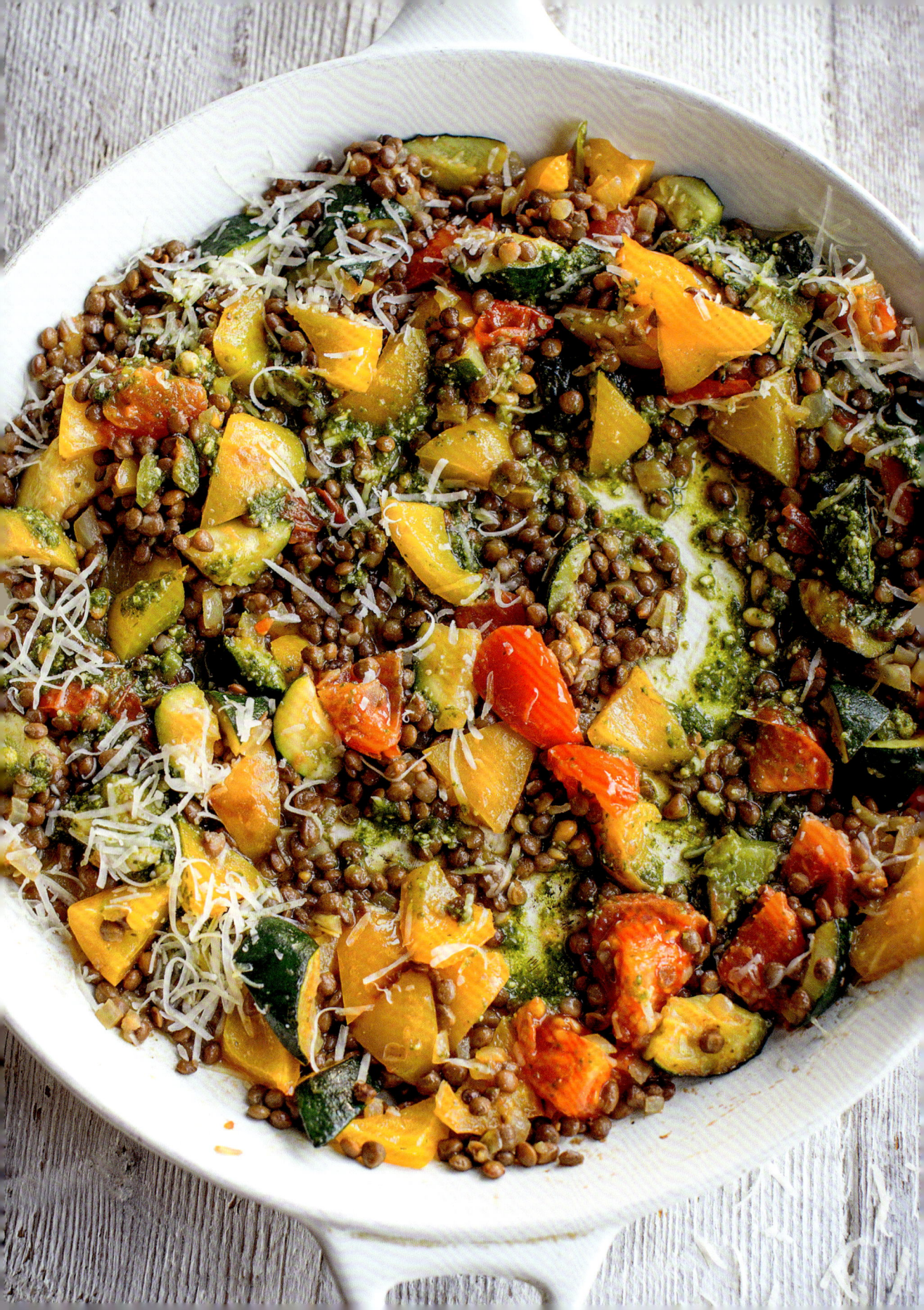

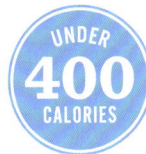

Pesto Lentils

SERVES	PREP	COOK
2	**10** mins	**11** mins

1 tbsp olive oil
½ onion, finely chopped
1 yellow or red pepper,
    deseeded and cut into
    roughly 2cm chunks
½ courgette, trimmed and cut
    into roughly 2cm chunks
2 tomatoes, roughly chopped
1 × 400g can lentils
    (any variety), drained
½ vegetable stock cube
2 tbsp basil pesto
20g Parmesan, finely grated

NON-FAST DAYS
Serve with some warmed
wholemeal pitta bread
and extra grated cheese.

COOK'S TIP
For a zingier dish, use fresh
basil pesto (found in tubs
in the chilled cabinet at the
supermarket). It keeps for
several days in the fridge
and can be frozen, too.

Canned lentils are versatile, cheap and convenient.
Cooked up with fresh veg and pesto, they make a
brilliant quick meal that's packed with fibre and
contains a good protein hit. Serve with a mixed salad.

1. Heat the oil in a large frying pan over a low heat. Add the
onion, pepper and courgette and fry gently for 5 minutes,
or until softened and beginning to brown, stirring regularly.

2. Add the tomatoes and cook for 2–3 minutes, or until
the tomatoes are softened, stirring constantly.

3. Add the lentils, crumbled stock cube and 2–3 tablespoons
water. Stir in the pesto and season with lots of freshly
ground black pepper. Cook for 2–3 minutes, or until
the lentils are hot, stirring constantly.

4. Remove from the heat and sprinkle with the Parmesan
to serve.

VEGGIE   GLUTEN FREE

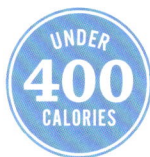

Tofu Mushroom Ramen

SERVES	PREP	COOK
2	**15** mins	**10** mins

10g dried mushrooms,
   mixed or porcini
2 tbsp red miso paste,
   or any other miso
2 tsp olive or rapeseed oil
150g extra-firm tofu,
   cut into 4 slices
25g cashew nuts,
   roughly chopped
40g dried wholewheat noodles
125g closed cup or shiitake
   mushrooms, sliced
1 pak choi, trimmed and
   thickly sliced, leaving
   any smaller leaves whole
100g bean sprouts,
   rinsed and drained
4 spring onions, trimmed
   and very finely sliced
freshly sliced red chilli or
   crushed dried chilli flakes,
   to serve (optional)

COOK'S TIP
You can also use silken
tofu instead of firm tofu
but don't fry it. Instead,
cut it into cubes and warm
through in the stock for
a couple of minutes
before serving.

Tofu is a great source of protein and helps make
this dish deliciously satisfying. Add finely sliced
fresh root ginger and garlic to the broth for extra
flavour, and season with a splash of soy sauce.

1. Place the dried mushrooms in a large wide-based
saucepan and add 1 litre of just-boiled water. Stir in
the miso paste to make a broth and leave to stand for
15 minutes.

2. Meanwhile, heat the oil in a large non-stick frying
pan, add the tofu slices and fry over a medium heat
for 2½ minutes, or until lightly browned. Turn the
tofu, add the nuts and fry for a further 2½ minutes,
stirring regularly.

3. Add the noodles, closed cup or shiitake mushrooms
and pak choi to the saucepan with the dried mushrooms
and miso. Bring to a simmer and cook for 3 minutes,
stirring to separate the noodles.

4. Stir in the bean sprouts and spring onions, and cook
for 1 minute.

5. Divide the noodles, mushrooms and vegetables
between two deep, wide bowls and top with the tofu.
Ladle over the broth and sprinkle with the chopped
nuts and chilli, if using, to serve.

VEGAN   DAIRY FREE

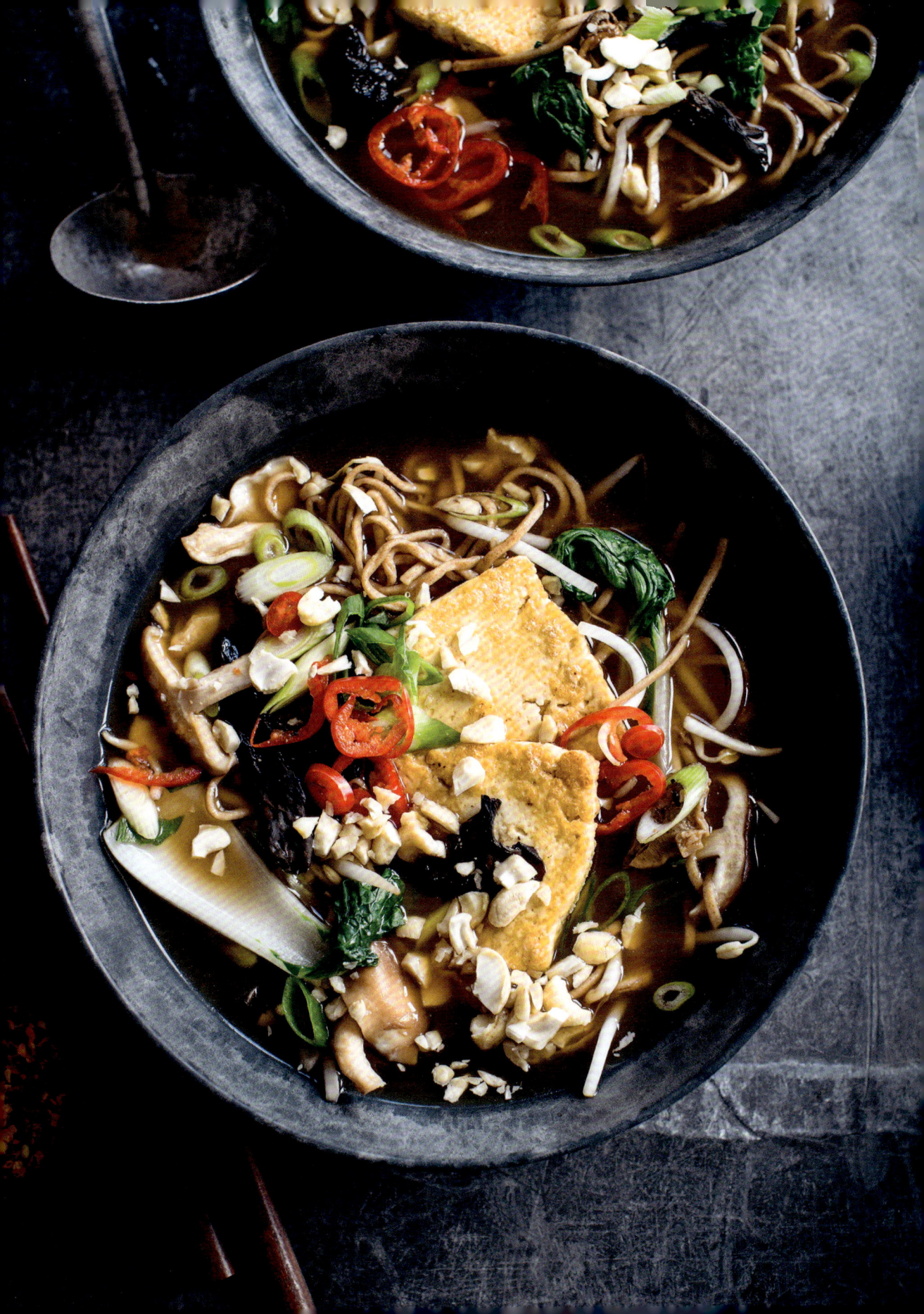

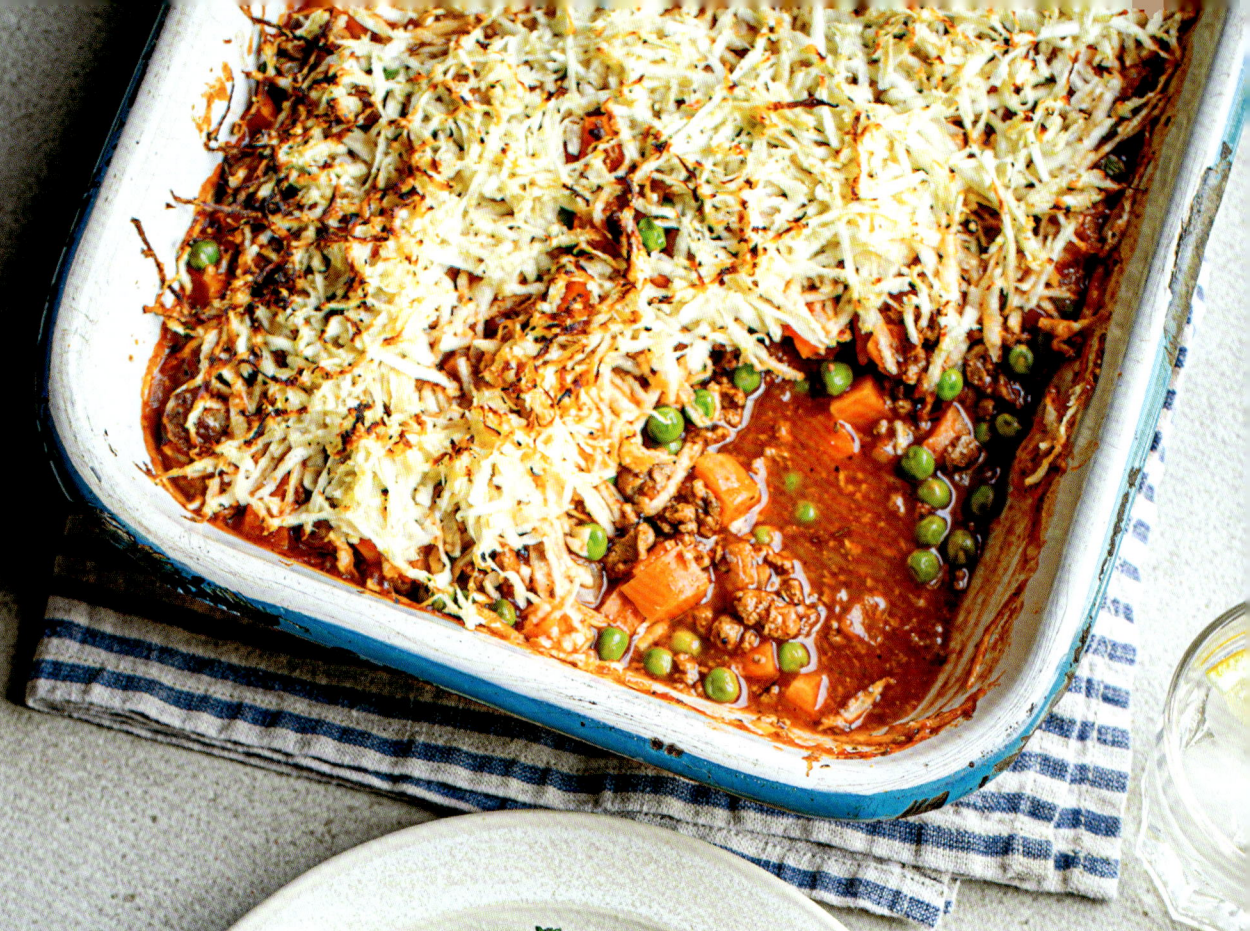

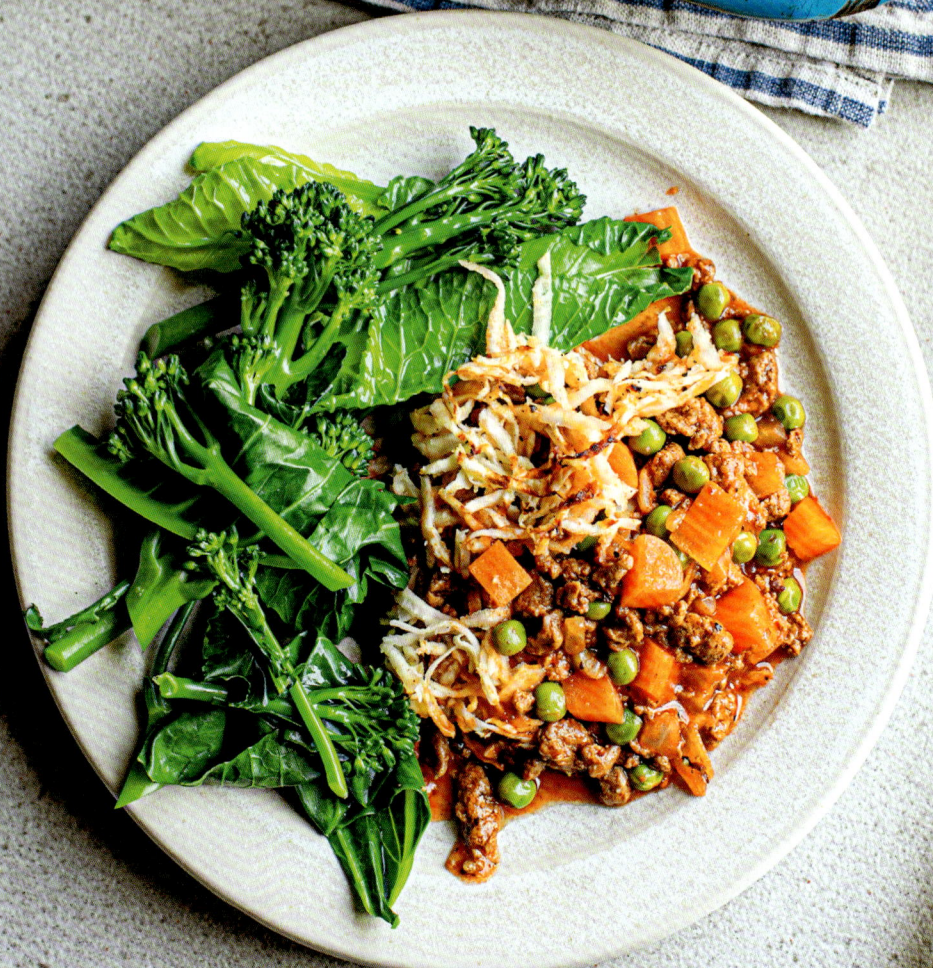

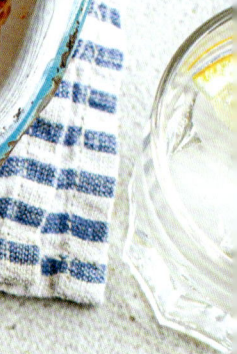

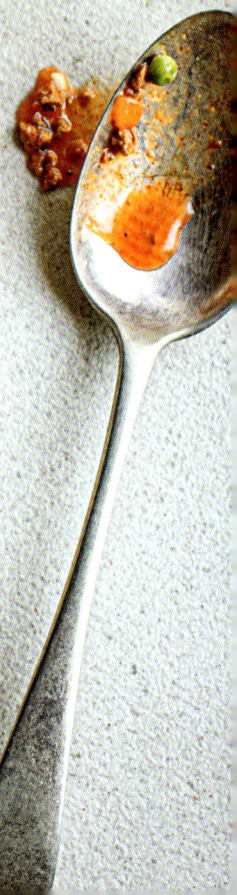

Veggie Cottage Pie

SERVES
4

PREP
15 mins

COOK
40 mins

1 tbsp olive oil
1 onion, finely chopped
200g carrots, trimmed
     and cut into 1cm chunks
350g Quorn mince
1 vegetable stock cube
2 tbsp tomato purée
1 tsp dried mixed herbs
2 tsp cornflour
150g frozen peas
225g celeriac, peeled and
     coarsely grated (around
     175g prepared weight)
20g Parmesan, finely grated

COOK'S TIP
If you don't want to use
Quorn, try 2 × 400g cans
lentils instead. Or make
the pie with minced chicken
or turkey. Without the Quorn,
the recipe contains 147cals
and 6g protein per serving.

One of of Michael's comfort dishes, this cottage pie
is made with Quorn mince, but you could use canned
or cooked lentils instead (see tip below). The grated
celeriac makes an easy alternative to mash and can
be used on top of any pie filling.

1. Heat the oil in a large, deep frying pan over a low–
medium heat. Add the onion and carrots, and fry for
5 minutes, or until the onion is softened, stirring regularly.

2. Add the mince, crumble the stock cube over the top and
stir in 650ml water. Add the tomato purée, herbs, a little
salt and lots of freshly ground black pepper. Bring to a
simmer and cook for 10 minutes, stirring occasionally.

3. Meanwhile, preheat the oven to 220°C/Fan 200°C/Gas 7.

4. Mix the cornflour with 1 tablespoon cold water in a small
bowl. Add to the mince with the peas and cook for about
2 minutes, stirring, until the sauce is slightly thickened
and glossy. Spoon into a 1.5-litre shallow ovenproof dish.

5. Place the grated celeriac and Parmesan in a large bowl,
season, then mix well. Scatter on top of the mince and bake
in the oven for about 20 minutes, or until the celeriac is
tipped with brown and the filling is bubbling.

6. Serve with lots of green vegetables.

AIR-FRYER TIP
Prepare the filling as instructed in Steps 1, 2 and 4.
Preheat the air fryer to 170°C, if needed. Prepare the
celeriac and Parmesan topping, season, then scatter
the mixture over the filling. Drizzle a little olive oil
over the top and air fry for 13–15 minutes until golden.

VEGGIE   NUT FREE

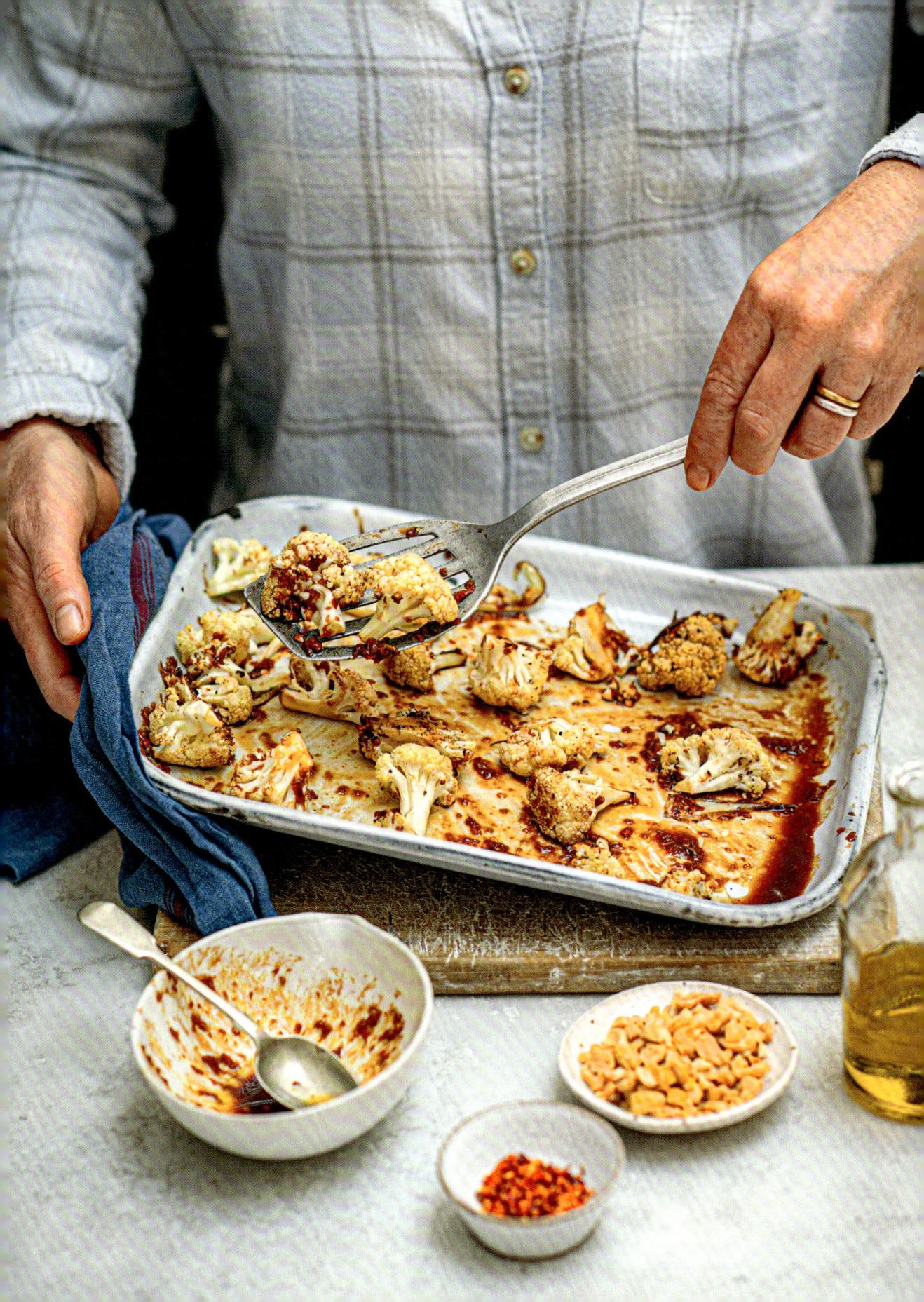

Vegetable Sides
and Snacks

Minty Yoghurt Raitha

Serve as a cooling accompaniment to curries, or as a dip with veg sticks.

SERVES 4
⅓ cucumber (around 135g)
150g full-fat live Greek yoghurt, or dairy-free alternative
3–4 tbsp finely chopped mint leaves

1. Cut the cucumber in half lengthways and scoop out the seeds with a teaspoon. Coarsely grate the flesh on to a board then transfer to a bowl.

2. Add the yoghurt and mint, and season with a good pinch of salt and lots of freshly ground black pepper. Mix well and leave for 20–30 minutes to allow the flavours to mingle.

3. Keep chilled until ready to serve.

NON-FAST DAYS
Serve with fingers of toasted wholemeal pitta bread or wholegrain seeded crackers.

COOK'S TIP
If using as a dip, add 1 green chilli, deseeded and finely chopped, for a bit more zing.

Minted Beetroot Hummus

A magnificent magenta-coloured hummus. Beetroot is surprisingly low in calories but high in nutrients. It can help reduce blood pressure and inflammation.

SERVES 6
300g cooked beetroot, drained and quartered
1 × 400g can chickpeas, drained and rinsed
1 garlic clove, peeled and halved
1 tsp ground coriander
2 tbsp finely chopped mint leaves
2 tbsp extra-virgin olive oil
2 tbsp fresh lemon juice
½ tsp flaked sea salt
2 tbsp mixed seeds

1. Put all the ingredients, except the seeds, in a food processor and season with freshly ground black pepper. Blitz until almost smooth. Adjust the seasoning and lightly blitz again. Spoon into a bowl.

2. Toast the mixed seeds in a small dry frying pan over a low heat for about 2 minutes, shaking the pan regularly.

3. Sprinkle the seeds over the hummus to serve.

NON-FAST DAYS
Drizzle with olive oil and top with an extra sprinkling of toasted mixed seeds. Serve with fingers of toasted wholemeal pitta bread or wholemeal crispbread.

COOK'S TIP
Keep covered in the fridge for up to 3 days or you can freeze for up to 1 month.

VEGAN · GLUTEN FREE · NUT FREE · DAIRY FREE

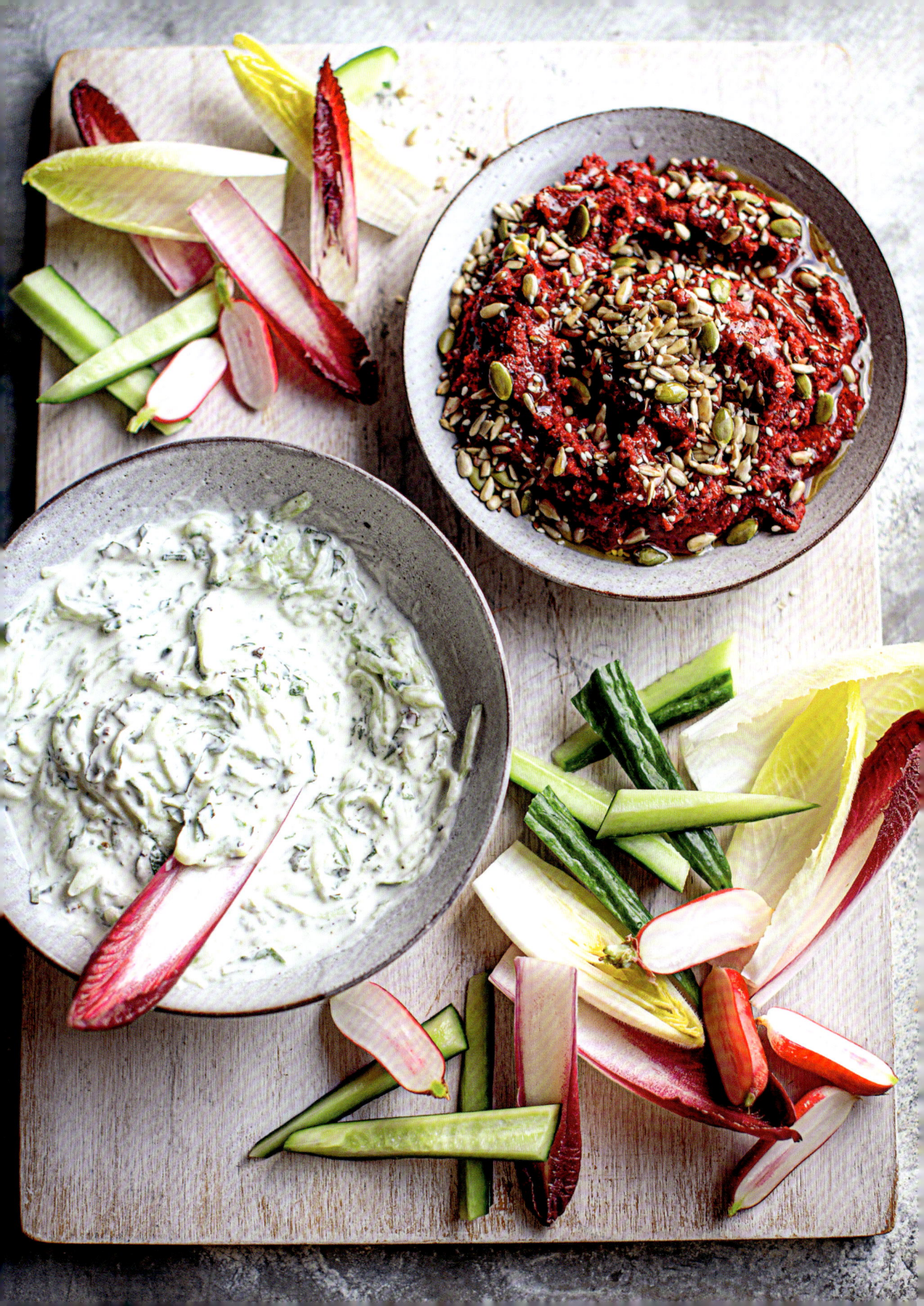

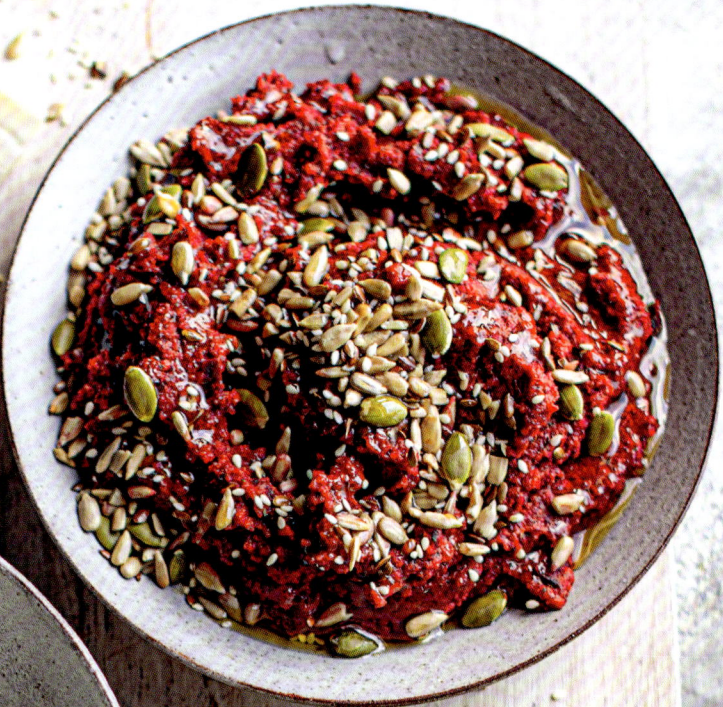

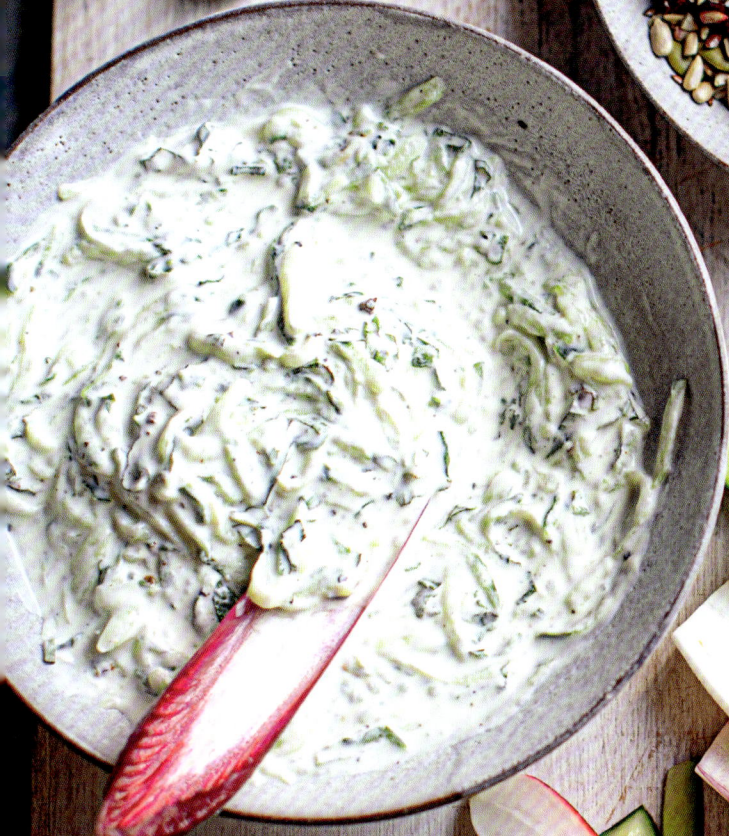

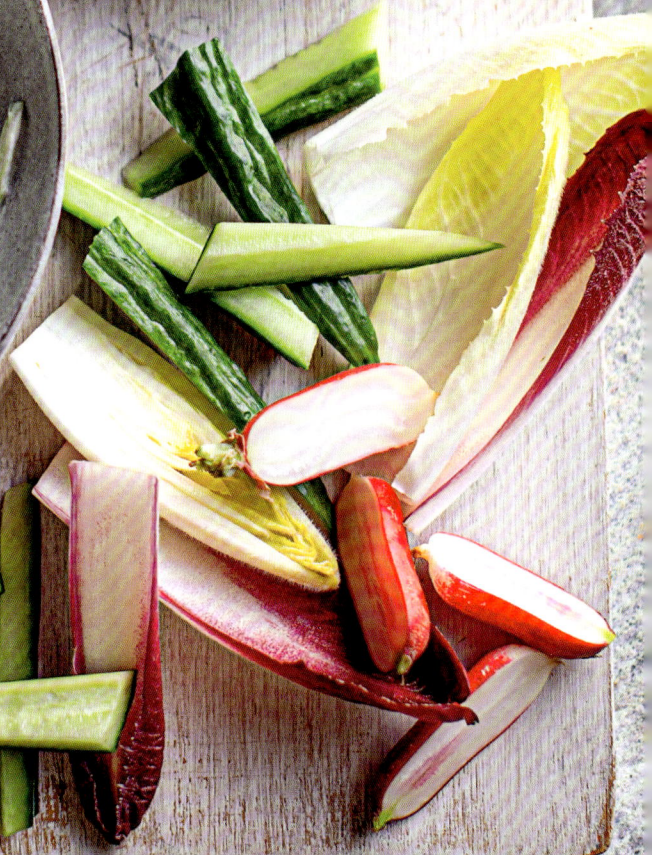

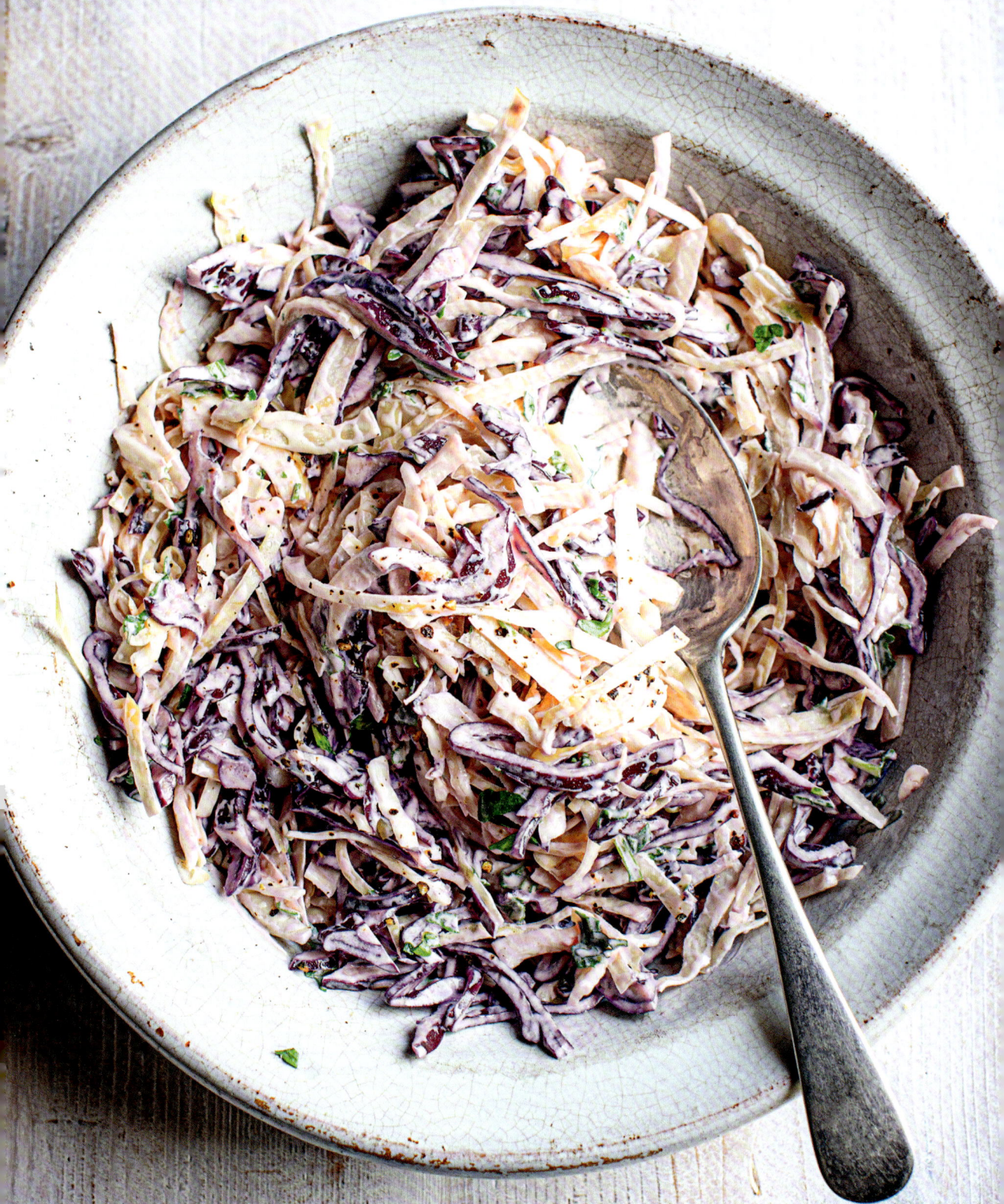

PER SERVING | **87cals** | PROTEIN **2.5g** | CARBS **5.6g**

UNDER 100 CALORIES

Simple Coleslaw

SERVES **4** | PREP **15** mins

2 tbsp full-fat live Greek yoghurt
1½ tbsp full-fat mayonnaise
1 tbsp English mustard
¼ white cabbage, finely sliced
¼ red cabbage, finely sliced

COOK'S TIP
A small handful of finely chopped rocket or spinach would make a lovely addition, if you have any in the fridge.

Michael was a huge fan of crunchy, multi-coloured coleslaw, rich in fibre and a boost to the gut microbes. He enjoyed it alongside lots of different meals. It will keep for up to 4 days in the fridge. The English mustard can be replaced by Dijon, if you prefer.

1. Mix the yoghurt, mayonnaise and mustard together in a large bowl.

2. Add the sliced cabbages and toss to coat thoroughly.

VEGGIE | NUT FREE

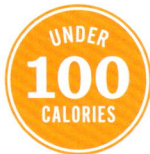

Halloumi Fries

SERVES **4** | **PREP** **5** mins | **COOK** **7** mins

1 tbsp olive oil
1 × 225g pack halloumi,
   cut into 8 chunky fries

COOK'S TIP
You can season the halloumi fries, if preferred. Sprinkle the fries with salt and freshly ground pepper, or add a squeeze of lemon juice, some roughly chopped parsley and crushed dried chilli flakes.

Halloumi fries were a perfect, protein-packed alternative to potatoes for Michael, a self-proclaimed chip addict.

1. Place the oil in a large frying pan over a high heat. When hot, add the halloumi and fry on each side until golden brown and crisp.

2. Transfer to a plate lined with kitchen paper to absorb the excess oil. Serve immediately.

AIR-FRYER TIP

Preheat the air fryer to 190°C, if needed. Carefully pat the halloumi fries dry with kitchen paper. Place the halloumi chips in the air fryer and brush the tops with a little oil. Air fry for 4–5 minutes, or until beginning to brown. Turn the halloumi and brush with more oil (you are unlikely to need the full quantity). Return the halloumi to the air fryer for another 4–5 minutes until golden and crisp.

VEGGIE · GLUTEN FREE · NUT FREE

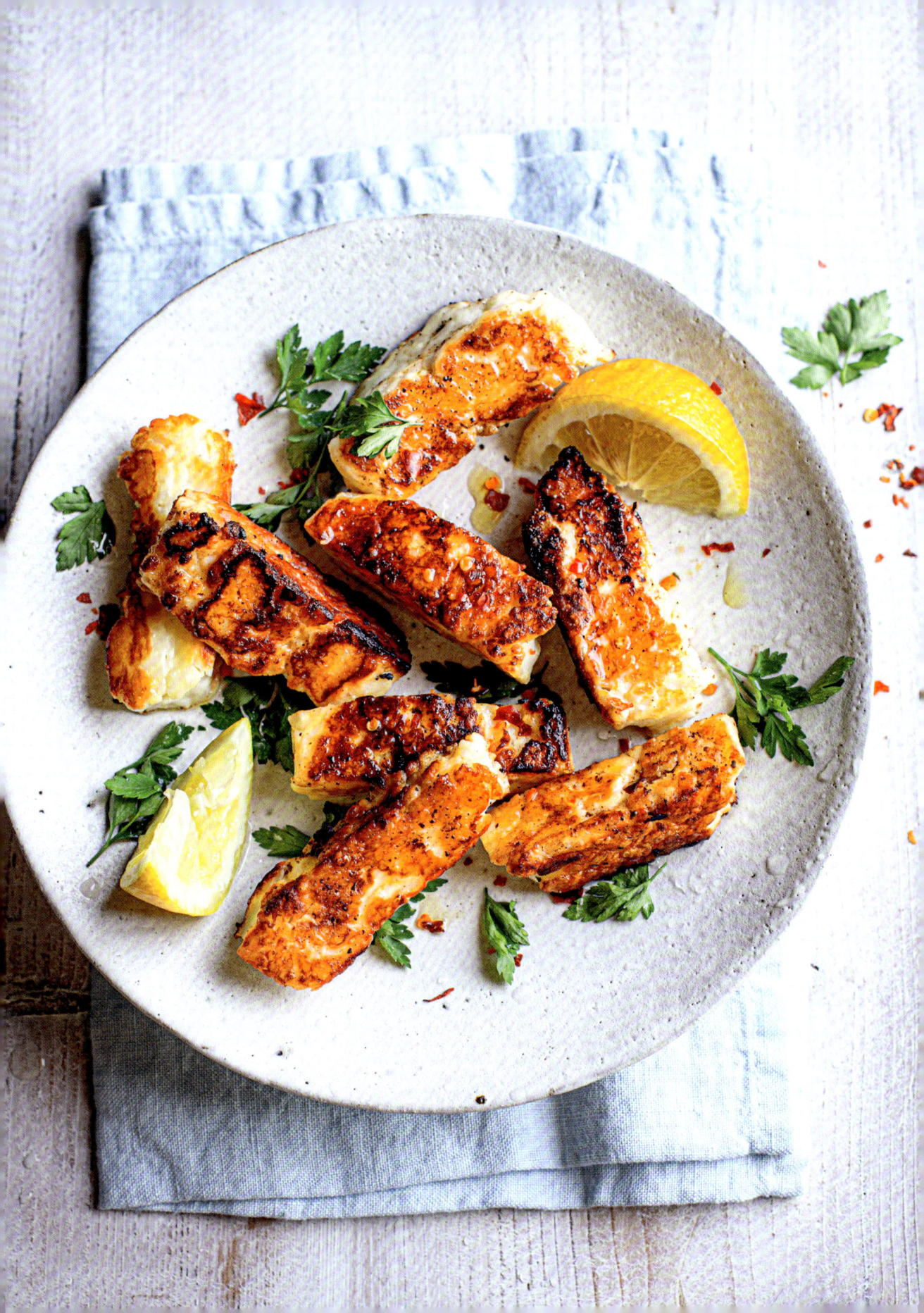

EASY WAYS WITH PICKLES & SAUERKRAUT

Fermentation is an ancient technique for preserving foods, using the natural healthy bacteria in the food (and is best done with organic veg, if available). The process encourages yeast and bacteria to break down the carbohydrates (sugars) in the vegetables. Fermentation also achieves another wonderful benefit: it produces natural probiotics, live micro-organisms, which support our gut microbiome and boost our immune system. Together, Michael and I sliced crunchy veg, massaged it with salt, burped, bottled and stored it in the fridge – then we scattered it on scrambled eggs, fish, salads and more. In doing so, we boosted our microbiome. These non-starchy veg, eaten in fairly small quantities, don't need calorie counting.

Build a Pickle

Pickles are cheap, quick and easy to make – they are ready to eat in just over a week but last for ages in the fridge.

MAKES 500G
1 tbsp sea salt
filtered water
1 × 500ml clean jam jar with tight-fitting lid

Add 500g veg	Add 2–4 tsp any spices:
beetroot	turmeric (ground or grated fresh)
cabbage	cumin seeds
carrots	coriander seeds
cauliflower	black peppercorns
courgette	grated fresh root ginger
cucumber	crushed dried chilli flakes
onion	mustard seeds

COOK'S TIPS
To keep the salty water topped up, make extra brine by dissolving 1 teaspoon salt in 200ml filtered water.

Keep an eye on your pickle or kraut and discard any vegetables that have blackened or turned mouldy.

1. Rinse the veg in filtered water. Depending on your choice, trim your carrots/cucumber/courgette, discard the outer leaves of your cauliflower and cabbage, and peel your onions. Slice the veg into 1–1.5cm cubes or batons, as appropriate, and place in a bowl.

2. Scatter with the salt and use your hands to rub the salt in. Leave the veg to soak for 30–60 minutes.

3. Stir in your choice of spices, then transfer the veg and juices to the jar, packing it in tightly.

4. Top up with filtered water so the veg are submerged – keep levels at least 2cm from the top of the jar.

5. Close the lid firmly and keep the pickle at room temperature for 5–10 days. Release the gases daily (burp them), especially in the first few days. Make sure the veg remain submerged and top the jar up with salty water (see cook's tip), if necessary.

6. Taste regularly and, when it tastes nicely sweet and sharp, store in the fridge and eat within 2–3 months.

Build a Kraut

Sauerkraut – fermented cabbage – goes well with almost any savoury food. We often have it with an omelette or scrambled eggs. This recipe is for turmeric and ginger sauerkraut but feel free to experiment with other spices, such as cumin, caraway, peppercorns, fennel, toasted coriander or mustard seeds.

MAKES 1 LITRE
½ medium white cabbage, quartered lengthways, hard core removed, finely sliced, or 1 small green pointed cabbage (about 600g)
2 large white onions, halved and sliced
1 heaped tbsp sea salt
2 tsp grated fresh ginger
1 tsp ground turmeric
2 × 500ml or 1 × 1 litre clean jam jars with tight-fitting lids

1. Combine the cabbage and onion in a large bowl, sprinkling the salt between the layers as you fill it. Massage the salt into the veg, then leave it for 1–2 hours to soften and release the liquor.

2. Stir in the ginger and turmeric. (This is the point to add other spices – see list opposite – if you want to flavour your kraut differently.)

3. Spoon the cabbage mixture and the juices into the jars. Pack the mixture down, pressing it firmly into the fluid – keep levels at least 2cm from the top of the jar. If there is not enough liquid to cover the mixture, top up with a few teaspoonfuls of filtered water. You can use a stone or piece of ceramic to keep the veg submerged.

4. Close the lid firmly, place the jars on a plate to catch any overflow and keep at room temperature, out of direct sunlight for 5–10 days. Release the gases daily (burp them), especially in the first few days. Make sure the veg remains submerged and top the jar up with salty filtered water (see cook's tip opposite), if necessary.

5. Sample regularly and, when it tastes good and tangy (usually 7–10 days), store in the fridge and eat within 2–3 months. Fermenting is a live process and occurs at different rates, according to the environment and temperature.

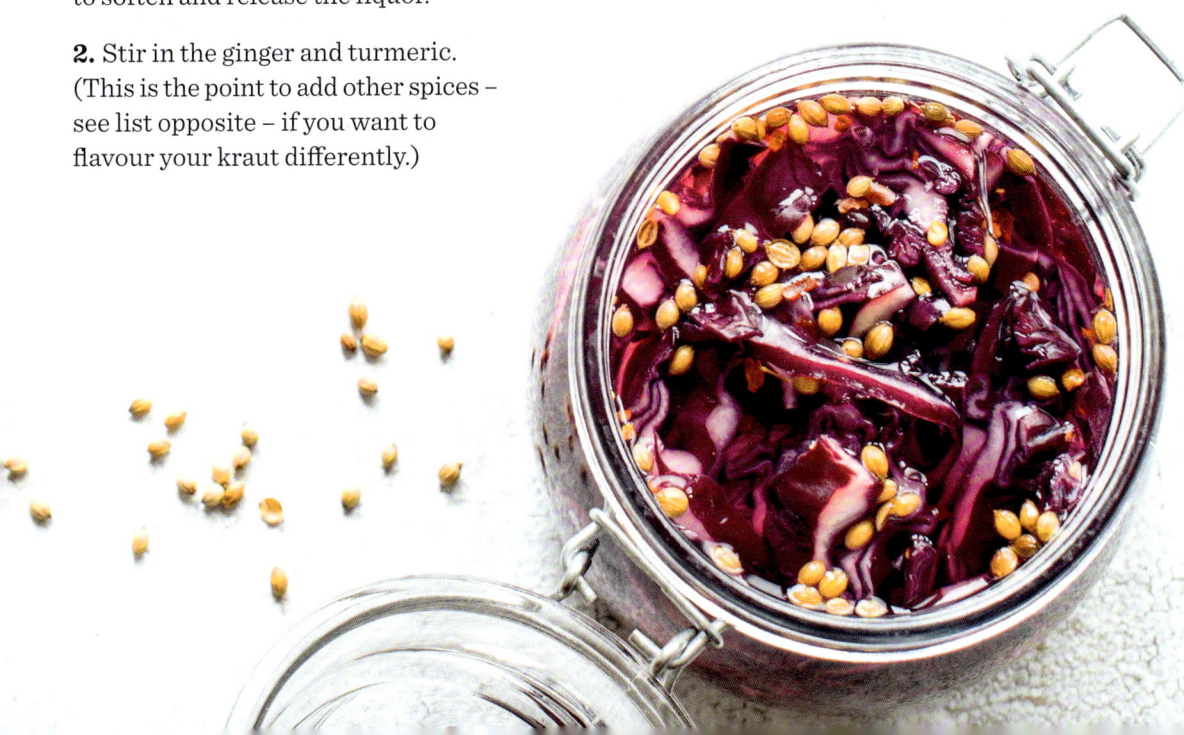

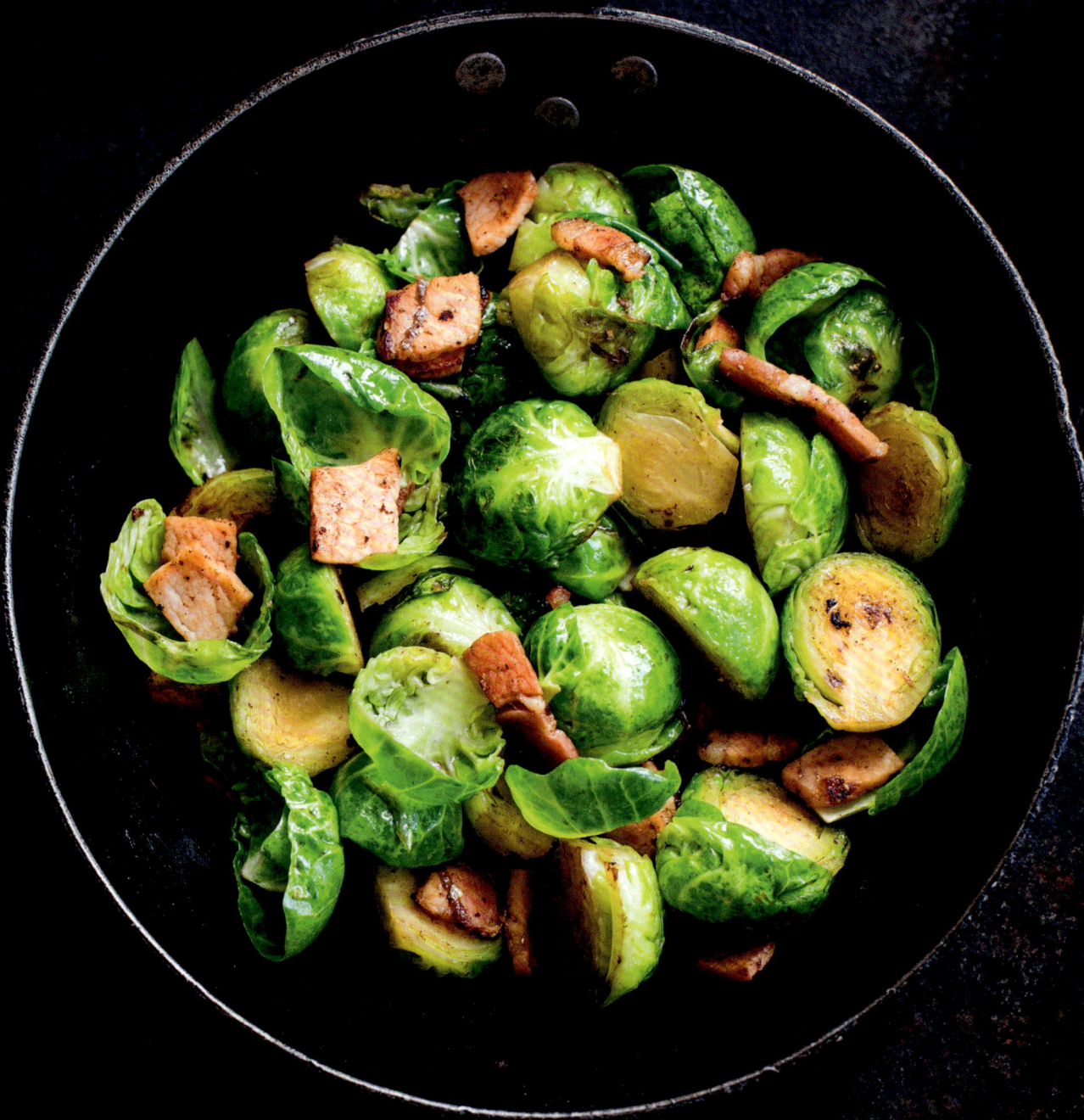

PER SERVING | **174cals** | PROTEIN **11g** | CARBS **5g**

UNDER
200
CALORIES

Brussels Sprouts with Bacon

SERVES | PREP | COOK
2 | **5** mins | **10** mins

2 tsp olive or rapeseed oil
2 rashers smoked back bacon,
   cut into 1–2cm pieces
250g small Brussels sprouts,
   trimmed and halved
2 tsp apple cider vinegar

COOK'S TIP
Try sprinkling with Parmesan,
or dotting with small chunks of
soft blue cheese at the end for
extra protein, but don't forget to
add the calories (see page 271).

This much-maligned vegetable needs to be given
another chance. The recipe here has converted most
of our family, although Michael remained on the fence.
When fried quickly to retain a bit of crunch, Brussels
sprouts have a wonderful, delicate flavour.

1. Heat 1 teaspoon of the oil in a large frying pan over
a medium heat. Add the bacon and fry for 2–3 minutes,
or until lightly browned, stirring regularly. Transfer to
a plate with a slotted spoon.

2. Add the remaining oil and Brussels sprouts to the pan,
reduce the heat slightly and fry gently for 4–6 minutes,
or until browned in places and just tender, stirring often.

3. Return the bacon to the pan, sprinkle in the vinegar,
and add a pinch of salt and lots of freshly ground
black pepper. Toss everything together for 1 minute
before serving.

GLUTEN FREE · NUT FREE · DAIRY FREE

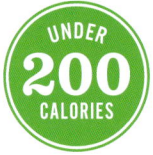

Creamy Beans

SERVES	PREP	COOK
4	**5** mins	**5** mins

2 × 400g cans butter beans in water
4 tbsp full-fat crème fraîche
1 tbsp finely snipped chives (optional), plus extra to garnish

COOK'S TIP
If you are cooking for two, simply halve the ingredients.

These make a wonderful alternative to mash. Serve them with any grilled or roasted meat or fish. These beans are great with casseroles, too.

1. Place the beans and their water in a saucepan and cook over a low heat for 3–4 minutes, or until hot, stirring regularly.

2. Drain the beans, then return them to the pan and add the crème fraîche and chives, if using. Season with salt and plenty of freshly ground black pepper, and toss everything together for 20–30 seconds, or until hot, stirring.

3. Remove from the heat and either leave whole or mash thoroughly with a potato masher, adding a splash of hot water, if needed, to loosen. You could also blitz the beans with a stick blender to achieve a smoother mash.

4. Serve the beans sprinkled with some more snipped chives, if using, and a drizzle of oil, if liked - but don't forget to add the extra calories (27cals for each teaspoon).

VEGGIE · GLUTEN FREE · NUT FREE

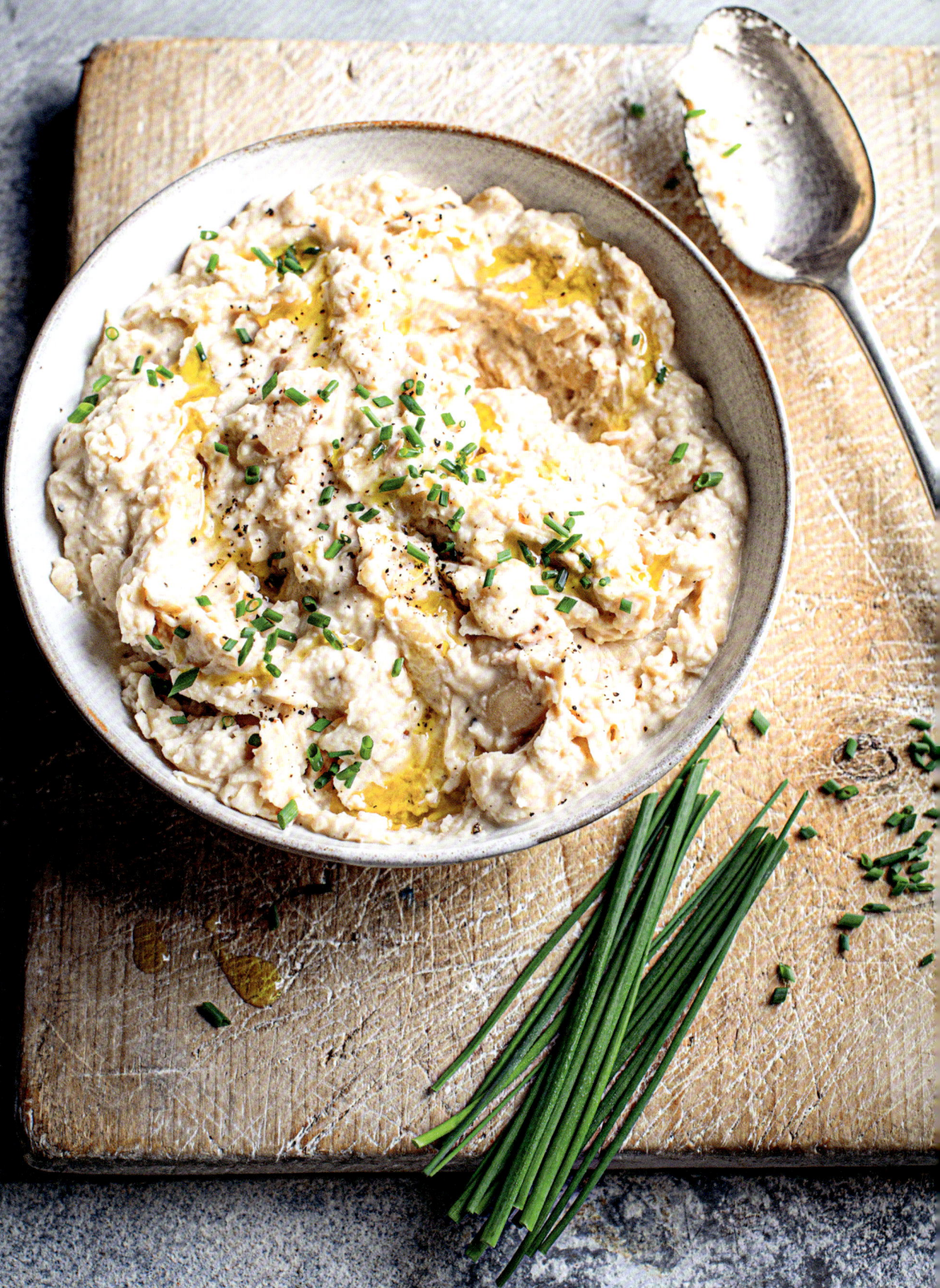

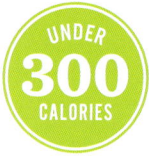

| PER SERVING | **255cals** | PROTEIN **10g** | CARBS **25g**

Simple Dahl

SERVES	PREP	COOK
4	**5** mins	**25** mins

4 tbsp rapeseed oil
1 large or 2 small onions
   (around 200g), thinly sliced
20g fresh root ginger,
   peeled and finely chopped,
   or 1 tsp ground ginger
2–3 tsp medium curry powder
150g dried split red lentils
juice of 1 small lemon
   (optional)

COOK'S TIP
To skip frying the onions
for the topping, cook the
full amount of onion in
2 tablespoons olive oil
until soft before adding the
ginger and curry powder.
The dahl will contain
205cals per serving.

Fast-cooking dried red lentils are invaluable to keep at hand for thickening stews, adding to soups and, of course, for making dahl. They add a bit of texture and plenty of gut-friendly fibre. You can throw in extra non-starchy veg, such as spinach, mushrooms, aubergine or cauliflower, or have them on the side, without counting the extra cals. To transform it into a main meal, serve it with one of the protein-rich additions on page 271. Michael made this regularly, as a versatile staple.

1. Pour the oil into a large saucepan and place over a high heat. Add half the sliced onion and fry for 2–3 minutes, or until lightly browned and crisp in places, stirring regularly. Remove with a slotted spoon and set aside on a plate lined with kitchen paper.

2. Reduce the heat, add the remaining onion, ginger and curry powder and fry gently for 1 minute, stirring.

3. Add the lentils and 750ml cold water. Bring to a simmer, then cover the pan, reduce the heat and cook for 15–20 minutes, or until the lentils are very soft, stirring regularly.

4. Season with salt and freshly ground black pepper, drizzle with lemon juice, if using, and scatter the crispy onions on top to serve. Add a tablespoon of full-fat live Greek yoghurt for 20cals.

VEGAN | GLUTEN FREE | NUT FREE | DAIRY FREE

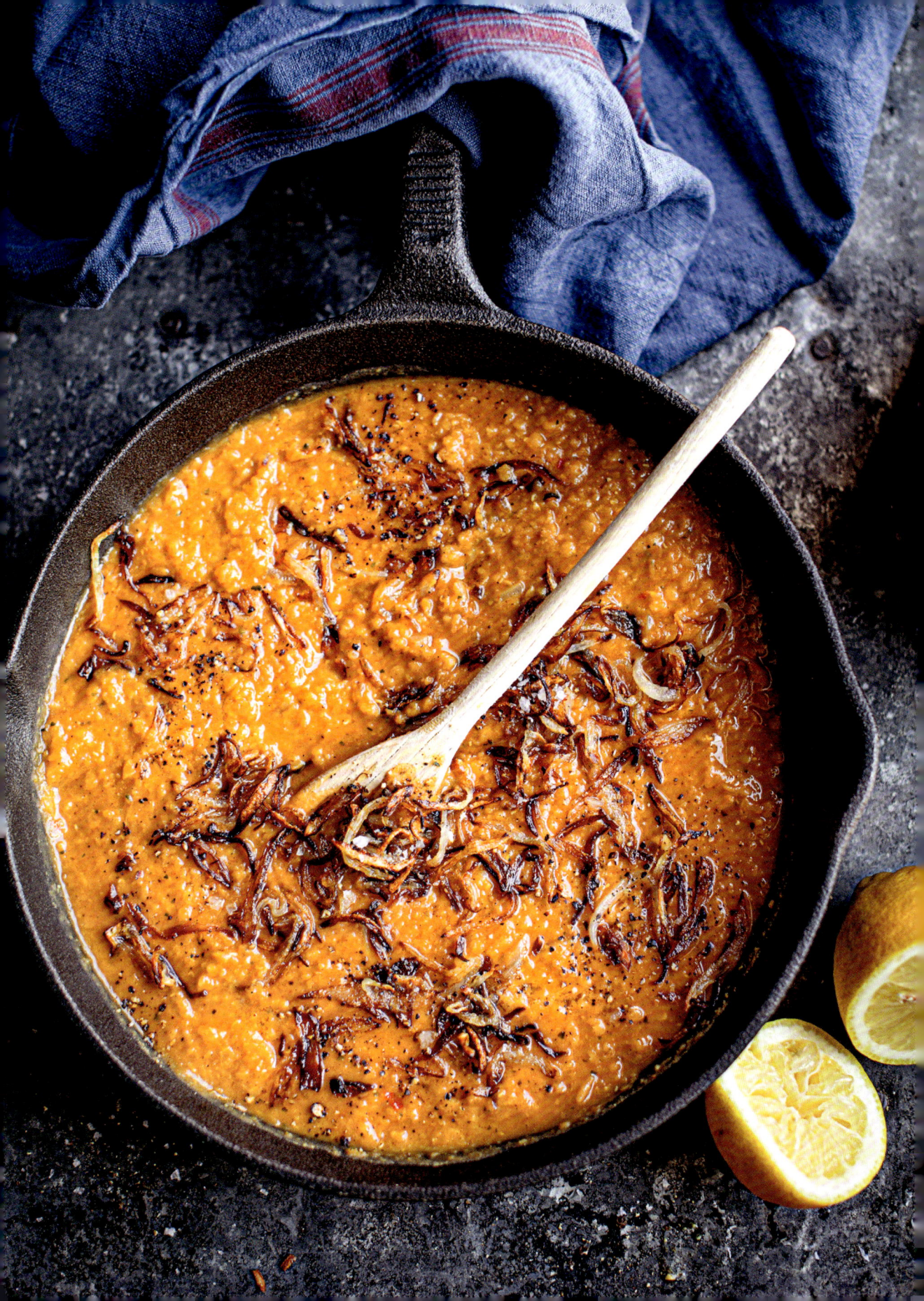

EASY WAYS WITH WITH CAULIFLOWER

Highly nutritious and surprisingly rich in vitamin C and fibre, cauliflower has become a popular substitute for many starchy foods, such as rice and potato. Here we suggest three great ways to cook it – as cauli-rice, mash and roasted. These were Michael's go-to recipes on a fast day – who would have guessed cauliflower could be so delicious and versatile?

UNDER 100 CALORIES | PER SERVING | **68cals** | PROTEIN **5g**

Cauli-rice

SERVES 1
½ small cauliflower (around 200g)

1. Hold the cauliflower at the stalk end and coarsely grate in short, sharp movements in a downward direction. You can also do this in a food processor but don't let the pieces get too small or they will turn to a paste.

2. Either **stir fry** with 1 teaspoon olive oil (27cals) in a large non-stick frying pan or wok over medium–high setting for 4–5 minutes, or **steam** in a saucepan over a medium–high heat for 3–4 minutes. You could also microwave on HIGH for 2–3 minutes. The rice should retain a bit of bite, like al-dente pasta.

3. Stir in some chopped parsley or coriander, or squeeze over some fresh lemon juice for added flavour.

UNDER 100 CALORIES | PER SERVING | **95cals** | PROTEIN **5g**

Cauliflower Mash

SERVES 1
½ small cauliflower (around 200g), trimmed, broken into small florets and stalk thinly sliced
1 tsp olive oil

1. Half fill a medium pan with water and bring to the boil. Add the cauliflower and return to the boil. Cook for 15–20 minutes or until very soft.

2. Drain, then return to the pan. Add the oil, a pinch of salt and lots of ground black pepper. Blitz with a stick blender, or cool slightly and blend in a food processor until smooth. (You can also mash vigorously with a potato masher.)

VEGAN · GLUTEN FREE · NUT FREE · DAIRY FREE

PER SERVING | **95cals** | PROTEIN **5g**

Roasted Cauliflower

SERVES 1

½ small cauliflower (around 200g),
  trimmed and broken into small florets,
  halving or quartering any large ones
1 tsp ground turmeric, or spices of your choice
1 tsp fresh lemon juice
1 tsp olive or rapeseed oil

1. Preheat the oven to 220°C/Fan 200°C/Gas 7.

2. Place the cauliflower, turmeric or other
spices and the lemon juice in a large bowl.
Drizzle with the oil and season with salt
and lots of freshly ground black pepper.
Toss together well, massaging the spice
into the florets.

3. Scatter the cauliflower over a large
baking tray and roast for 10–15 minutes,
or until just tender and browning in places.

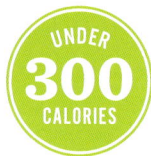

Hoisin Roasted Cauliflower with Peanuts

SERVES **2**

PREP **10** mins

COOK **15** mins

½ cauliflower, trimmed and cut into small florets (around 300g prepared weight)
1 tbsp olive or rapeseed oil
1 tbsp hoisin or plum sauce
½–1 tsp crushed dried chilli flakes
1 tsp finely grated fresh root ginger or ½ tsp ground ginger
1 tbsp apple cider vinegar
25g unsalted peanuts, finely chopped
handful roughly chopped coriander leaves, to serve

A tasty side dish, which works well with some added protein for a light lunch (see page 271). For extra flavour, serve with a portion of sauerkraut (see page 225) or kimchi – no need to count the calories.

1. Preheat the oven to 200°C/Fan 180°C/Gas 6.

2. Place the cauliflower florets on a large baking tray and season generously with salt and lots of freshly ground black pepper. Roast for 10 minutes, until starting to brown.

3. Meanwhile, place the oil, hoisin or plum sauce, chilli flakes, ginger and cider vinegar in a large bowl and mix well.

4. Remove the tray from the oven and carefully transfer the hot cauliflower to the bowl to coat in the dressing. Return to the baking tray and scatter with the peanuts. Place back in the oven for another 5 minutes, until the cauliflower is starting to soften but still has a firm texture.

5. Scatter with the coriander to serve.

AIR-FRYER TIP

Preheat the air fryer to 180°C, if needed. Season the cauliflower florets and air fry for 8 minutes. Prepare the hoisin or plum sauce mixture as Step 3 and use to coat the cauliflower as Step 4. Return the cauliflower to the air fryer for 4–5 minutes, turning halfway, until softened and golden. Scatter with coriander to serve.

VEGAN   DAIRY FREE

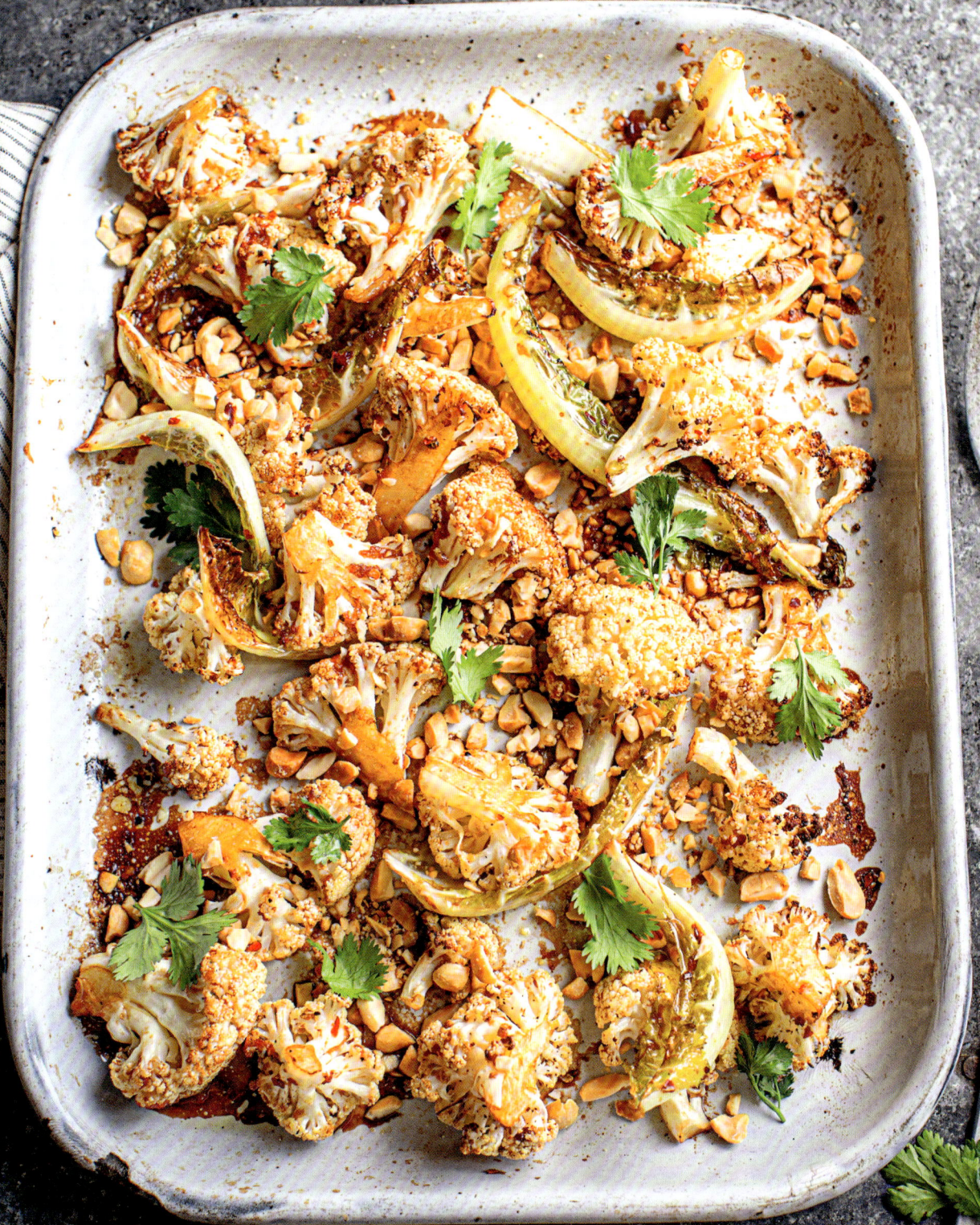

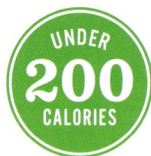

Steamed Broccoli and Edamame Beans with Soy and Chilli

SERVES	PREP	COOK
1	**2** mins	**5** mins

130g tenderstem broccoli, trimmed
50g frozen edamame beans
1 tbsp light soy sauce
pinch crushed dried chilli flakes (optional)

NON-FAST DAY
Increase the portion size, add a protein top-up (see intro) and serve with some non-starchy carbs.

This simple green dish pings with flavour and is high in protein and fibre, too. Add protein top-ups such as cheese, toasted nuts, cooked chicken or tofu (see page 271) for a light meal.

1. Place the broccoli in a colander set over a pan of boiling water and cover. Steam for 2 minutes. Add the edamame beans and steam for a further 2 minutes.

2. Transfer to a plate, drizzle the soy sauce all over and sprinkle with chilli flakes, if using. Season generously with freshly ground black pepper to serve.

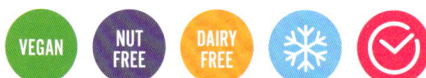

VEGAN · NUT FREE · DAIRY FREE

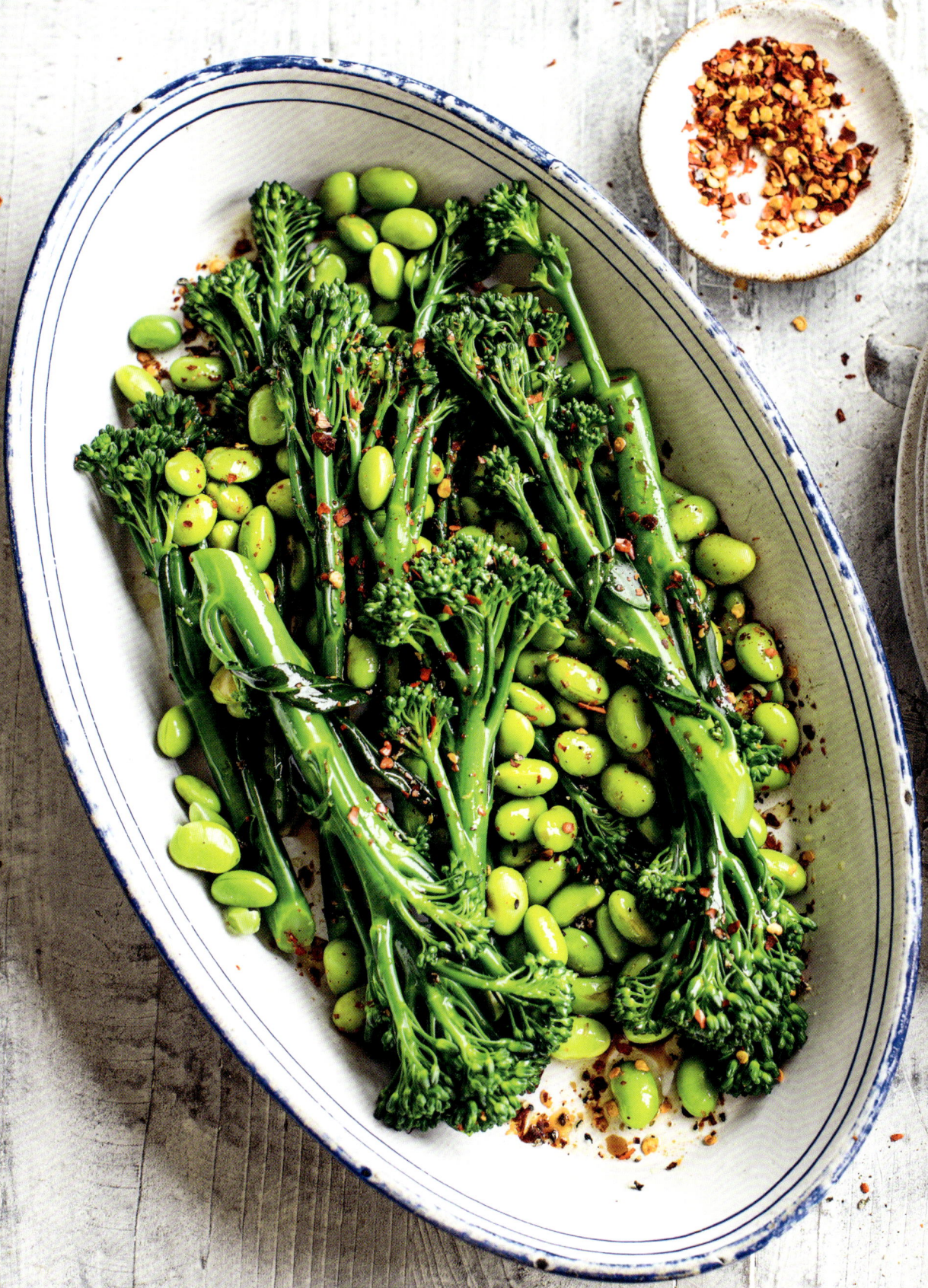

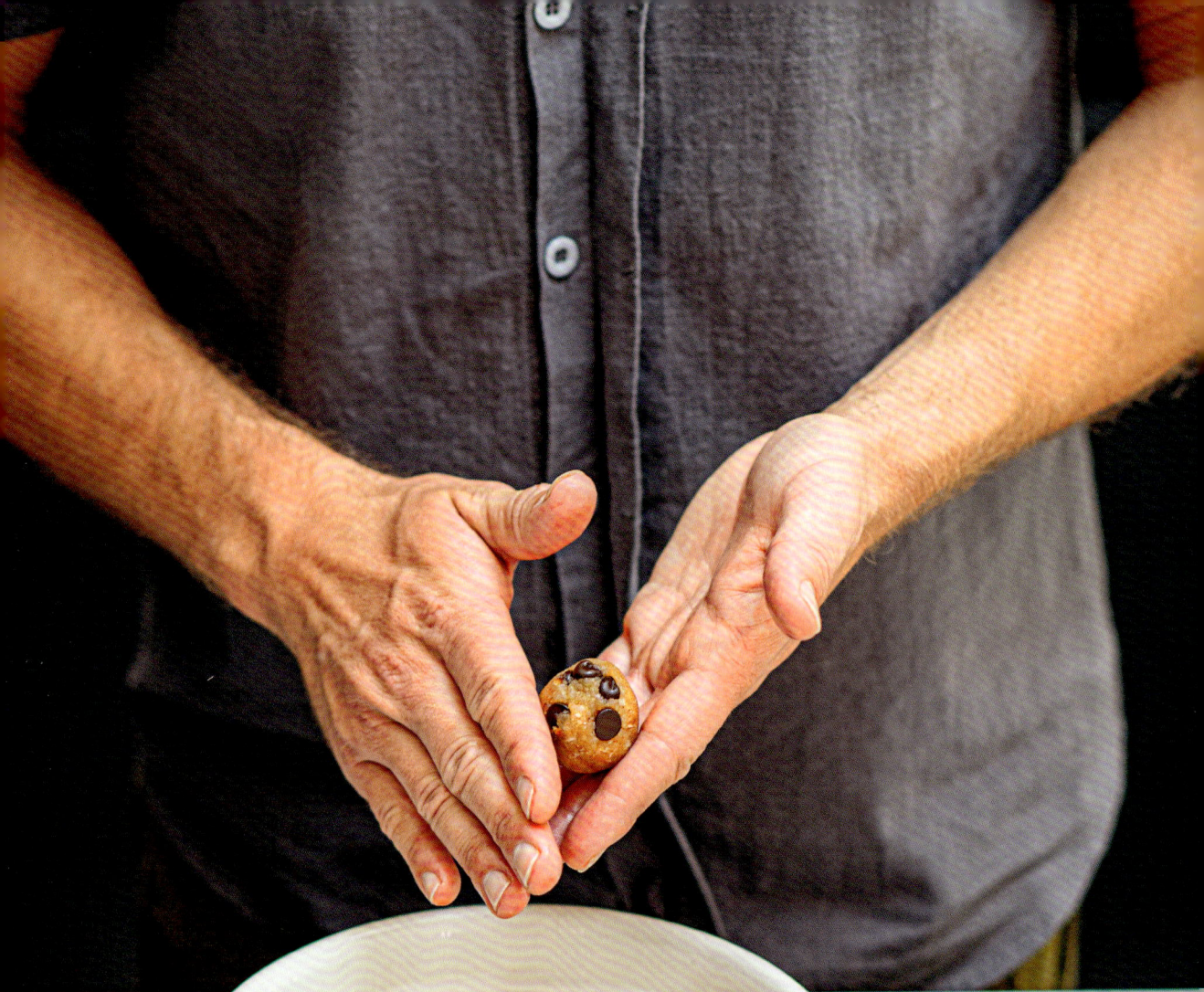

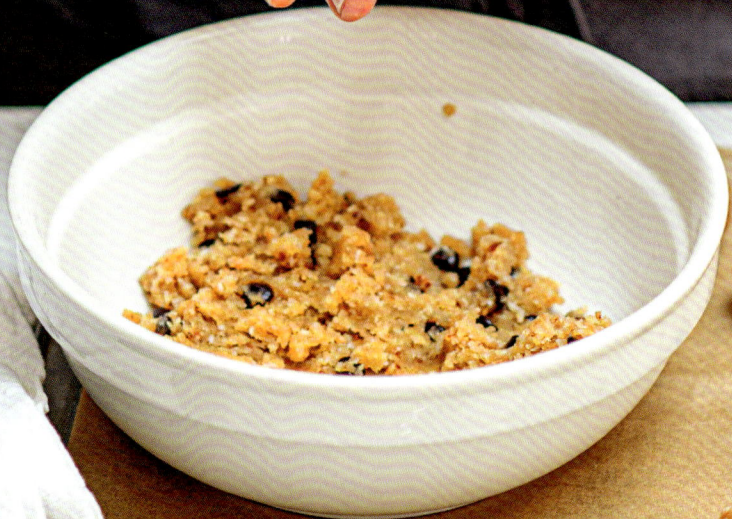

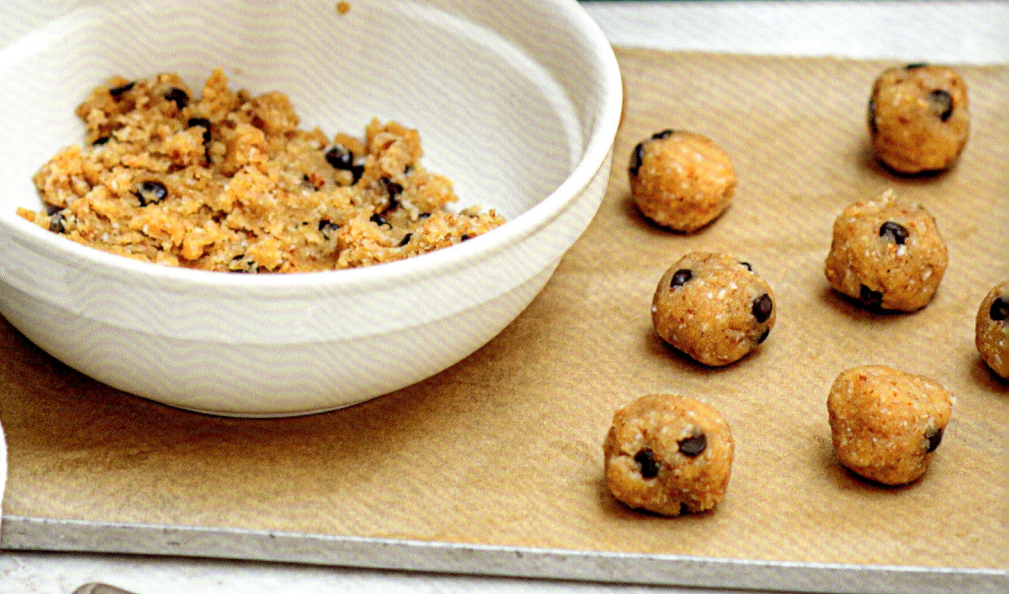

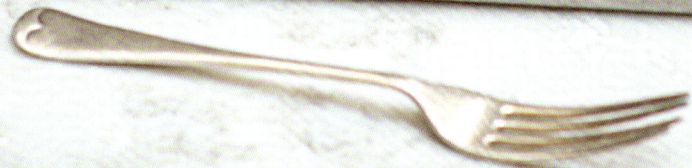

Occasional Treats

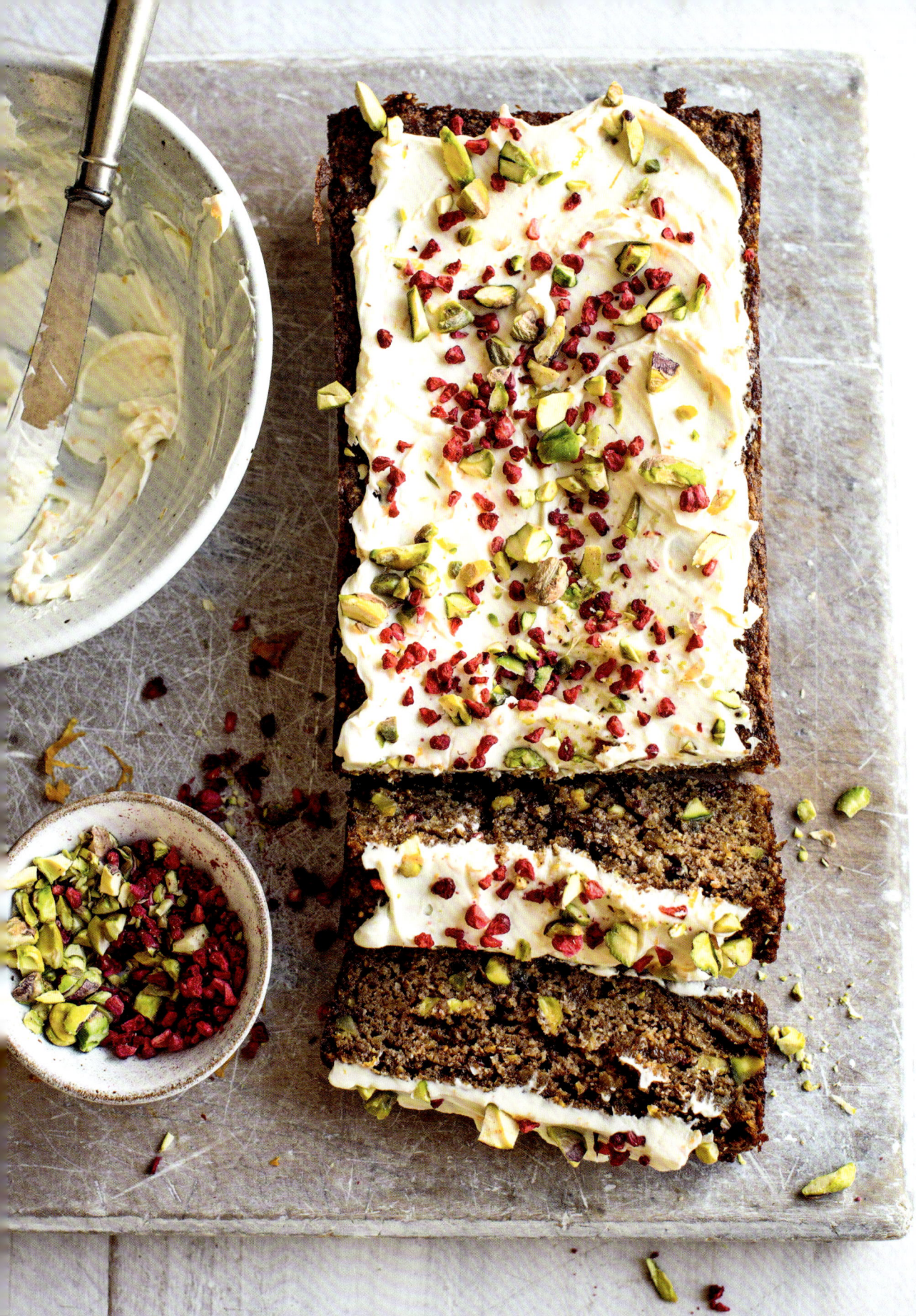

Persian Love Cake

SERVES 8 | **PREP** 30 mins | **COOK** 30 mins

100g dried figs, finely chopped
60g coconut oil or butter
2 medium free-range eggs
60g shelled pistachio nuts, roughly chopped
finely grated zest and juice of 2 oranges
100g ground almonds
1 tsp ground cinnamon
1 tsp ground cardamom
1 tsp bicarbonate of soda
2 tbsp freeze-dried raspberries
1 tbsp apple cider vinegar

For the icing
60g full-fat cream cheese
1 tsp honey
1 tsp finely grated lemon zest

COOK'S TIP
This freezes well (so you don't need to eat it all at once, as Michael was frequently tempted to do). You could use a loaf tin liner if you have one.

PER SERVING | **273cals** | PROTEIN **8g** | CARBS **9.8g** | SUGAR **10.5g** — UNDER 300 CALORIES

For lovely Michael, this enchantingly exotic concoction lives up to its name. Not sure I do it justice, but it certainly goes down well, with its tangy, orange-flavoured topping, and rich, nutty base. High in protein and nutrients, it has no added sugar, is low carb and feels like a real treat... Enjoy!

1. Preheat the oven to 180°C/Fan 160°C/Gas 4. Line the base of a 20 × 10cm loaf tin with non-stick baking paper.

2. Place the figs, coconut oil or butter and eggs in a bowl and blitz with a stick blender for about 1 minute, until creamy but retaining some texture.

3. Stir in 40g of the pistachios, half the orange zest, the orange juice, ground almonds, cinnamon, cardamom, bicarbonate of soda, half the dried raspberries and a generous pinch of salt. Mix well, then add the cider vinegar and mix again.

4. Pour the mixture into the prepared loaf tin and bake for about 30 minutes, until cooked through and a skewer inserted into the centre comes out clean. Turn out of the tin and leave to cool on a wire rack.

5. To make the topping, mix the remaining orange zest with the cream cheese, honey and lemon zest in a small bowl. Spread it on to the cooled cake, then sprinkle the remaining chopped pistachios and dried raspberries on top.

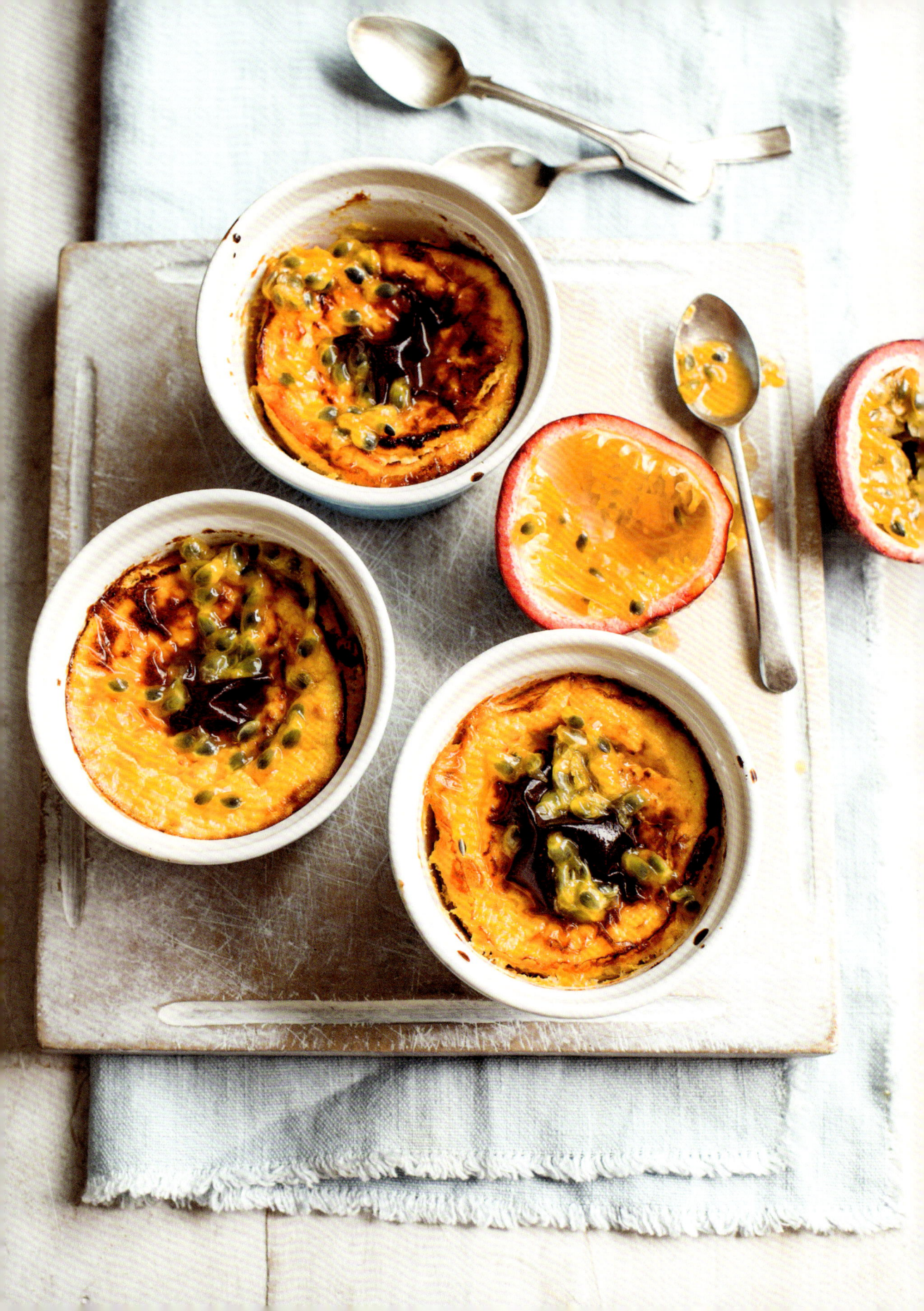

Peach, Passionfruit and Vanilla Mini Basque Cheesecakes

SERVES | PREP | COOK
4 | **5** mins | **20** mins

coconut oil, for greasing
160g full-fat cream cheese
½ × 415g can peaches
 in juice, drained
 (125g drained weight)
½ tbsp vanilla extract
1 medium free-range egg
2 medium free-range egg yolks
1 large or 2 small passionfruit

COOK'S TIP
If you don't have ramekin dishes you can use a muffin tin lined with 6 muffin cases. Keep any leftovers in the fridge for up to 3 days.

These delightful little cheesecakes come out of the oven with a deep golden, almost burnt-looking surface and are light and delicate inside. Spices, such as ground cardamom or cinnamon, would make a lovely addition.

1. Preheat the oven to 240°C/Fan 220°C/Gas 9 and grease 6 × 8cm ramekins with a little coconut oil.

2. Place the cream cheese, peaches, vanilla extract, egg and egg yolks in a jug and blitz with a stick blender until smooth.

3. Pour into the ramekins and bake in the oven for 20 minutes, or until the tops are golden brown. Set aside to cool.

4. Cut a passionfruit in half and scrape out the seeds with a teaspoon. Spoon over the cheesecakes to serve.

AIR-FRYER TIP

Preheat the air fryer to 190°C, if needed. Grease 4 x 8cm ramekins with a little coconut oil. Prepare the cheesecake mixture as Step 2 and pour into the prepared ramekins. Air fry for 13–15 minutes, until the tops are golden brown. Allow to cool and serve as above.

VEGGIE   GLUTEN FREE   NUT FREE

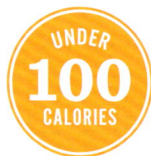

Mango and Lime Semifreddo

SERVES | PREP | FREEZE
6 | **15** mins | **6** hours

250g full-fat live Greek yoghurt
finely grated zest of 1 lime
1 tbsp vanilla extract
2 medium free-range
   eggs, separated
1 × 425g can mangoes in juice,
   drained and blitzed until
   smooth (around 230g
   drained weight)

A simple but indulgent frozen dessert. A very ripe fresh mango could be used here instead of canned, but the beauty of using canned is that you can have it on hand, ready to pull together whenever you fancy. As an ice cream lover, this was a great recipe for Michael and it didn't raise his sugars.

1. Line 1 × 450g loaf tin with 2 large sheets of clingfilm, leaving the excess hanging over the sides of the tin.

2. Place the yoghurt, lime zest, vanilla and egg yolks in a bowl and whisk until smooth. Stir in three-quarters of the blitzed mango.

3. Place the egg whites in a separate bowl and whisk until very stiff.

4. Gently fold the egg whites into the yoghurt mixture until fully incorporated.

5. Transfer to the lined tin and swirl the remaining mango on top. Fold the clingfilm over the tin and place in the freezer for 4–6 hours or overnight.

6. Remove from the freezer about 30 minutes before you are ready to serve.

VEGGIE | GLUTEN FREE | NUT FREE

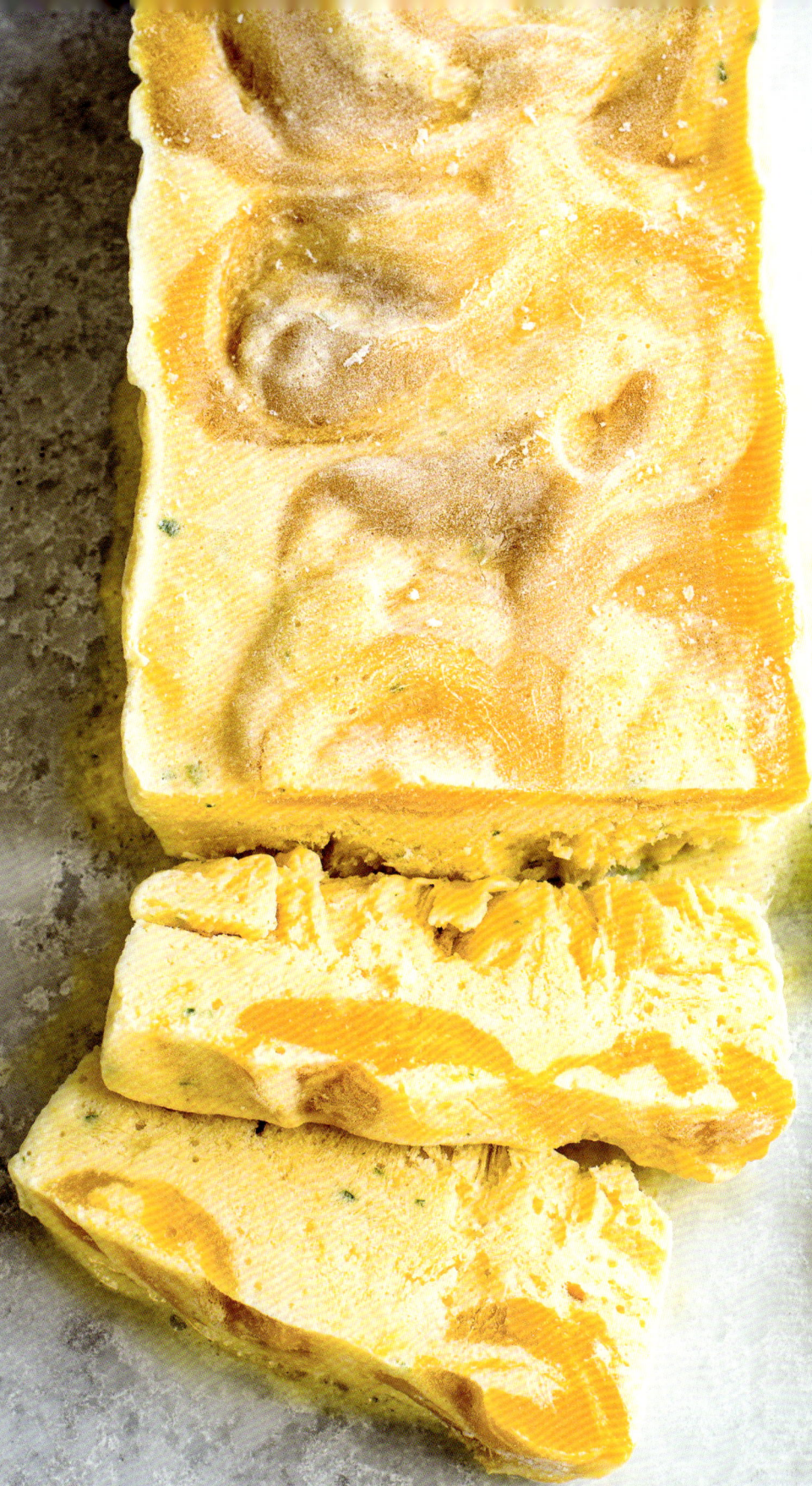

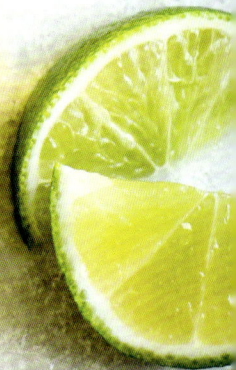

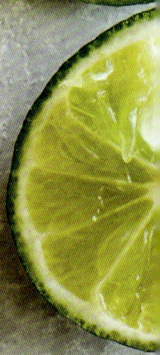

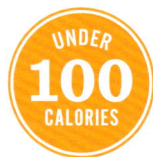

PER SERVING | **84cals** | PROTEIN **1.5g** | CARBS **6g** | SUGAR **3g**

Ginger Cookies

SERVES	PREP	COOK
14	**10** mins	**25** mins

2 medium free-range
  egg whites
50g ground almonds
50g porridge oats
  (not jumbo oats)
50g coconut oil (or butter)
2 balls of stem ginger in syrup,
  drained and finely chopped
2 tbsp stem ginger syrup
  from the jar

COOK'S TIP
If you have a mini food
processor, you can halve
the quantity to make
7 cookies instead.

Crunchy on the outside and soft and chewy on the inside, these delicious mini biscuits are surprisingly guilt free. They contain a decent hit of protein and fibre, are lovely as an after-dinner treat, or you can enjoy them crumbled in yoghurt with a handful of berries. In the past, Michael could eat almost a whole packet of biscuits. These simple ginger cookies were plentifully satisfying, but not addictive.

1. Preheat the oven to 180°C/Fan 160°C/Gas 4 and line a large baking tray with non-stick baking paper.

2. Combine all the ingredients in a large bowl and mix together using a stick blender. You could also tip them into a food processor and blitz briefly to combine. The dough should be fairly soft. Alternatively, mix together by hand.

3. Use two dessertspoons to drop the dough on to the lined tray. Press down into roughly 4cm rounds with the back of the spoon. Make all 14 cookies in the same way. Bake for about 22–25 minutes, or until golden brown.

4. Cool for a few minutes before serving. Store excess cookies in an airtight container in the freezer.

AIR-FRYER TIP
Preheat the air fryer to 160°C, if needed. Prepare and shape the cookies as Steps 2–3. Air fry (in batches) for 15 minutes, then turn over and cook for another 5–6 minutes, until golden brown.

VEGGIE · GLUTEN FREE · DAIRY FREE

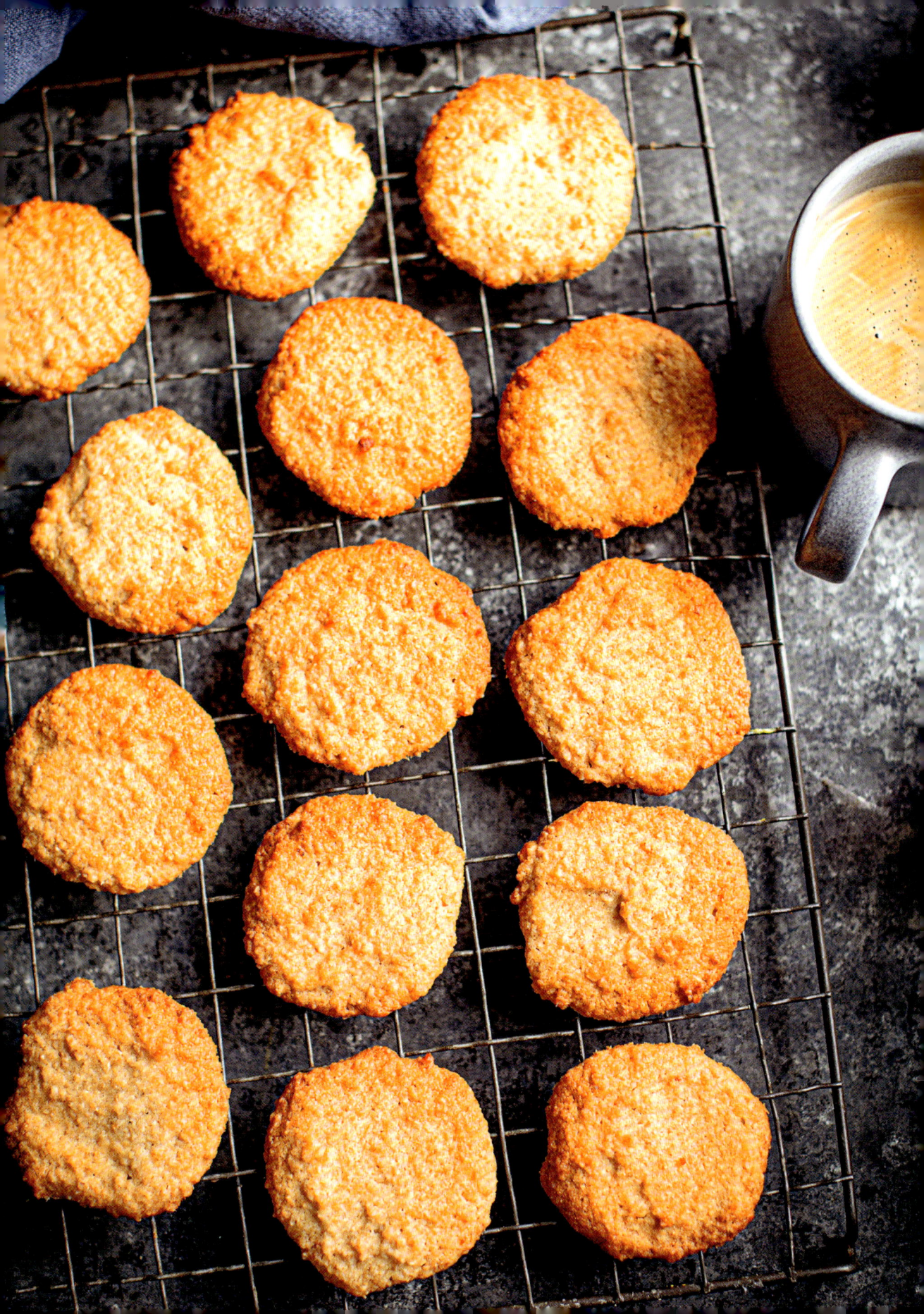

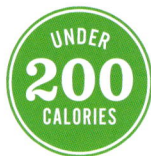

PER SERVING | **102cals** | PROTEIN **3g** | CARBS **15g** | SUGAR **15g**

Baked Nectarines with Blackberries

SERVES	PREP	COOK
4	**5** mins	**40** mins

4 ripe nectarines or peaches,
   halved and stoned
150g fresh or frozen
   blackberries
2 tbsp flaked almonds
   (around 15g)

COOK'S TIP
If you don't have blackberries,
use raspberries instead.

This is one of our favourite summer desserts. It's incredibly easy to make and can be served warm or cold. It also makes a lovely, fruity breakfast, served with yoghurt and a sprinkling of sugar-free granola.

1. Preheat the oven to 200°C/Fan 180°C/Gas 6.

2. Place the nectarine or peach halves in a small, shallow ovenproof dish or tin, cut-side up. Sprinkle over 6 tablespoons of cold water, then scatter over the blackberries and flaked almonds. Cover the dish with foil and bake in the oven for 30 minutes.

3. Remove the foil and bake for a further 5–10 minutes, or until the almonds are lightly toasted and the nectarines are very soft.

4. Serve warm or cold with full-fat live Greek yoghurt (20cals per tablespoon).

AIR-FRYER TIP

Preheat the air fryer to 160°C, if needed. Place the nectarines, cut-side down, in an even layer in a baking dish or directly in the air fryer. Pour in 150ml water. Air fry for 15 minutes, turning halfway and spooning the juices over the nectarines (add a splash more water if dry). Add the blackberries (with more water, if needed) and scatter over the almonds. Air fry for another 5–8 minutes, until the nectarines are soft and the almonds lightly toasted.

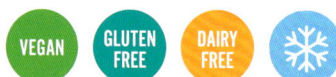

VEGAN | GLUTEN FREE | DAIRY FREE | ❄

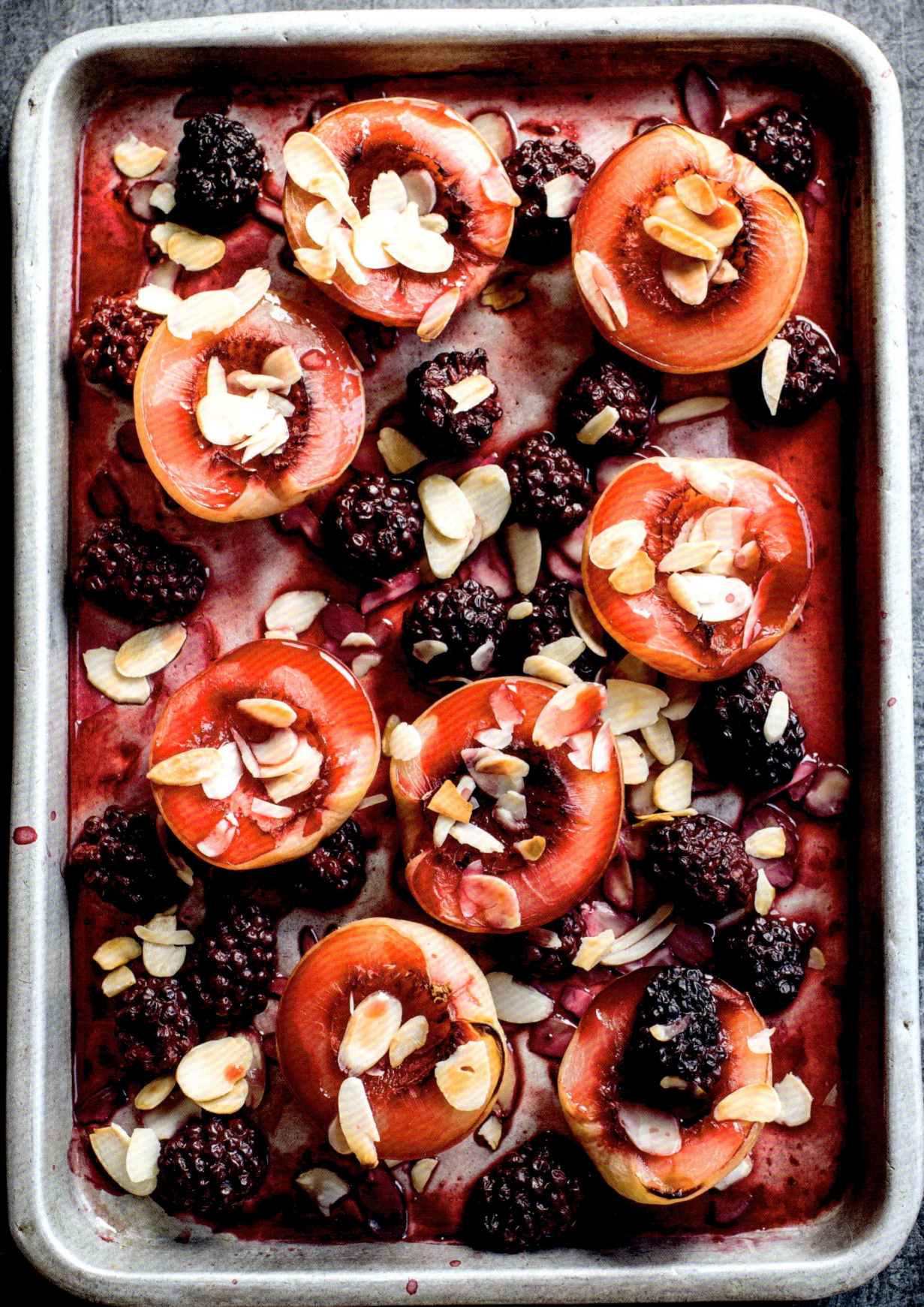

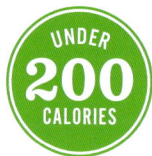

PER SERVING | **187cals** | PROTEIN **4.5g** | CARBS **13.5g** | SUGAR **10g**

Chocolate and Black Bean Torte

SERVES **12** | PREP **25** mins | COOK **25** mins

100g dark chocolate
    (at least 70% cocoa solids),
    broken into squares
100g coconut oil,
    plus extra for greasing
100g soft pitted dates
1 × 400g can black beans,
    drained and rinsed
3 large free-range eggs,
    separated
¼ tsp unsweetened cocoa
    powder, for dusting

COOK'S TIP
Keep in the fridge and
eat within a couple of
days, or freeze in slices.

This light chocolate cake is gluten free and tastes luxurious without being too rich. Serve in small wedges with a handful of raspberries.

1. Melt the chocolate in a heatproof bowl over a pan of gently simmering water – make sure the bowl isn't touching the water. (You can also melt the chocolate in a microwave.) Remove from the heat and leave to cool for 20 minutes.

2. Preheat the oven to 190°C/Fan 170°C/Gas 5 and grease and line the base of a 20cm loose-bottomed cake tin with non-stick baking paper.

3. Place the dates, oil and black beans in a food processor and blitz until well combined. Add the egg yolks and blend until as creamy and smooth as possible. You may need to remove the lid and push the mixture down a couple of times. Add the cooled, melted chocolate, followed by 100ml cold water, in slow steady streams, until thoroughly combined.

4. Next, whisk the egg whites in a large clean bowl with an electric whisk until stiff but not dry.

5. Stir a heaped tablespoon of the egg whites gently into the chocolate mixture to soften, then transfer the chocolate mixture to the bowl with the rest of the egg whites and fold in gently using a large metal spoon, until thoroughly combined. Spoon the mixture into the prepared cake tin and spread to the sides. Bake in the centre of the oven for 25 minutes, or until risen and firm to the touch.

6. Cool for 30 minutes, then remove from the tin. Sift over the cocoa powder to dust and cut into small wedges to serve.

VEGGIE · GLUTEN FREE · NUT FREE · DAIRY FREE

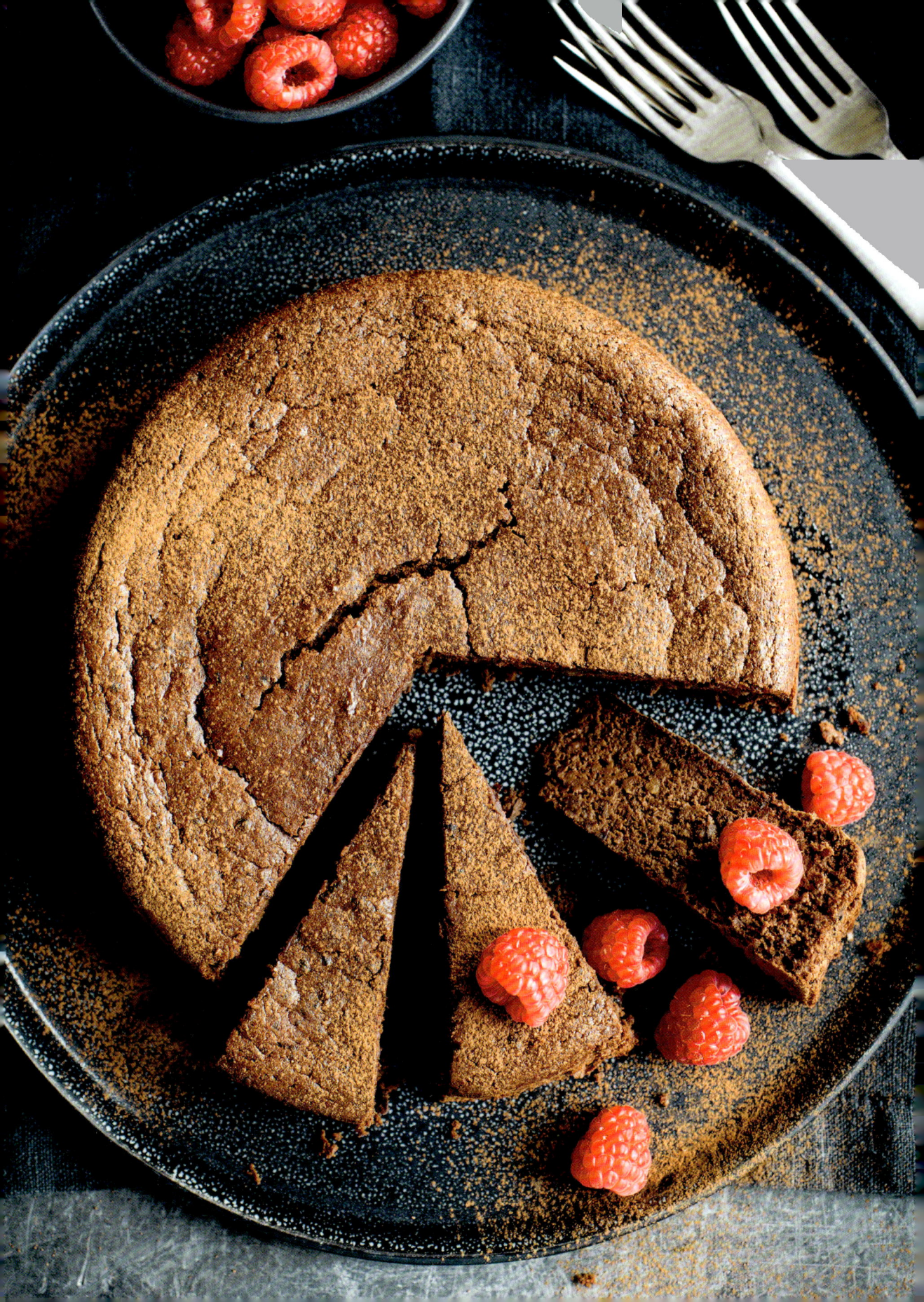

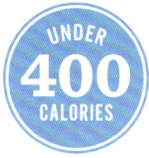

| PER SERVING | **301cals** | PROTEIN **11.1g** | CARBS **6.6g** | SUGAR **5.6g**

Orange and Pistachio Upside-down Cake

SERVES	PREP	COOK
8	**15** mins	**25** mins

½ tsp coconut oil, melted
1 large orange, peeled
    and cut into 5 slices
25g shelled pistachios,
    roughly chopped
6 dried apricots,
    roughly chopped
3 medium free-range eggs
100g full-fat live Greek
    yoghurt, or dairy-free
    alternative
70ml olive oil
1 tsp almond extract
2 tsp vanilla extract
200g ground almonds
2 tsp baking powder

COOK'S TIP
The cake freezes well.
When cooled, just cut it
into slices before freezing.

There is something magical about an upside-down cake. There's also a hint of jeopardy! With the base of ground almonds, eggs and nuts, this indulgent high-protein cake will leave you satisfyingly full without spiking sugars.

1. Preheat the oven to 200°C/Fan 180°C/Gas 6. Line a 20cm square baking dish with non-stick baking paper.

2. Brush the non-stick baking paper all over with the melted coconut oil, then lay the orange slices on the base of the tin. Scatter the pistachios around the orange slices and set the tin aside.

3. Place the dried apricots, eggs, yoghurt, olive oil and almond and vanilla extracts in a food processor or blender and blitz until the apricots are broken up and the mixture is smooth.

4. Add the ground almonds, baking powder and a pinch of salt and mix until combined.

5. Pour into the prepared tin and smooth the surface. Bake in the oven for 20–25 minutes, or until golden and a skewer inserted into the centre comes out clean. Allow to cool slightly and tip out on to wire rack. Carefully remove the non-stick baking paper.

6. Slice and serve with full-fat live Greek yoghurt (20cals per tablespoon).

VEGGIE   DAIRY FREE

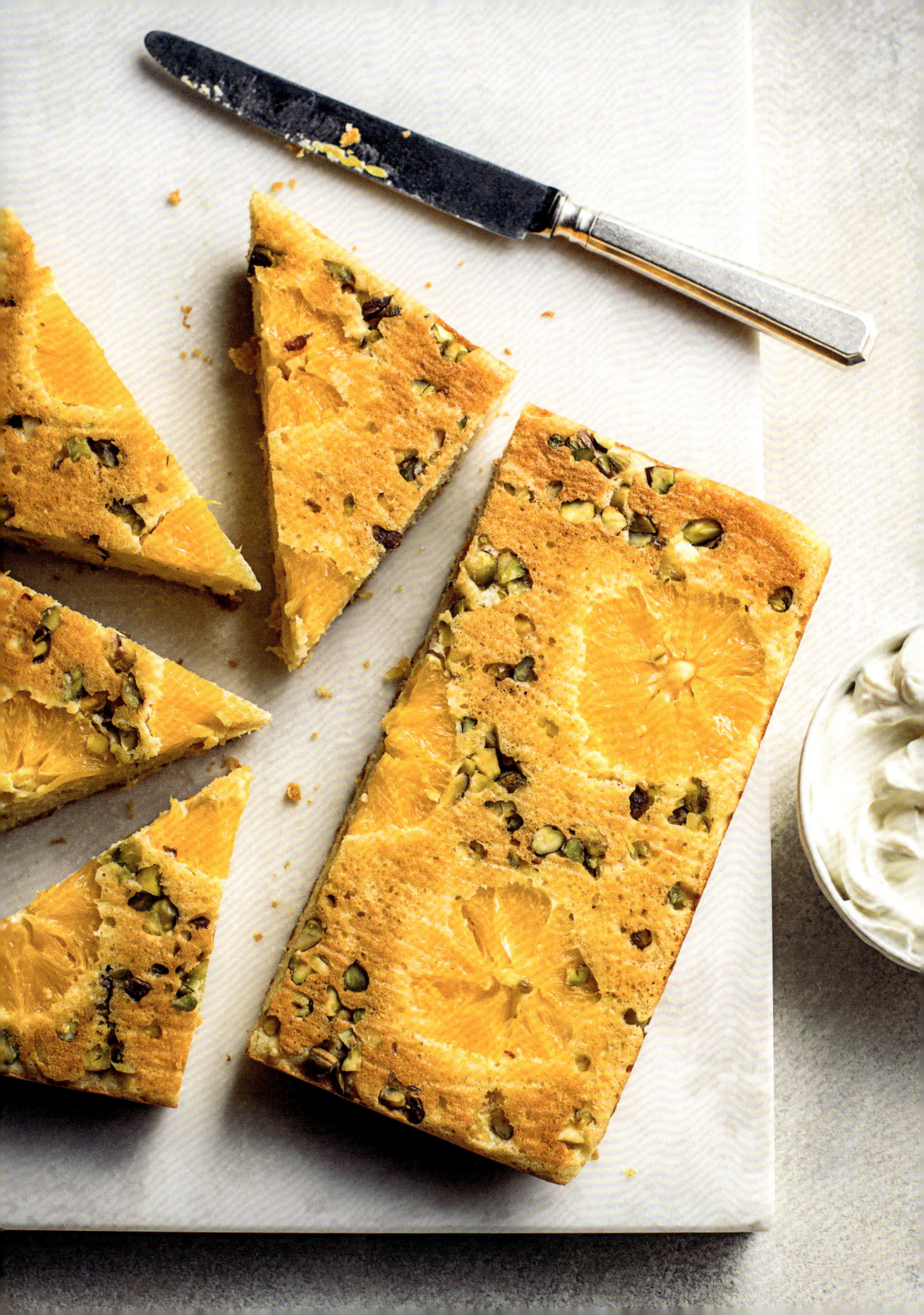

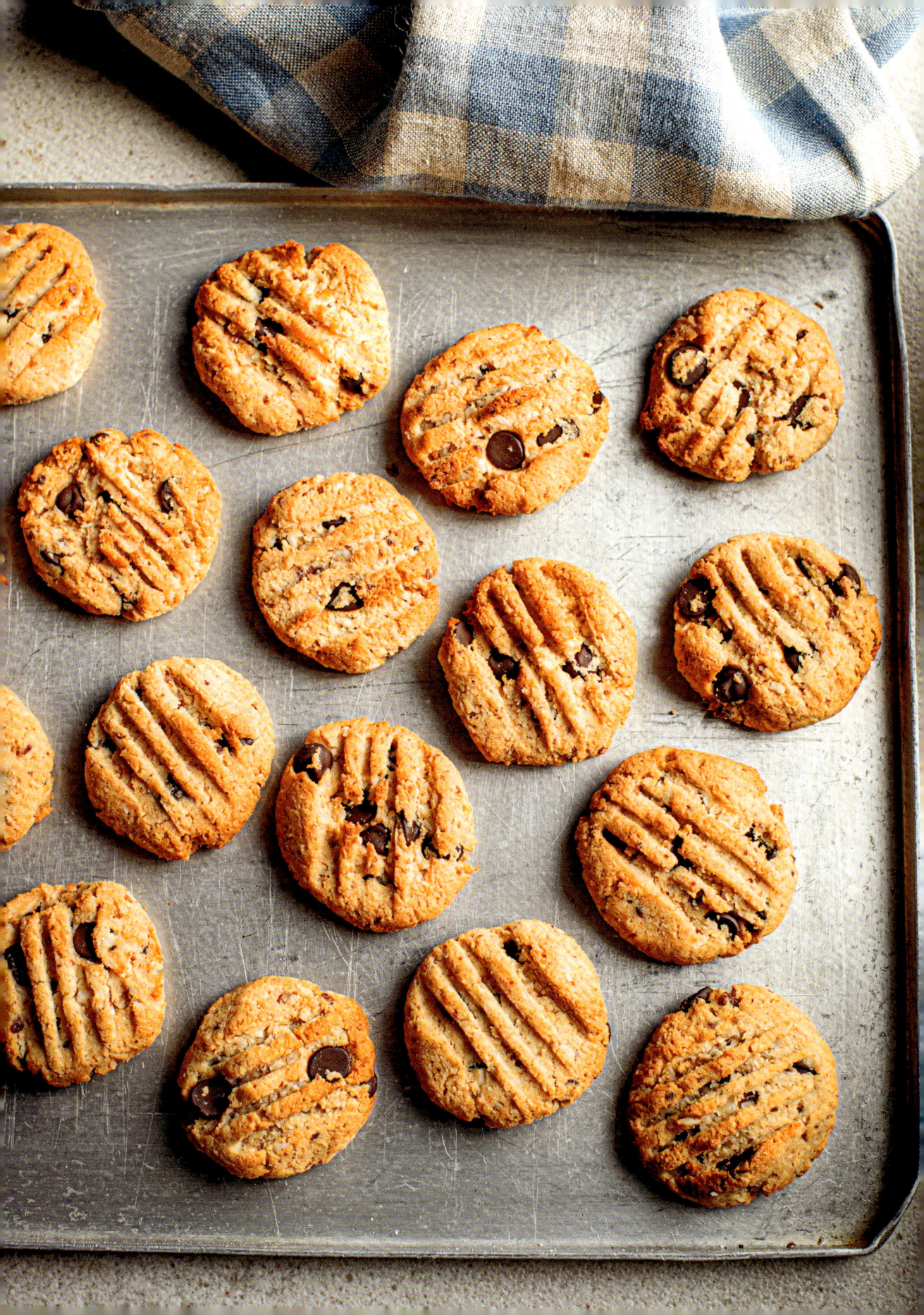

No-added-sugar Coconut and Choc-chip Cookies

SERVES | **PREP** | **COOK**
20 | **15** mins | **15** mins

½ tsp rapeseed or coconut oil
120g ground almonds
30g desiccated coconut
   (unsweetened)
60g coconut oil
1 large egg
½ tsp baking powder
½ tsp vanilla extract
40g soft pitted dates,
   finely chopped
40g dark chocolate chips
   (at least 70% cocoa solids)

COOK'S TIP
If you don't have dark chocolate chips, use any dark chocolate – as long as it contains over 70% cocoa solids – and chop it into small pieces.

Light and chewy, these coconut-flavoured biscuits have a satisfying burst of chocolate. Another family favourite, they are so easy to make.

1. Preheat the oven to 180°C/Fan 160°C/Gas 4 and grease a large baking tray with the oil.

2. Place all the ingredients, except the chocolate chips, in a medium bowl, add a generous pinch of salt and blitz briefly with a stick blender or in a food processor to make a slightly sticky dough. You may need to add ½ tablespoon water, if the mixture is a bit crumbly. Alternatively, mix together by hand. Stir in the chocolate until well combined.

3. Roll the mixture into 20 small balls and place on the greased tray. Flatten each of them with a fork, until around 1cm thick. Bake in the oven for about 15 minutes, or until firm and turning deep golden brown around the edges.

4. Leave to cool on the tray for a few minutes, then transfer to a wire rack. Store excess cookies in an airtight container in the freezer.

AIR-FRYER TIP
Preheat the air fryer to 160°C, if needed. Prepare and shape the cookies as Steps 2–4. Air fry (in batches) for 10 minutes, or until firm and turning deep golden brown around the edges.

VEGGIE   DAIRY FREE

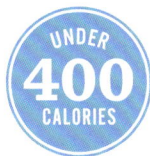

PER SERVING | **325cals** | PROTEIN **8.2g** | CARBS **12g** | SUGAR **8.2g**

Almond and Plum Sponge Pudding

SERVES	PREP	COOK
8	**15** mins	**40** mins

4 medium plums,
  quartered and stoned
  (350g prepared weight)
125g coconut oil (or butter)
150g ground almonds
3 medium free-range eggs
2 tsp baking powder
100g soft pitted dates,
  roughly chopped
1 tsp almond extract (optional)

COOK'S TIP
This pudding freezes
well, just divide into
portions before freezing.

Almonds and plums are a classic combination, making an ideal autumn pudding to use up those abundant plums. This also works well with defrosted or even canned plums (in juice, not syrup). Although we suggest removing the stones, we often decide to leave them in as it's less fiddly to prepare – just remember to warn people to look out for them!

1. Preheat the oven to 190°C/Fan 170°C/Gas 5. Line a 20cm square baking dish with non-stick baking paper.

2. Lay two thirds of the plums in the prepared baking dish and set aside.

3. Place the coconut oil, ground almonds, eggs, baking powder, dates, almond extract, if using, and a pinch of salt in a food processor or blender and blitz to combine.

4. Pour the mixture over the plums, then press the remaining plums on to the surface for decoration. Bake in the centre of the oven for 30–40 minutes, or until turning golden on top.

5. Serve with full-fat live Greek yoghurt (20cals per tablespoon).

VEGGIE   DAIRY FREE

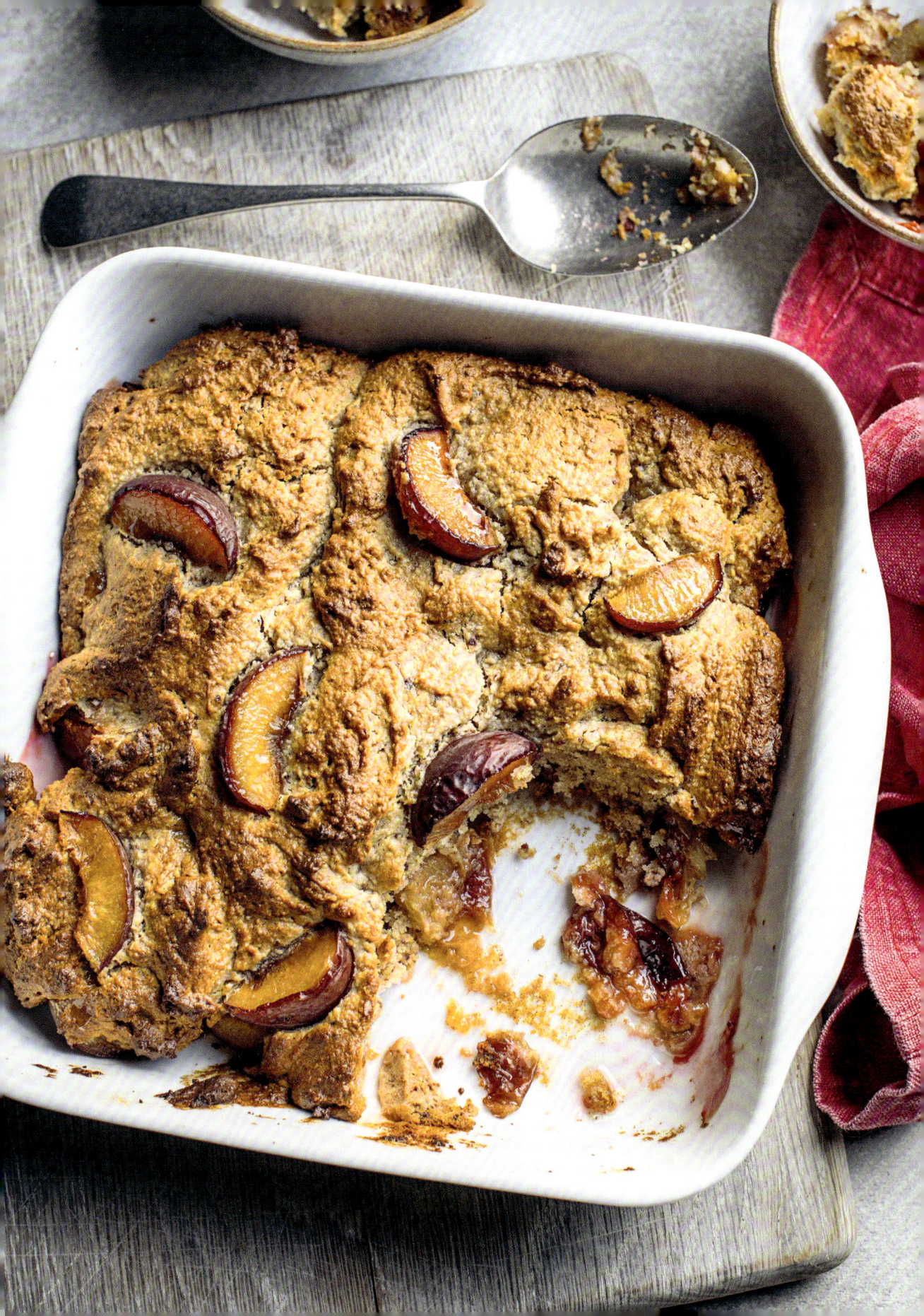

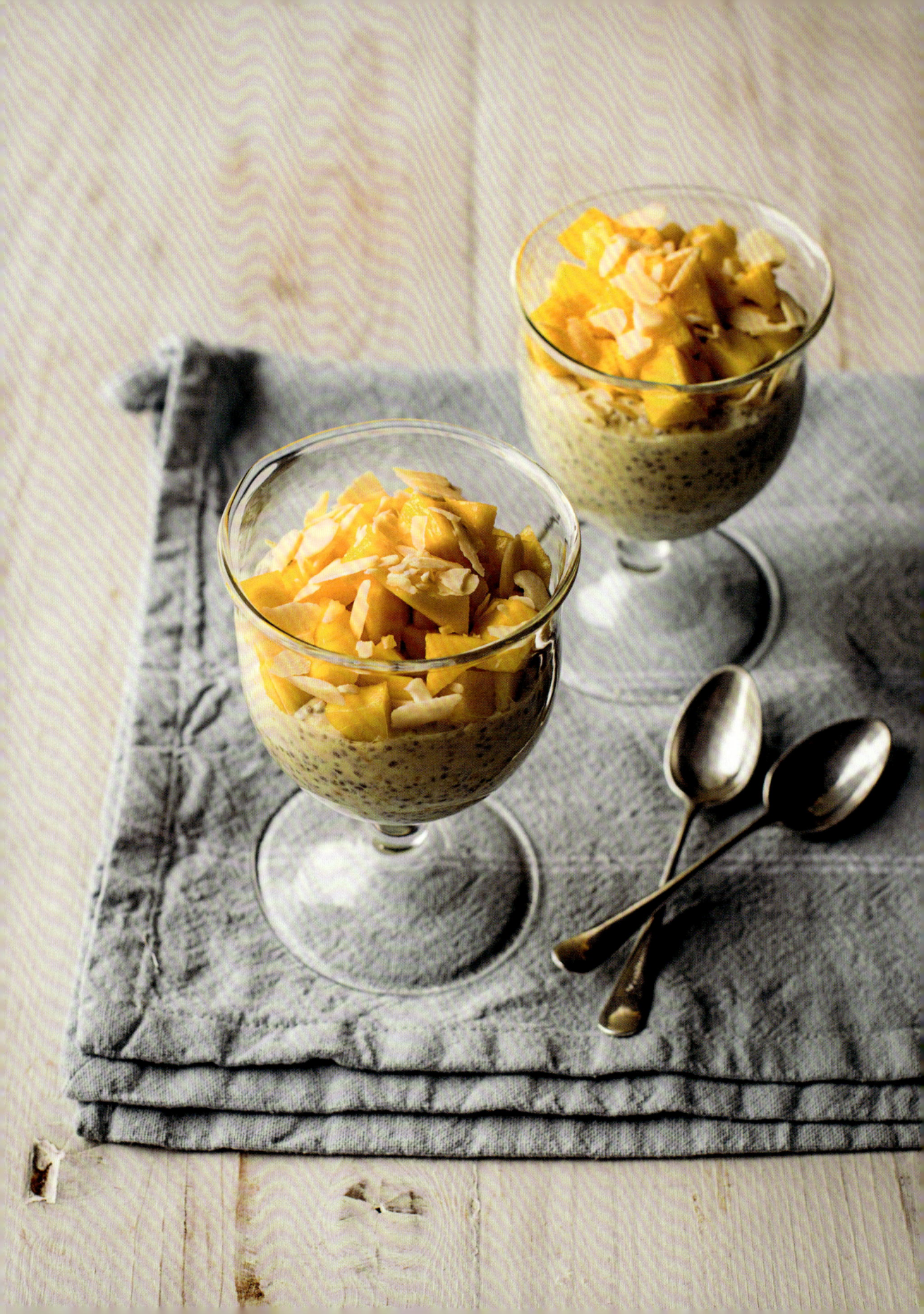

Mango and Lime Chia Pots

SERVES | PREP | CHILL
2 | **5** mins | **30** mins

30g chia seeds
100g full-fat live Greek yoghurt
120ml full-fat milk
1 tsp vanilla extract
finely grated zest of ½ lime
100g mango
   (roughly 1 small mango),
   roughly chopped
1 tbsp flaked almonds

This luxurious and zingy mango recipe serves two, but the pots will keep for a few days in the fridge, making it a good dessert to prepare ahead. I am a big fan of chia seeds as they have interesting properties. An unassuming little seed, it produces a flavourless gel when soaked in water, making the pudding thicker and creamier. It also packs a punch when it comes to its impressive nutritional credentials, as it is high in protein, fibre and much-needed omega-3.

1. Place the chia seeds, yoghurt, milk, vanilla extract, lime zest and half the mango in a medium bowl and blitz for about 30 seconds with a hand-held blender. You want to retain some of the texture of the chia seeds.

2. Divide the mixture between two glasses and scatter the remaining mango on top.

3. Leave to set in the fridge for about 30 minutes. Top with the flaked almonds just before serving.

VEGGIE | GLUTEN FREE

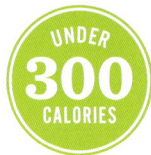

PER SERVING | **224cals** | PROTEIN **2.2g** | CARBS **22.2g** | SUGAR **19.2g**

Chocolate Coconut Pudding with Pear

SERVES	PREP	CHILL
4	**10** mins	**60** mins

**4 soft pitted dates,
    roughly chopped**
160ml coconut cream
½ tsp vanilla extract
**75g dark chocolate (at least
    70% cocoa solids), broken
    into pieces**
2 small pears

COOK'S TIP
Coconut or full-fat live
Greek yoghurt would
make a nice addition
to this dessert; allow
½ tablespoon per person.
You could also serve this
with 50g raspberries
per person instead of
the pears, if you prefer.

**A rich and creamy mousse with a delicate fruity tang.
This is a perfect indulgence to round off a meal.**

1. Place the dates, coconut cream and vanilla extract in
a small saucepan over a medium heat. Bring to the boil
and simmer for 30 seconds.

2. Remove from the heat, add the chocolate and a pinch
of salt and stir until melted.

3. Blitz the mixture with a hand-held blender until
smooth. Divide between four small glasses and
refrigerate for 1 hour until set.

4. Meanwhile, core and slice the pears (you don't want
to do this too much in advance or the fruit will brown).
Divide the slices between the puddings to serve.

VEGAN   GLUTEN FREE   NUT FREE   DAIRY FREE

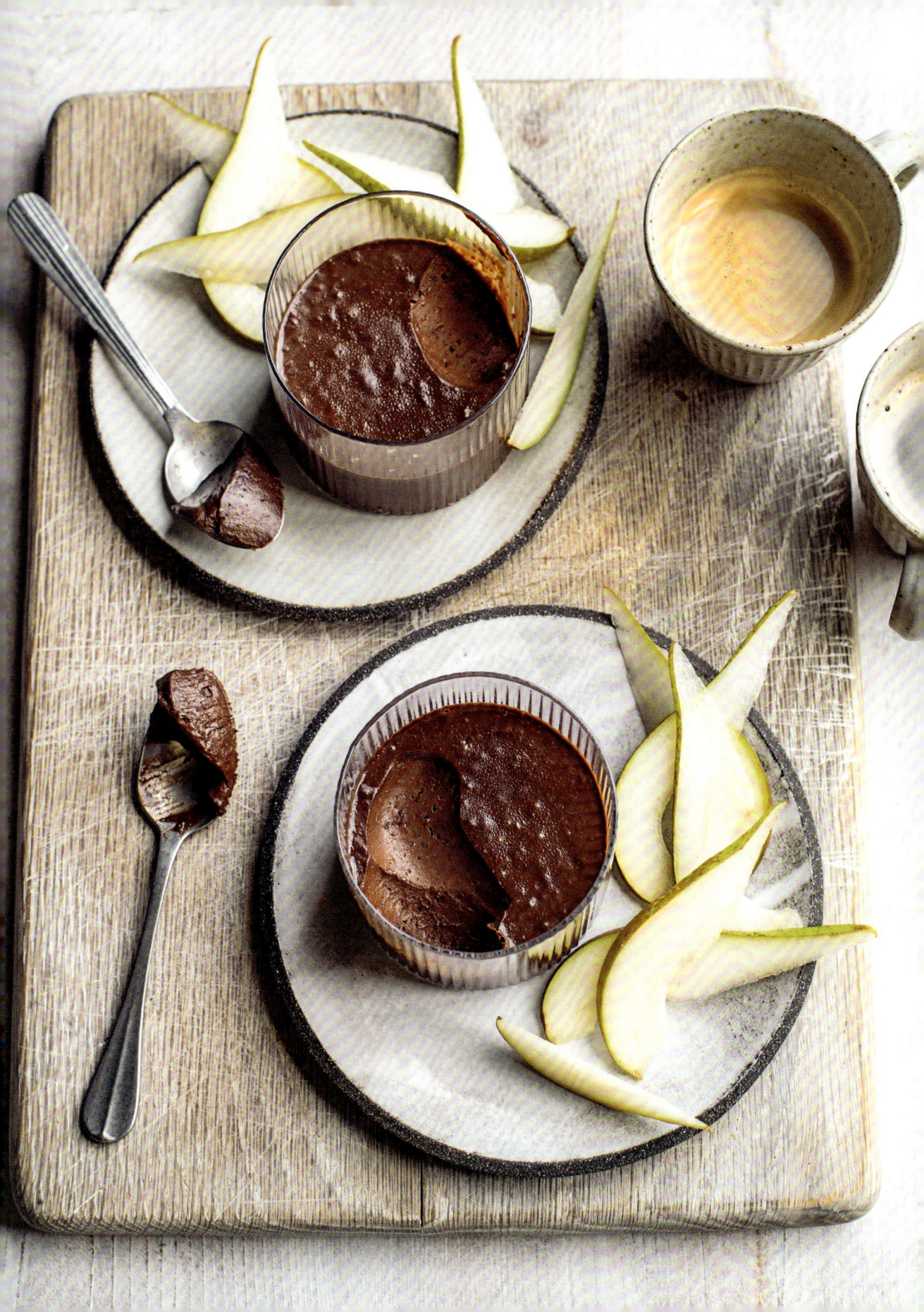

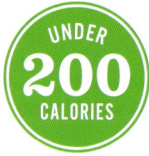

PER SERVING | **140cals** | PROTEIN **3.1g** | CARBS **14.6g** | SUGAR **8.4g**

Rustic Filo Plum Tart

SERVES	PREP	COOK
4	**15** mins	**20** mins

1 sheet filo pastry, halved
1 tbsp olive oil
1 tbsp vanilla extract
2 tbsp ground almonds
2 large plums, halved,
    stoned and thinly sliced
    (200g prepared weight)
1 tbsp honey

The joy of filo pastry is that the delicate thin layers give a taste of pastry indulgence without the sugar-spiking effect of thicker pastry. This is a serious treat, yet it's easy to make. Heating the baking tray in the oven first helps the pastry to crisp on the base.

1. Preheat the oven to 200°C/Fan 180°C/Gas 6. Place a baking tray in the oven to get hot.

2. Lay a piece of non-stick baking paper the same size as the baking tray on a flat surface.

3. Brush each half of filo pastry with olive oil, then layer one on top of the other on the non-stick baking paper.

4. Mix the vanilla extract and ground almonds together to form a crumbly paste. Spread this on the pastry, leaving a 2.5cm border around the edge.

5. Arrange the sliced plums on top of the almond paste in a single layer. Drizzle the honey all over. Fold the edges of the pastry over the plums, creating a square-shaped tart with the plums exposed in the centre.

6. Remove the hot baking tray from the oven and carefully slide the tart and its non-stick baking paper on to the hot tray. Bake in the oven for 15–20 minutes, or until the edges are golden and crisp.

7. Slice in four and serve immediately with full-fat live Greek yoghurt (20cals per tablespoon).

VEGGIE   DAIRY FREE

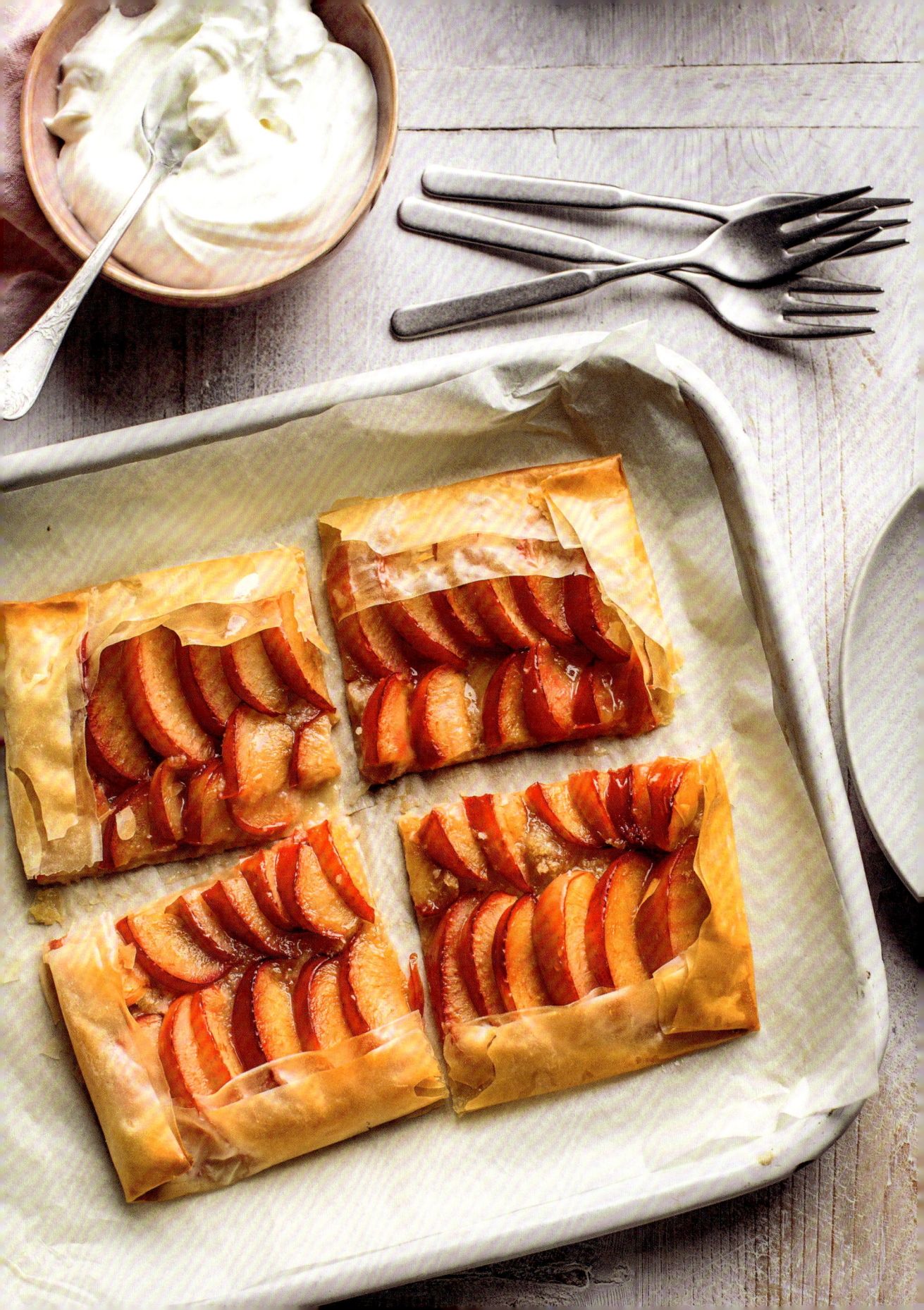

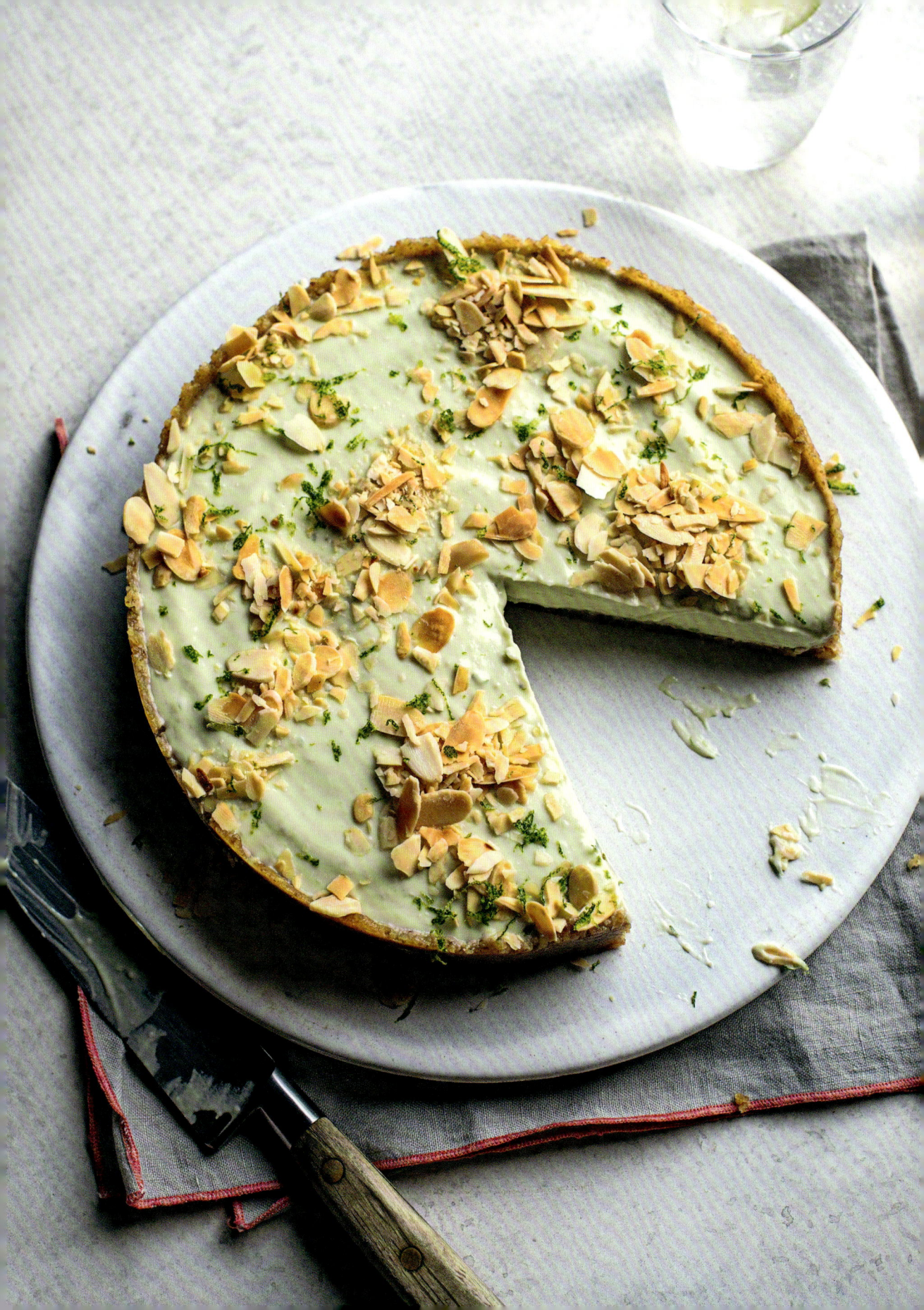

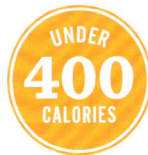

Avocado Lime Tart

SERVES	PREP	CHILL
6	**20** mins	**3** hours

80g soft pitted dates
130g walnuts
2 tbsp coconut oil, melted
2 medium ripe avocados,
   peeled and stoned
finely grated zest and juice
   of 2 limes, plus extra to serve
½ × 400ml can full-fat
   coconut milk
2 balls of stem ginger in syrup,
   drained and finely chopped
20g toasted flaked almonds

COOK'S TIP
The tart will keep for
2 days in the fridge.

There is something special about tucking into a tart, but if you don't have time for the base, you can just enjoy the delicious green mousse on its own. It sets beautifully in glasses, making it a refreshing and light dessert. Halve the recipe to make a mousse for two.

1. Line a 20cm round loose-bottomed cake tin with non-stick baking paper.

2. Place the dates and walnuts in a food processor or blender and blitz until finely chopped. Add the melted coconut oil and blitz again until the mixture is clumping together.

3. Tip the nutty mixture into the prepared tin and use the back of a spoon to press the mixture firmly into the base and sides. Set aside.

4. Place the avocados, lime zest and juice, coconut milk and stem ginger in a bowl and blitz with a hand-held stick blender until smooth. You could also make this in a food processor or blender.

5. Pour the avocado mixture into the tart case and smooth the surface. Refrigerate for at least 3 hours.

6. Decorate with the toasted almonds and some finely grated lime zest to serve.

VEGAN GLUTEN FREE DAIRY FREE

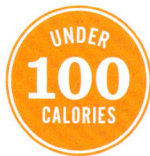

PER SERVING | **66cals** | PROTEIN **1.8g** | CARBS **5g** | SUGAR **10g**

Astonishingly Simple Creamy Tangerine Sorbet

SERVES **2** | **PREP** **2** mins | **CHILL** **1** hour

4 medium tangerines (mandarins), peeled and segments separated
2 tbsp full-fat live Greek yoghurt, or dairy-free alternative

An elegantly simple sorbet based on blitzing frozen tangerine (mandarin) segments. It's sweet and tart with a creamy orange flavour. Fun to make with the help of little ones – kids will love to eat it, too. Michael loved the fun and simplicity of this zingy, creamy sorbet.

1. Put the tangerine (mandarin) pieces on a small tray or plate and place in the freezer for 1 hour at least.

2. Place the frozen segments in a food processor or blender with the yoghurt and blitz to make a creamy, tangy sorbet.

3. Share between two bowls to serve.

VEGAN · GLUTEN FREE · NUT FREE · DAIRY FREE

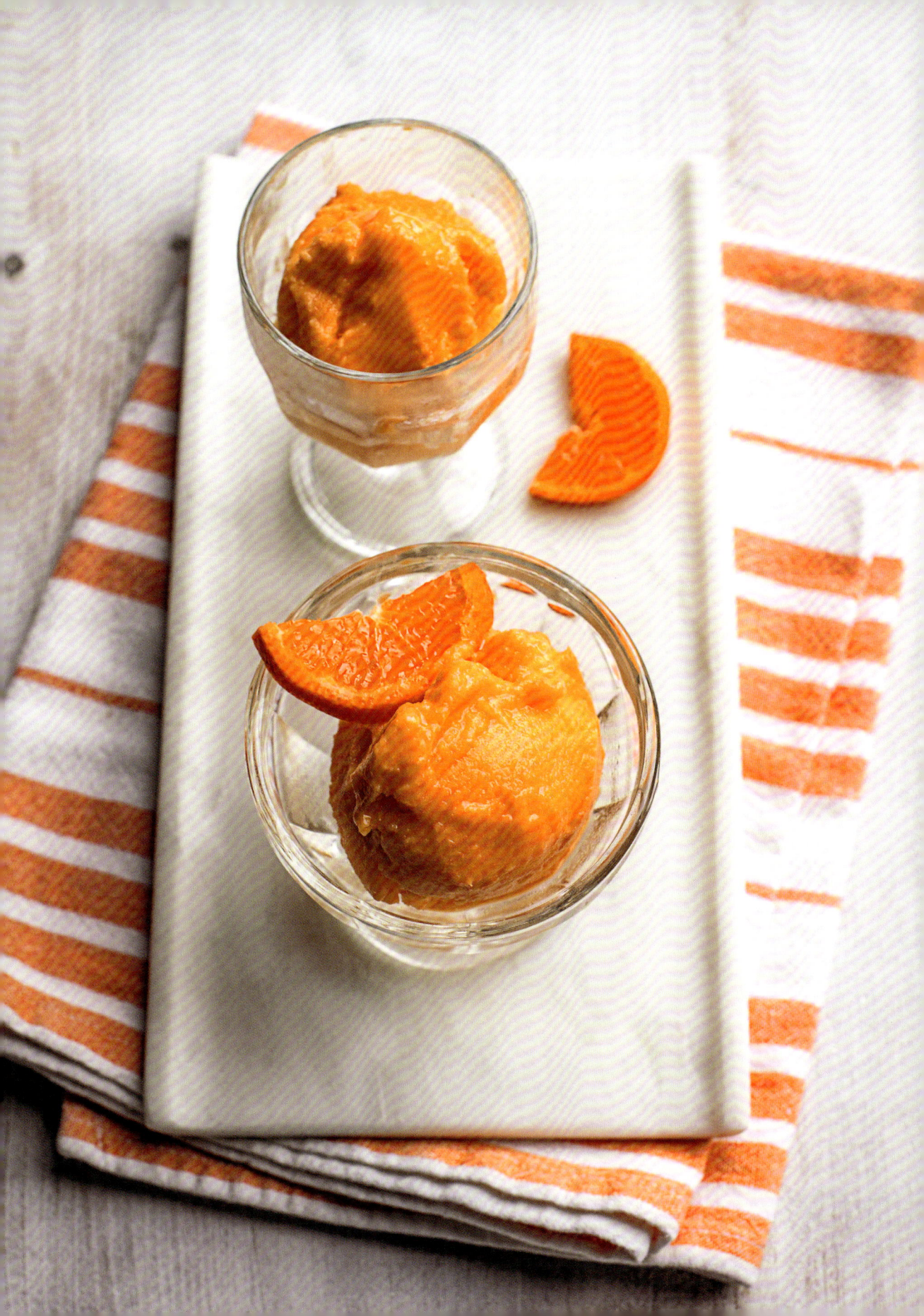

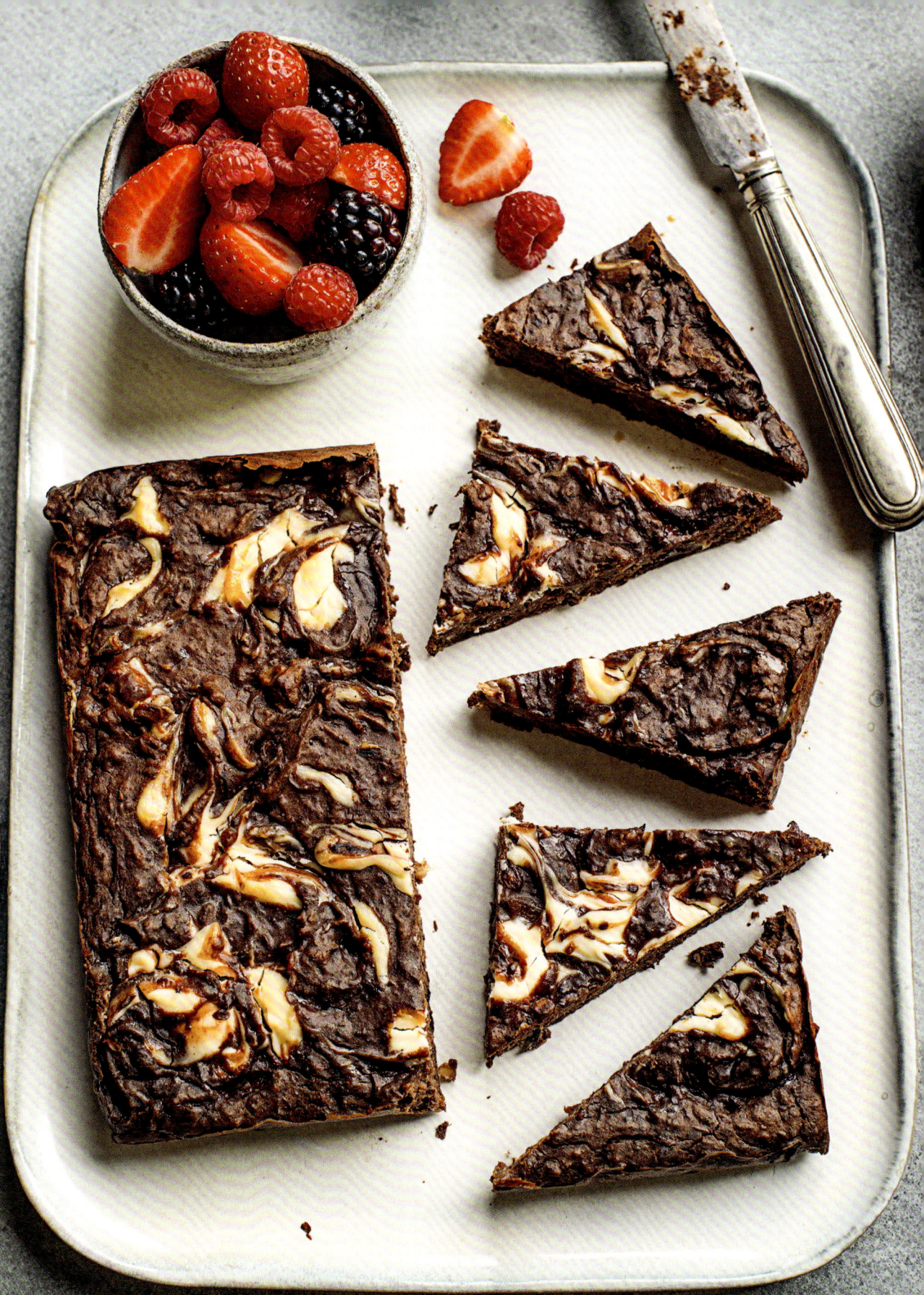

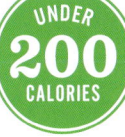

Chocolate Cheesecake Black Bean Brownies

SERVES | **PREP** | **COOK**
12 | **10** mins | **20** mins

1 × 400g can black beans, drained and rinsed
3 medium free-range eggs
100g soft pitted dates
3 tbsp unsweetened cocoa powder
3 tbsp coconut oil
2 tsp vanilla extract
30g dark chocolate chips (at least 70% cocoa solids)
2 tbsp full-fat cream cheese, or dairy-free alternative
1 tbsp honey

These brownies are dense and gooey in the centre and topped with a delicious cheesecake swirl. We both loved these super-healthy and scrumptious brownies, and the fact that no-one could guess the main ingredient – black beans! An easy variation would be to stir in some nuts at the last moment, this would also increase the protein.

1. Preheat the oven to 190°C/Fan 170°C/Gas 5. Line a 20cm square cake tin with non-stick baking paper.

2. Place the black beans, eggs, dates, cocoa powder, coconut oil, 1 teaspoon of the vanilla extract and a pinch of salt in a food processor or blender and blitz for about 2 minutes, until really smooth.

3. Stir in the chocolate chips and pour the mixture into the prepared tin.

4. Mix the cream cheese, remaining vanilla extract and honey together in a small bowl until smooth. Swirl into the surface of the brownie mixture, creating a marbled effect. Bake in the oven for 20 minutes.

5. Leave to cool in the tin, then slice into 12 to serve.

VEGGIE · GLUTEN FREE · NUT FREE · DAIRY FREE

Your Fast 800 toolkit

Traffic lights quick food check

A guide to help you see at a glance which foods are to be encouraged, which eaten in moderation and which to avoid. This is a rough guide only, as people respond differently to different foods.

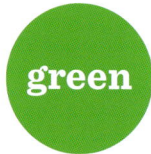

green

Foods you can eat freely – calories still to be counted on fasting days on all but the non-starchy veg
- Non-starchy vegetables, including salad, leafy greens, broccoli, courgettes, onions and mushrooms
- Fish
- Nuts and seeds
- Tofu
- White meat
- Extra-virgin olive oil and rapeseed oil
- Herbs and spices
- Tomatoes, peppers, peas and aubergines
- Full-fat fermented dairy, including cheese, yoghurt and fromage frais (these are borderline orange – enjoy in moderation)
- Lowish-sugar fruit, including berries and hard fruits (e.g. apples and pears) and citrus fruits – preferably at the end of a meal

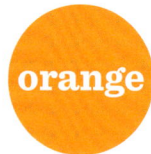

orange

Foods you can eat in moderation or occasionally
- Full-fat dairy, such as milk and butter
- Coconut oil or coconut milk
- Diced bacon or chorizo for garnish or flavour
- Eggs
- Beans, lentil and quinoa (NB these are in the green category if you are vegetarian)
- Whole grains
- Wholegrain seeded or sourdough bread
- Wholemeal/seeded pitta or flatbread
- Wholemeal pasta
- Wholemeal/stoneground flour
- Unprocessed, unsweetened cereals
- Red meat (up to two times a week)
- Moderately starchy root veg, such as swede, parsnip and sweetcorn
- Butternut squash and pumpkin
- Sweet tropical fruits (e.g. mango and pineapple)

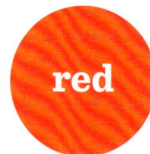

red

Foods to avoid if possible
- Most pastries, cakes, snacks and biscuits
- White pasta/bread/rice
- White flour
- Highly processed foods
- Low-fat dairy products
- Highly processed oils, especially anything with trans fats
- Pre-prepared convenience food with lots of unrecognisable ingredients!
- Sugars and sweets

Easy ways to add protein

New research points to the importance of eating adequate amounts of protein – ideally at least 50g a day. It's harder for vegetarians to achieve their daily protein requirement on 800cals, so they may need to increase their intake to over 800–1000cals. Using a high-protein shake can help you stick to 800cals (see thefast800.com for more info on meal replacement shakes). These simple, calorie-counted solutions are particularly useful if you haven't got time to cook a full recipe or you just want to beef up a plate of non-starchy veg.

Meat
75g cooked chicken breast
    (115cals, 22.5g protein)
2 slices roast turkey breast, around 50g
    (76cals, 17g protein)
1 tbsp diced chorizo, around 10g
    (40cals, 2.5g protein)
1 tbsp chopped fried back bacon, around 7g
    (24cals, 1.5g protein)
2 thin slices ham, around 40g
    (43cals, 7g protein)
2 slices roast beef, around 80g
    (140cals, 26g protein)
4 slices salami or cured chorizo, around 20g
    (88cals, 4g protein)
1 rasher cooked back bacon, around 20g
    (61cals, 5g protein)

Fish
75g frozen cooked prawns, defrosted
    (52cals, 11.5g protein)
45g tuna, canned in oil (72cals, 11.5g protein)
3 drained anchovies in oil (17cals, 2g protein)
1 smoked mackerel fillet, around 70g
    (211cals, 15g protein)
2 slices smoked salmon, around 50g in total
    (92cals, 11.5g protein)
100g roasted or poached salmon
    (239cals, 24.5g protein)

Dairy & egg
1 medium boiled egg (78cals, 7g protein)
1 tbsp grated cheese, around 10g
    (41cals, 2.5g protein)
30g mature Cheddar (124cals, 7.5g protein)
30g halloumi, sliced, lightly fried in 1 tsp
    olive oil for 4–5 mins (130cals, 6g protein)
40g Greek-style yoghurt (53cals, 2g protein)
50g feta (124cals, 7.5g protein)
20g Parmesan (82cals, 7g protein)
50g soft blue cheese, such as Roquefort,
    (187cals, 10g protein)
50g soft cheese, such as Brie
    (171cals, 10g protein)

Vegetarian
Handful of nuts, around 10g total weight,
    e.g. walnuts, pecans, hazelnuts
    (71cals, 2g protein)
15g almonds (95cals, 4g protein)
2 tsp sesame seeds, around 10g
    (63cals, 2g protein)
2 tbsp mixed seeds, around 20g
    (122cals, 5.4g protein)
100g tofu (123cals, 12.5g protein)
80g cooked edamame beans
(110cals, 9g protein) 100g cooked puy lentils
    (143cals, 11g protein)
40g mushrooms fried in 1 tsp olive oil
    (33cals, 1g protein)
2 tbsp hummus, around 50g
    (160cals, 3.5g protein)
100g canned beans (109cals, 7g protein)
100g cooked lentils (143cals, 11g protein)
100g cooked quinoa (185cals, 6g protein)

How to make your greens even tastier

Green and non-starchy vegetables are so healthy and such an important part of the Fast 800 that we encourage you to eat these freely, filling half your plate at each meal. Steam, boil or microwave them, and then try some of the following ideas to make them taste even better. We list both 'no-calorie counting' options, for when you are at your 800cals limit, and low-calorie options for when you've got some calories going spare.

Examples of non-starchy greens and veg:
Cabbage, spring greens, chard, kale, pak choi, cavolo nero and spinach; as well as fine green beans, mangetout, sliced courgette or broccoli. And salad leaves of all colours – the more colourful, the better the nutritional value (and they look so enticing too).

Ways to add flavour with insignificant calories:
- Flaked sea salt and a generous amount of black pepper
- A pinch of crushed dried chilli flakes
- A pinch of crushed garlic
- 1 tbsp soy sauce
- A squeeze of lemon or lime, e.g. on cabbage, broccoli or cauliflower
- 1 tbsp apple cider vinegar or balsamic vinegar, e.g. on spinach or cavolo nero
- A pinch of herbs
- I like to scatter little black nigella seeds on steamed veg, salads and slaws

Low-calorie ways to add flavour:
- 1 tsp butter – good on any veg (25cals)
- 1 tsp extra-virgin olive oil – good on any veg (27cals)
- 1 tsp hoisin sauce, e.g. on wilted spinach or cabbage (12cals)
- 1 tsp sesame or nigella seeds, e.g. on fine green beans or cabbage (32cals)
- 1 tsp grated Parmesan scattered on top, e.g. steamed broccoli (8cals)
- Jazz up greens by frying the veg in ½ tbsp olive oil with ½ garlic clove (you could add 1 tsp light soy sauce, if you like), e.g. cabbage, mange tout, broccoli or chard (52cals)
- Drizzle dressing on a large green or mixed salad

Enjoy healthy complex carbs

Ditch the empty white stuff – white bread, pasta, potatoes and rice – and embrace complex carbs instead, which contain important nutrients and are an excellent source of fibre.

Healthy wholegrains, beans and lentils

As these foods often take longer to cook, you can save yourself time by cooking larger quantities and freeze them in portions. Try crumbling in half a stock cube during cooking for added flavour. Beans and pulses are a particularly good source of protein for vegetarians and, like wholegrains, they are good for gut bacteria, too. We have included some wholegrains in small quantities in some of our recipes. But if you have calories to spare you might add 1 or possibly 2 tablespoons to a dish. On a non-fasting day, you can add 2–3 heaped tablespoons to your meal without counting. Here are a few options:

- 1 tbsp cooked brown rice (21cals)
- 1 tbsp cooked quinoa (18cals)
- 1 tbsp cooked bulgur wheat (13cals)
- 1 tbsp cooked puy lentils (18cals)
- 1 tbsp cooked pearl barley (19cals)

Other low-carb swaps

- **Cauliflower** makes an excellent swap as it's very low in calories and high in nutrients. It's also remarkably flexible. We love it.
- **Cauli-rice** Make cauli-rice by grating or quickly blitzing half a cauliflower, or buy it ready-made from the supermarket freezer cabinet.
- **Courgetti spaghetti** (100g) 20kcals. Allow 1 courgette per person.
- **Squash Mash** (see page 156)
- **Crushed Minted Peas** (see page 158)
- **Celeriac Chips** (see page 168)
- **Ratatouille** (see page 192)
- **Roasted vegetable wedges** Choose non-starchy veg, such as cabbage, courgette, aubergine, asparagus, beetroot, Brussels sprouts and peppers. Toss the veg in a small amount of extra-virgin olive oil before roasting (also see page 134).
- **Halloumi Fries** (see page 222)
- **Creamy Beans** (see page 228)
- **Cabbage linguine** Use ½ Savoy cabbage for 2 people. Remove the core, finely slice the cabbage then steam for about 5 minutes or in the microwave for less. You want it to be al dente.
- **Konjak 'Zero' noodles or spaghetti (Shiritaki).** Originally from Japan, these contain remarkably few calories and plenty of fibre. They are available in most large supermarkets.

The Fast 800 stores

As I said in my introduction, fresh meat and fruit and veg may be nice to have, but I'm also a big fan of cooking from stores. Frozen veg, such as peas, spinach or cauliflower florets, are already conveniently prepared and chopped; they provide high-quality nutrients and, because they last for many weeks in the freezer, you know they're always available. Likewise, tins of chickpeas, tomatoes, tuna or jars of red peppers are brilliant staples, sitting there, ready to be pulled out of the cupboard and thrown together for a quick meal. Remember, if you have the right foods to hand, you are much less likely to get sidetracked or tempted by unhealthy ones. This list is intended as a guide. Please don't feel you have to go out and buy every item on it! Be selective and start with the foods you think you are most likely to eat.

Oils & vinegars
Extra-virgin olive oil, or the least refined oil you can afford
Cold-pressed rapeseed (for high-temperature frying)
Coconut oil
Apple cider vinegar
Balsamic vinegar

Canned
Tomatoes
Chickpeas
Coconut milk
Beans: kidney, mixed beans, haricot, butter beans, black beans
Puy lentils
Fish: tuna, sardines, salmon, mackerel, anchovies

Dried
Stock cubes
Wholemeal flour
Baking powder
Wholegrains
Oats
Brown/red/black or wild rice
Pearl barley
Quinoa
Puy lentils, red lentils

Jars & bottles
Red peppers
Piquant peppadew peppers
Capers
Jalapeños
Stem ginger in syrup

Herbs & spices
Oregano or mixed herbs
Thyme
Medium curry powder
Cumin seeds
Ground turmeric
Smoked paprika
Black pepper
Chilli flakes
Sea salt

Nuts & seeds
Mixed unsalted nuts
Ground almonds
Flaked almonds
Cashews
Walnuts
Pecans
Mixed seeds

Flavourings, sauces & pastes
Harissa paste
Pesto
Thai red or green curry paste
Medium curry paste
Dark soy sauce
Tomato purée
Plum sauce
Light soy or tamari sauce
Hoisin sauce
Miso paste

Frozen
Chicken breasts
Prawns
Spinach
Peas
Edamame
Mixed veg
Raspberries, mixed berries
Broccoli, cauliflower

Fridge
Eggs
Full-fat live Greek yoghurt
Cheese – mature Cheddar, goat's cheese, feta, Parmesan, halloumi
Leafy greens and salad
Fresh garlic
Fresh ginger
Parsley
Coriander
Cooked chicken
Chorizo
Bacon
Smoked mackerel
Lemons and limes
Full-fat mayo
Mustard
Sauerkraut

Sweet things
Soft pitted dates
Maple syrup
Vanilla extract
Dark plain chocolate (ideally 70% cocoa solids or higher)

Making meals work for the whole family

Because the Fast 800 programme is based on a healthy, lowish-carb Mediterranean-style diet, it is extremely flexible – whether you want to bump up a low-calorie recipe to eat on a non-fasting day or to feed other members of your household. While Michael was doing some 800–1000 calorie days during lockdown, we all ate together, often using the recipes in this book as I was testing them – the children and I eating freely, while Michael skipped any starchy carbs, like bread or potatoes, and occasionally ate a couple of tablespoons of brown rice, quinoa or puy lentils. The simple message is that you can expand the portion sizes of our recipes and add in extras where and how you wish.

When you are making a meal such as a stew, curry or a substantial salad, simply double up portions and/or add a veg side dish (see pages 216–38) and/or extra protein (see page 271). Breakfast may be doubled up, too, or become a brunch or lunch. Soups are wonderfully adaptable – add toasted seeds, bacon, chorizo or grated cheese (see page 271 for more tasty and high-protein toppings) and/or a slice of wholemeal seeded bread.

Increase your complex carbs, such as beans, lentils and wholegrains, by adding an extra 2–3 heaped tablespoons of these foods on a non-fasting day, and encourage the rest of the family to eat these, too. When it comes to bread, it's about choosing carefully, as white bread and a slice of seeded wholemeal sourdough are two entirely different species, and this is also true for your non-dieting family. Encourage them to choose wholegrain, seeded or sourdough wherever possible. Equally, urge all the family to choose fruit which is moderately low in sugar, like berries, apples and pears, and to enjoy these with full-fat live Greek yoghurt.

Common chronic conditions caused by poor metabolic health include

- Type 2 diabetes
- Heart disease (e.g., coronary artery disease and heart failure)
- Stroke
- Hypertension (high blood pressure)
- Non-alcoholic fatty liver disease (NAFLD)
- Polycystic ovary syndrome (PCOS)
- Chronic kidney disease (CKD)
- Obesity and its complications
- Certain cancers (e.g., breast, colon and pancreatic)
- Sleep apnoea
- Cognitive decline / Alzheimer's (sometimes called 'Type 3 diabetes')
- Gout
- Depression and anxiety (linked via inflammation and insulin resistance)
- Osteoarthritis (via weight-related joint stress and inflammation)
- Retinopathy and vision loss (especially in diabetes)

7-day meal plans

These meal plans are intended to give you a taste of how the different options might work. Do feel free to use up your leftovers and swap in different recipes you like the look of and to repeat days, so you don't have to cook two days in a row – whatever best suits you. Just keep an eye on the nutritional information on the recipe pages to make sure you are keeping protein high (more than 50g daily if you can) and starchy carbs and sugar lowish (try not to go over 75g carbs on most days and ideally keep it below 50g).

Remember, the 800–1000cals a day is just a ballpark figure. Calories, although useful, are not an accurate science and there is considerable variation between calorie counters. So, going over by 50cals here and there is not going to make a significant difference to your rate of weight loss. Just remind yourself that any reduction below 1,000cals a day is going to have a substantial impact. And beyond that, it's the quality of the food that really matters. Eating 800cals of pastries is going to be far worse for you than 1000cals on a Med-style diet!

You will see that in the meat-free plan the daily calorie totals tend to be higher, which is fine. This is to ensure adequate daily protein is included. If you are vegetarian, you may wish to swap in a suitable high-protein shake to top up your protein (see thefast800.com for options); and if you are vegan, adding in high-protein shakes may be the only way to do this diet.

On days when you have calories to spare, you might want to choose a dressing for your salad or try some of the other ideas on page 272 to jazz up your non-starchy vegetables. You can also include a portion of hard fruit, such as an apple or pear, or a handful of berries, to take you just over the 800cals – eat this either with breakfast or straight after a meal. You will see that on some days in the 3-meal plans, the daily calorie quota falls far enough below the 800cals mark for you to have a treat (see pages 238–69). The important thing, if you want to encourage fat-burning, is to stick to a lowish-carb diet, avoid snacking between meals, and ideally add in some Time Restricted Eating (see page 12 for more on this).

2 meals a day

Monday	Protein	Carbs	Cals
1. Blueberry and Chocolate Protein Smoothie	17.6	22.9	251
2. Simple Steak with Salad	30	5	346
protein top up: 40g mixed seeds	10.8	3.2	244
	58.4	**31.1**	**841**

Tuesday			
1. Salmon Salad Bowl	33	20	542
2. Classic Burger with Celeriac Chips	24	6	259
	57	**26**	**801**

Wednesday			
1. Harissa Yoghurt with Soft-boiled Eggs and Spinach	20.6	2.1	228
2. Lamb Saag	29	10.5	361
side dish: Simple Dahl	10	25	255
	59.6	**37.6**	**844**

Thursday			
1. Chicken Satay	36	3	264
2. Beef and Black Bean Stir Fry	30.5	14.5	294
occasional treat: Mango and Lime Chia Pot	18.3	11.3	255
	84.8	**28.8**	**813**

Friday			
1. Pesto Chicken Traybake	14	40	333
2. Pork with Mustard and Cider Vinegar	34	1	288
side dish: Creamy Beans	9	18	184
	57	**59**	**805**

Saturday			
1. Chinese-style Drumsticks	33	3	238
2. Navarin of Lamb with Mangetout	39.6	19.3	582
	72.6	**22.3**	**820**

Sunday			
1. One-pan Breakfast: *double portion*	31.4	4.2	454
2. Tandoori Lamb Cutlets with Garlic and Ginger Spinach	28.9	6.8	415
	60.3	**11**	**869**

3 meals a day

Monday	Protein	Carbs	Cals
1. Chorizo and Parsley Muffins	11.4	1.2	181
2. Warm Crispy Kale Salad with Mushrooms and Bacon	13.4	1.3	285
3. Roast Chicken Thighs with Lemon	58	0	385
	82.8	**2.5**	**851**
Tuesday			
1. Blueberry Protein Pancakes	3.4	1.4	79
2. Salmon Salad Bowl	33	20	542
3. Satay Chicken	36	3	264
	72.4	**24.4**	**885**
Wednesday			
1. Harissa Yoghurt with Soft-boiled Eggs and Spinach	20.6	2.1	228
2. Chorizo and Bean Salad	15	20.5	349
3. Pan-fried Fish with Lemon and Parsley	33	0.5	369
	68.6	**23.1**	**946**
Thursday			
1. Chorizo Omlette	19.4	2.8	269
2. Chinese-style Drumsticks	33	3	238
3. Roasted Fish with a Cheese and Parsley Crumb	24	8	349
	76.4	**13.8**	**856**
Friday			
1. Sardines with Tomatoes on Sourdough	15.5	18.4	239
2. Chicken Ceasar-ish Salad	32	5.5	300
3. Made-in-Minutes Prawn Curry	20.4	5.2	396
	67.9	**29.1**	**935**
Saturday			
1. Breakfast Burrito	17.1	4.8	316
2. Miso Soup with Mushrooms and Prawns	12	3.5	69
3. Lamb Chops with Crushed Minted Peas and Feta	47	12	542
	76.1	**20.3**	**927**
Sunday			
1. One-pan Breakfast	15.7	2.1	227
2. Piri Piri Roast Chicken	56.9	4.4	377
3. Salmon Burgers	25	3	304
	97.6	**9.5**	**908**

3 meals a day, vegetarian

Monday	Protein	Carbs	Cals
1. Harissa Yoghurt with Soft-boiled Eggs and Spinach	20.6	2.1	228
2. Black Bean and Mango Slaw	11.3	27.5	332
side dish: Halloumi Fries	4.7	0.1	99
3. Egg-fried Cauli and Broccoli Rice	14.3	15.8	258
	50.9	**45.5**	**917**
Tuesday			
1. Blueberry Protein Pancakes	3.4	1.4	79
2. Spicy Bean Chilli	18	26	346
protein top up: 30g Cheddar	7.5	0.4	124
3. One-pan Miso Aubergine with Peanuts	21.3	28.2	421
	50.2	**56**	**970**
Wednesday			
1. Poached Eggs with Mushroom and Spinach	21	0.5	241
2. Harissa Lentil and Chickpea Soup with Spinach	10	19	206
3. Cauli Cheese with Jalapeno Peppers	20.5	13.7	467
	51.5	**33.2**	**914**
Thursday			
1. Smashed Avocado on Toast	6	10.5	289
protein top up: 40g mixed seeds	10.8	3.2	244
2. Tofu Mushroom Ramen	21.5	24	339
3. Halloumi Skewers	13.8	14	304
	52.1	**51.7**	**1176**
Friday			
1. Harissa Yoghurt with Soft-boiled Eggs and Spinach	20.6	2.1	228
2. Creamy Cashew and Tofu Curry	22	28.5	570
3. Ratatouille and Halloumi Bake	16	12	321
	58.6	**42.6**	**1119**
Saturday			
1. Poached Eggs with Mushroom and Spinach	21	0.5	241
2. French Bean Bowl with Feta and Pine Nuts	12.7	7.6	328
3. Pesto Lentils	14.5	24	331
protein top up: 40g mixed seeds	10.8	3.2	244
	59	**35.3**	**1144**
Sunday			
1. Shakshuka	19.5	17.5	312
2. Ratatouille and Halloumi Bake	16	12	321
3. Veggie Cottage Pie	19	17.5	238
side dish: Peach, Passionfruit and Vanilla Mini Basque Cheesecake	5.9	5	159
	60.4	**52**	**1030**

*Vegetarians may need to add protein top ups (see page 271) and aim for 1000 calories or more to ensure they get enough protein.

Index by calories

UNDER 400 CALORIES

UNDER 500 CALORIES

UNDER 600 CALORIES

Index

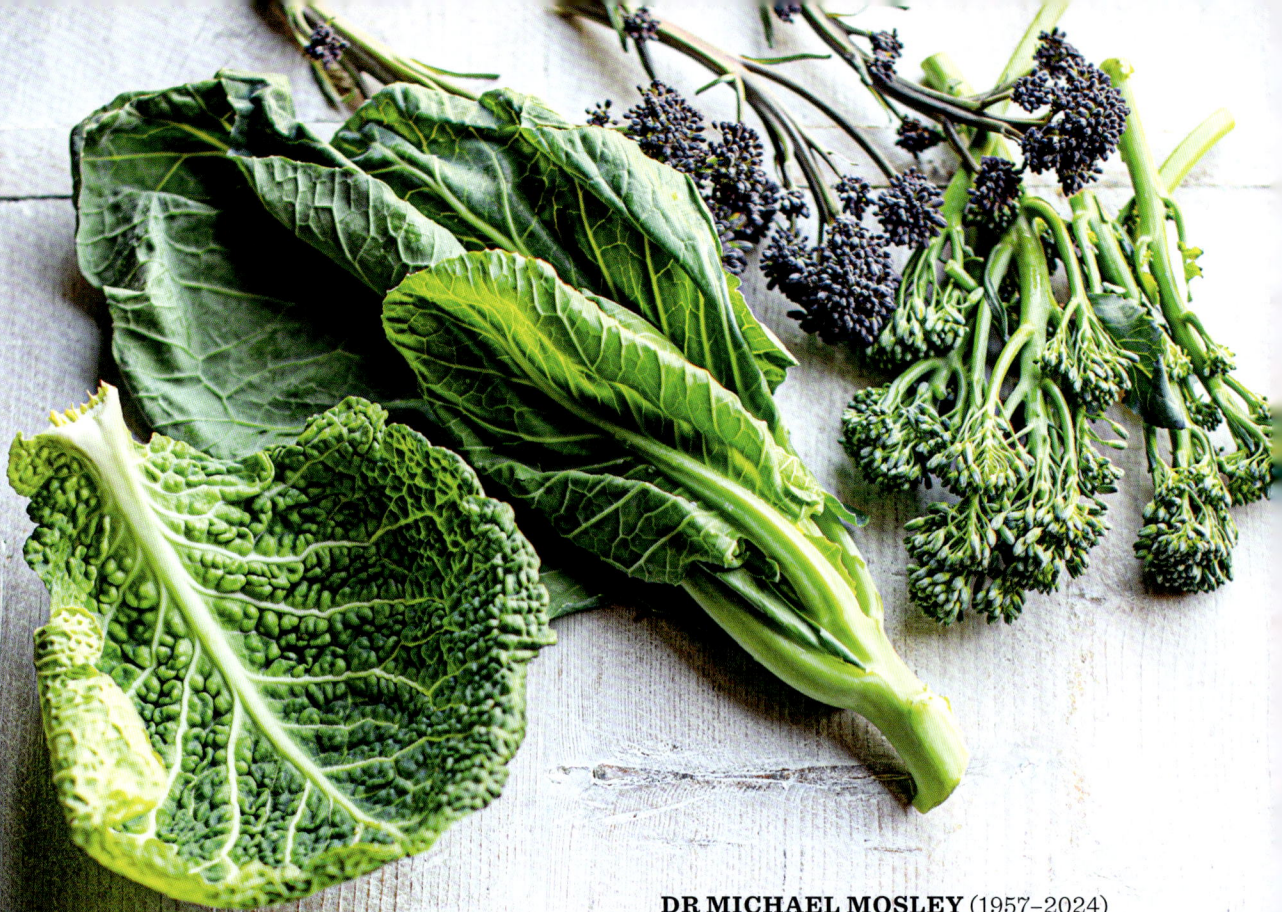

DR MICHAEL MOSLEY (1957–2024) was a much-loved author, journalist, podcast host and television presenter. Michael pioneered the Fast 800 programme, which helped countless people improve their health, particularly those with type 2 diabetes. His bestselling books include *The Fast Diet, The 8-Week Blood Sugar Diet, The Clever Guts Diet, The Fast 800, The Fast 800 Keto, Just One Thing* and *4 Weeks to Better Sleep*. He and his wife, Dr Clare Bailey Mosley, have four children.

DR CLARE BAILEY MOSLEY is a GP who has supported hundreds of patients to lose weight, reduce their blood sugar levels and put their diabetes in remission at her surgery in Buckinghamshire. She is the author of the bestselling *8-Week Blood Sugar Diet Recipe Book, The Clever Guts Diet Recipe Book, The Fast 800 Recipe Book, The Fast 800 Easy, The Fast 800 Treats Recipe Book* and *Eating Together: A Recipe for Healthier, Happier Families*.